Creating Modern Neuroscience

Creating Modern Neuroscience
The Revolutionary 1950s

Gordon M. Shepherd, MD, DPhil

Department of Neurobiology
Yale University School of Medicine
New Haven, CT

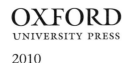

UNIVERSITY PRESS

2010

OXFORD
UNIVERSITY PRESS

Oxford University Press, Inc., publishes works that further
Oxford University's objective of excellence
in research, scholarship, and education.

Oxford   New York
Auckland   Cape Town   Dar es Salaam   Hong Kong   Karachi
Kuala Lumpur   Madrid   Melbourne   Mexico City   Nairobi
New Delhi   Shanghai   Taipei   Toronto

With offices in
Argentina   Austria   Brazil   Chile   Czech Republic   France   Greece
Guatemala   Hungary   Italy   Japan   Poland   Portugal   Singapore
South Korea   Switzerland   Thailand   Turkey   Ukraine   Vietnam

Copyright © 2010 by Oxford University Press, Inc.

Published by Oxford University Press, Inc.
198 Madison Avenue, New York, New York 10016

www.oup.com

Oxford is a registered trademark of Oxford University Press

Library of Congress Cataloging-in-Publication Data
Shepherd, Gordon M., 1933–
Creating modern neuroscience : the revolutionary 1950s /
Gordon M. Shepherd.
p. ; cm.
Includes bibliographical references and index.
ISBN: 978-0-19-539150-3
1. Neurosciences—History—20th century. I. Title.
[DNLM: 1. Neurosciences—history.   2. Brain—physiology.
3. History, 20th Century.
WL 11.1 S548c 2010]
RC338.S54 2010
616.8—dc22
2009005360

9 8 7 6 5 4 3 2 1

Printed in the United States of America
on acid-free paper

For Grethe

Preface

This account has many origins.

Early in my career as a neurophysiologist I became curious about the discoveries made by Camillo Golgi and Santiago Ramón y Cajal and their contemporaries in the late nineteenth century, from which emerged the "neuron doctrine" as the basis for the eventual rise of modern neuroscience. Both the technical innovations and the strong intellects of that time established a high level for the founding of this new field. This history was covered in my *Foundations of the Neuron Doctrine*, published in 1991, on the centenary of the neuron doctrine. The centenary of the synapse was commemorated in an article in 1997 with my late colleague Sol Erulkar, as well as an exhibit in the rotunda of the Whitney/Cushing Medical Library at Yale.

Meanwhile, the Society for Neuroscience was established, in 1971, and soon burgeoned with thousands of investigators from many disciplines. In 1985 I suggested to then President William Willis that this new field needed to take responsibility for its own history with a history committee. The Committee on the History of Neuroscience was duly formed, in which I was joined by Ted Jones, Albert Aguayo, and Louise Marshall. With the Council's support, we set up the Lecture on the History of Neuroscience at the annual meeting of the Society for Neuroscience. The first speakers included Andrew Huxley, Viktor Hamburger, and Francis Crick and many others who have played key roles in the early events chronicled here. As the society has grown to its present nearly 40,000 members, the lectures have remained among the most popular, with up to several thousand in the audience, belying the idea that the present generation has no interest in history.

In 2002 I was invited to give one of those lectures. In preparing "The Origins of Modern Neuroscience" I took the opportunity to review the breadth and depth of our field. It was striking, first, how many different fields combined under the rubric of "neuroscience," making it in my view the most multidisciplinary field in all of science. To grasp this vast range of knowledge, it was necessary to see it in terms of levels of organization, a concept I had discussed in an article on revising the neuron doctrine in 1972. Also striking was the fact that in most of these fields the origins for modern methods and concepts traced back to the mid-twentieth century, particularly the 1950s. All of these strands seemed to come together to begin to give some coherence to the rise of neuroscience as a scientific discipline.

A final step occurred in 2004, at the end of the graduate course I have taught at Yale since the 1970s on the synaptic organization of the nervous system, in recent years with my colleague Anne Williamson. It is based on my *The Synaptic Organization of the Brain*, then in its fifth edition. The book and the course provide an extensive historical background on the development of methods and concepts in understanding the brain at the microcircuit level. It was a great class with lively discussions, not only on the science but also on the creative process that produces the science. At the end, two of the students, Arjun Masurkar and Bilal Haider, suggested that it would be interesting to have a course that focused on the history.

I responded I would be happy to do it and challenged them with two conditions. First, we would focus on the 1950s, to test the proposition that it was the greatest decade in the history of modern biology and neuroscience and the source for much of the origins of modern neuroscience. Second, they would help with the assembly of historical materials and the teaching of the course entirely from the Internet. They enthusiastically agreed. As a consequence, we had a highly successful course, "History of Modern Neuroscience," in winter 2005 followed by 2007 and 2009. As far as I know, these have been the first courses to attempt to cover the origins of all of neuroscience in the modern era. A special thanks go to Arjun and Bilal and the students who have enthusiastically responded to the challenge.

The present account therefore represents a half-century of gestation, a series of articles and books, a long period of teaching classes, and the experience that derives from actually formulating and testing the best ways to teach a scientific field through examination of the creative process within a historical context. I hope the reader can feel a sense of participation in this stimulating enterprise. For the general reader, the historical development is one of the best ways to be introduced to neuroscience. For the modern expert, it will open doors to a deeper understanding and appreciation of the creative process in this field.

In teaching the course we have identified and used a wealth of materials on the Web which is now available. At Yale, these materials, together with the instructor's notes, are posted on the course site on Blackboard so that each class can be taught entirely from the Web. These materials are now gathered in the Appendix to this volume. In our course, we meet for a 2-hour session each week (that is a big slot in a graduate student or postdoctoral fellow's time, so we focus on the essentials). We take up a chapter in each session. The first hour I spend leading a discussion on an overview of the key issues faced by the investigators at that time in the field of the relevant chapter. In the second hour the students take over and discuss the key paper or papers, much as in a journal club, with no holds barred on exploring strengths and weaknesses.

In particular, we explore the creative process: the investigators, the new concepts, how graduate students and postdoctoral fellows were involved in the discoveries, and how credit was distributed, rightly or wrongly. Issues of gender and ethical concerns regarding credit make the course less of a history and more of a probing analysis of the creative process. Finally, how did these early discoveries lay the basis for our present research? What are the current research issues in these fields? How much of an advance have we made over the initial insights? What can we learn from how the initial discoveries were made to enhance and guide our current research efforts?

The book attempts to convey this range of issues that characterizes the history of modern neuroscience and how this history should be seen through the lens of intellectual history, focused on this most exciting of scientific enterprises: to know ourselves through understanding our brains.

In preparing this book I have many to thank. Kenny Marone, head of the Yale Medical Library, and Toby Appel, head of the Medical Historical Library, have generously provided space, materials, and support for this and other historical pursuits. John Warner, head of the Section of the History of Medicine at the medical school at Yale, has provided warm support and counsel. My chair, Pasko Rakic, and the late Patricia Goldman-Rakic, have given unstinting support for over 30 years. I'm particularly grateful to my long-time colleague Charles Greer and my students and colleagues in the laboratory for the experimental and computational studies that are the basis for any useful insights into the creative process that I've been able to glimpse. These studies have been made possible by a half-century of continuous research support from the National Institutes of Health.

I'm grateful to my mentors, Charles Phillips and Wilfrid Rall, for providing a rich training experience that included historical perspectives on their own seminal discoveries. The book is dedicated to them and the other giants of the time who trained and inspired me and my generation. Jeffrey House and Fiona Stevens of Oxford University Press have given me wonderful support in publishing the early historical accounts. Craig Panner, my current editor, has been enthusiastic from the start to see this volume into publication. Special thanks to Jonathan Yeh and Katherine Xie for expert assistance in the final gathering of the materials. Finally, David D'Addona, Lynda Crawford, and Andrew Pachuta have seen the book through to production with extraordinary patience and expertise.

A number of colleagues have read chapters and provided valuable advice, with special thanks to Peter Lengyel, Dale Purves, Larry Swanson, Ted Jones, Richard Mattson, Dennis Spencer, Gordon M.G. Shepherd, George Heninger, Dexter Easton, Wilfrid Rall, and Sol Snyder. Finally, as always, Grethe, who has made it all possible.

Hamden, Connecticut
April 27, 2009

Contents

Creating Modern Neuroscience

Chapter 1

Introduction: Why Study History?
Why the 1940s and 1950s?

Neuroscience is the study of the nervous system, in general, and the human brain, in particular. For neuroscience to mature as a discipline, it needs an understanding of its historical origins and development. This is a unique challenge in the history of science. It is not one discipline but many, spanning virtually every field of learning, from physics and chemistry to psychology and sociology to philosophy, politics, and religion. The history must therefore embrace many disciplines. It must include all species, not just a few model species. It must involve all nervous systems and their adaptations during evolution. It must involve all hierarchical levels of organization in those systems, from the single molecule to the most complex psychological states. Here, we review the origin and development of our knowledge across all these areas in order to understand the nature of the key discoveries and how they are the products of the people, the technical means, and the creative process that drove them. We also consider the ethical issues in the competition between leaders in the fields and how this has enhanced as well as distorted the advances. All of these facets constitute the foundations of our modern understanding of the nature of the brain and human existence and define the core concepts behind much of the research carried out today. Many surprises are in store, not least the fact that modern neuroscience has much of its origins in the mid-twentieth century, especially the 1950s.

Neuroscience embraces all of the scientific disciplines which contribute to revealing the mechanisms of the nervous system and their role in behavior. The last half of the twentieth century saw the rise of what we now recognize to be the modern era, when the full arsenal of experimental and theoretical methods available to biologists could be applied to this most complex of all the body organs. The mid-twentieth century is therefore a critical starting point for understanding the foundations of modern neuroscience.

Why Study History?

With so many challenges of modern research one may wonder why anyone would divert time to exploring these origins. Indeed, the opportunities for developing and applying the new methods have been so exciting, so all-absorbing, that it has led to an increasing tendency for today's neuroscientists to focus on the present and reject the past as irrelevant—the past rendered obsolete by the latest new method, the past that is not digitally accessible.

This is a mistake on several counts. It ignores Newton's dictum, that we stand on the shoulders of giants. It magnifies any new advance, however trivial. It encourages a drift from doing paradigm-shifting scholarly science to doing incremental technical or commercial development. An exclusive focus on the present deprives us of insights into the fundamental nature of the creative process in science. A historical perspective provides an education in how scientists are able to push past the limits of current concepts in order to fashion a new and more comprehensive understanding of the laws of nature. The 1950s was particularly rich in those examples. This book will therefore use this period as a laboratory for understanding the creative process in one of its most productive eras.

Finally, modern neuroscientists increasingly deplore the mass of data that engulfs us without giving the understanding we seek. A better perspective on the origins of our current concepts, their strengths and their limitations, can be a powerful aid in advancing toward that understanding.

The History of Neuroscience Embraces Many Disciplines

Historically, until well into the twentieth century the study of the nervous system was carried out within different disciplines. These included primarily neuroanatomy, neurophysiology, pharmacology, neurology, and psychiatry. Neurochemistry hardly existed. The word "neuroscience" did not gain use until The Neuroscience Program was formed by Francis Schmitt in the 1960s, and did not gain currency until the Society for Neuroscience was formed in 1971. This should be understood when we refer to the origins of neuroscience in discussing developments in the 1950s and earlier.

A big problem in learning about the history of neuroscience is the multiple disciplines it embraces. In addition to the traditional fields mentioned above, others, such as molecular biology, biochemistry, cell biology, and genetics, cover all body organs and only lately have come to apply directly to the nervous system. Still other fields, such as physics, chemistry, engineering, and computer science, have had powerful influences on neuroscience through the development of new methodologies and instrumentation. It is, in fact, this

Table 1.1 Fields of Neuroscience

Nervous system fields
  Neuroanatomy
  Neurochemistry
  Neurophysiology
  Neuropharmacology
  Neurology
  Psychiatry

Biology fields
  Molecular biology
  Biochemistry
  Biophysics
  Cell biology
  Genetics
  Developmental biology
  Evolution

Physical science fields
  Physics
  Chemistry
  Engineering
  Computer science

Behavior fields
  Ethology
  Psychology
  Sociology
  Neuroeconomics

Humanities fields
  Linguistics
  Neurophilosophy
  Neuropolitics
  Neuroreligion

rich mixture of disciplines that has fueled the rise of modern neuroscience and is one of the main themes of its development. A list of the many fields is given in Table 1.1.

The History of Neuroscience Extends Across All Species

Advances in neuroscience have been motivated by two interests: to understand the biological world, which is embedded in the conceptual framework of evolutionary theory, and to understand the human, which is embedded in, on the one hand, a desire to understand human nature and, on the other, a desire to understand and treat human diseases. In both endeavors, experiments on a wide range of animal species are critical.

The major share of work in modern neuroscience is carried out in vertebrates and, of this, most is in mammals, particularly laboratory animals such as the mouse and the rat. However, it is extremely dangerous to limit the view of the nervous system or any other system to a few model species. Our review of history therefore recognizes that essential contributions to neuroscience have come from research across many different species. Among the vertebrates, the

Table 1.2 Species Investigated in Neuroscience

Invertebrate
Bacteria
Worms
Insects
Arthropods
Molluscs
Limulus
Squid
Aplysia
Vertebrate
Fish
Amphibians
Reptiles
Birds
Mammals
Hedgehogs
Rabbits
Rats
Mice
Cats
Dogs
Subhuman primates
Humans

human is, of course, of overriding interest; but much of our understanding of the human nervous system has come from basic research on other vertebrate species. Similarly, many principles that have applied across vertebrate species have come from basic research on invertebrates, and many practical applications to fighting human disease have of necessity required analysis of invertebrates. In our historical review we will include the major discoveries in all of these species that have contributed to the core of general principles. The main species utilized in research through the 1950s are indicated in Table 1.2.

The History of Neuroscience Extends Across All Systems

In the study of nervous organization it is useful to think in terms of a simple division into three great systems. One comprises all of the different sensory systems, another all of the specific motor systems, and the remainder the specific central systems. A list of the main systems and subsystems is provided in Table 1.3.

Historically, knowledge of neural mechanisms has been built on those systems accessible to study by the methods at the time. In the nineteenth century and well into the twentieth century knowledge was dominated by work on vision among sensory systems, spinal reflexes among motor systems, and visual perception and learning among central behavioral systems.

Beginning with the period under study, nervous system studies expanded dramatically across all major systems. Knowledge burst forth so rapidly that we

Table 1.3 Systems Studied in Neuroscience

Sensory systems
  Smell
  Taste
  Touch
  Hearing
  Vision

Motor systems
  Autonomic
  Posture
  Reflexes
  Central pattern generation
  Spinal cord
  Higher motor centers

Central systems
  Neuroendocrine
  Circadian rhythms
  Feeding
  Mating and reproduction
  Motivation
  Perception
  Learning and memory
  Human higher cognitive functions

---

are still catching up with developments in systems we scarcely knew existed. This presents an enormous challenge in keeping the focus on the main advances that have formed modern neuroscience because each of the specific systems has its own special sets of operating principles that can be highly technical and specific for that system. For the purposes of our history we will identify only the main organizing principles that have been identified in each of these specific systems, especially those that can be compared across the different systems, to give insight into general principles. For greater depth and detail, there is an increasing number of excellent historical reviews of different specific fields which the student can access through the Internet.

The History of Neuroscience Extends Across All Hierarchical Levels of Organization

The strategy of this book in dealing with the history of all these fields, species, and systems in a systematic way is to recognize a fundamental principle, that biological organization involves a *hierarchy of levels*. As summarized in Table 1.4, this hierarchy begins with the genes and the proteins that the genes encode and builds up successively higher levels from macromolecules and molecular signaling pathways through organelles, microcircuits, whole cells, local regional circuits, and specific neural pathways and systems to the coordinated multiple systems that underlie behavior. This hierarchy allows the function at any one level to be understood as a part of the organization at higher levels. Conversely,

Table 1.4 Hierarchy of Levels in Nervous Organization

Higher cognitive and social functions
Clinical disorders: neurology, neurosurgery, psychiatry
Systems for behavior
Circuits of specific systems
Dendritic integration
Cellular functional properties: synaptic potentials and action potentials
Synapses
Molecules in development and neurotransmission
Genes

the neural basis of the function at any level is understood in terms of the mechanisms mediated by the lower levels.

The additional advantage of this conceptual framework is that it reflects in large part the way that experimental studies focus on the properties of the nervous system at one or another of the levels as determined by the methodology being used.

What Are the Factors that Produce the Discoveries?

As already indicated, our interest in history is much more than a recounting of what was discovered when. This is only the starting point for what we are really interested in: the creative process. What are the factors that produce the great leaps forward in science? One of the most rewarding insights to be gained from the study of history is to see how advances in our knowledge have depended on the convergence of different factors. It is by a deeper understanding of these factors that young investigators can pursue their own careers more effectively. For our purpose, six factors seem to be most critical (summarized in Table 1.5.)

First is the *methodology*, as expressed in the dictum of the nineteenth century, "Teknik ist alles." To paraphrase a modern quotation, "Methods are not everything, they are the only thing." To modern scientists, this increasingly means the newest sophisticated equipment. But the opposite view dominated much of the early experimental work in electrophysiology. This view has been eloquently explained by Alan Hodgkin (1992, 66–67), who with Andrew Huxley revealed the nature of the nerve impulse:

Table 1.5 Factors in Discovery in Neuroscience

Methodology
Biological preparation
Investigator
Theoretical framework
Chance
Support

Nowadays...it is regarded as somewhat unscientific to carry out experiments with anything but the best equipment. This certainly wasn't my feeling when I started research...all that mattered was that one should have enough equipment to do something new. [The example from physics at the Cavendish was that] an elegant piece of apparatus or an elegant experiment meant one that could be built or carried out very cheaply.

For neuroscience, we will see that technology often is critical, but even then it is not everything because it depends on the other components.

Second is the biological *preparation* to which the technique is applied. Biological preparations come in an almost infinite variety; the trick is to find a "model system" that will enable something new to be discovered. For Hodgkin, it was the squid giant axon, first described by J. Z. Young a few years earlier (see Chapter 6). The adroit matching of technique to a model system, whether it be a region, slice of region, or isolated cell or part of a cell, has been the key to most advances.

Third is the *investigator*, with his or her own unique blend of skills, personality, and insights. Hodgkin's memoirs give a wonderfully clear account of how the steps in his education and training led to the great result. He and his colleagues also demonstrate how the investigator often must have the ability to interact effectively with others and to persevere in developing and applying the new technology to the model system.

Fourth is the *theoretical framework* of the time, which explains what is known and what is not known, points to the need for new methodologies, and generates the hypotheses and predictions to be tested. It is an old observation in physics (at least by theoretical physicists) that "You can't explain a fact without a theory." Hodgkin and his colleagues went through several theories of the action potential before coming to the right one. Experimentalists often prioritize experiments over theory, but the importance of a strong theoretical foundation for the development of a field cannot be overemphasized. We recognize this by discussing specific advances in each chapter, with a separate chapter on the role of theory in neuroscience later in the book.

Fifth is the inevitable factor of *chance*, the fortuitous coming together of these components in unpredictable ways, as summarized in Louis Pasteur's (Bartlett, 591) famous axiom: "Dans les champs de l'observation le hazard ne favorise que les esprits prepare" (In the fields of observation chance favors only the prepared mind). The confluence of these components in an endless variety of circumstances lies at the heart of the scientific enterprise and gives a never-ending fascination to our story.

Finally, a scientist, like an artist or other creative worker, needs *support*. With the rise of technically sophisticated science in the late nineteenth century, this need for funds stimulated new philanthropic institutions such as the Rockefeller Foundation in the United States. But it was not until the vast demands of the Second World War that science became organized on a large scale, carrying over after the war to greatly expanded support that drove the rise of modern biology, in general, and modern neuroscience, in particular. The critical role this support played in the revolutionary advances in the late 1940s and 1950s deserves a book of its own, and is recognized in most of the chapters.

The History of Neuroscience Includes Ethical Issues

A new factor in science today is the ethics of how research is carried out. It is not enough to leave one's mark by one's discoveries; the legacy also includes whether it met ethical standards in the interactions between the investigators. These interactions take place along different axes (Table 1.6).

One is across generations, between a mentor and a student. Historically, there has been a tendency for the mentor to be recognized more than the student. We will identify these cases and see that this issue can cut both ways.

Another axis of interactions is across genders, between, usually, senior men and junior women in training with them. The difficulties of women in making careers in science, and in receiving credit for their contributions, are increasingly recognized. We will identify many of these cases.

A third axis is between laboratories, especially in cases of intense competition for making a discovery. To what extent is it unethical to obtain clues or data from your competitors in order to be the first to publish? Priority in discovery drives most scientists, but does it drive them across the border of collegiality and responsible behavior? Our history must identify these dilemmas if our field is to have an ethical foundation.

A fourth axis is between research focused within a single field and that which crosses different fields. Most advances involve a single discovery in a single field. There is an increasing concern that in addition to more data we need more integration, but science is not organized to recognize across-field integration. We will address this and related issues in characterizing each advance.

A fifth axis is between racial and ethnic groups. Racial bias against blacks and ethnic bias against Jews in Western culture was a fact of life during this period, to a degree beyond what most young people can imagine today.

A sixth axis is political. Science thrives when scientists can function free of any political intrusion or coercion. Lack of this freedom drove Jewish scientists from Germany in the thirties. The United States also experienced an unpleasant

Table 1.6 Ethical Issues in Neuroscience

Recognition between mentor and student
Recognition between male and female
Recognition in competition between laboratories
Recognition between single-discipline and multidisciplinary studies
Bias on the basis of race and ethnic group
Political intrusion and coercion
Nationalities and language

form of intrusion during the McCarthy era in the early 1950s. But for the most part this period in the United States is regarded as culturally bland: see for example Halberstam (1993). Those of us growing up in this period might disagree. The apparent blandness can be seen as crucial in allowing the greatest freedom for the scientific endeavor, producing a constant stream of major discoveries.

A final axis is between nationalities. In the years after the Second World War that are the focus of this book, American neuroscience enjoyed the greatest support and English became the international language of science. To what extent did this cause inadequate recognition of advances made in other countries and in other languages? We will attempt to give credit for advances across national and linguistic boundaries.

These and other ethical issues are coming to the fore in carrying out modern research in all areas of biology. With the perspective of history, we can assess these issues in a more objective fashion and include them in assessing the work in the period under review.

Why Focus on the 1950s?

The overall aim of this book is to provide a history of the origins of modern neuroscience. The sheer number of great breakthroughs quickly focused my research on the 1950s. What is so special about this decade? Wasn't it a boring time of a static conformist society in the United States and a period of struggling recovery in the rest of the world from the ravages of the 1939–45 world war?

Perhaps, but for those of us growing up in that period, it was also a time of rapidly shifting world events. In our science courses there was much that was new; but of course we had no way to compare it with other times, and we were aware of only a small part of all that was happening. My recent research into that period gave mounting evidence of so many advances in so many areas that I came to the conviction that the 1950s can be considered the greatest decade in the history not only of neuroscience but also of biology. The discovery of DNA is alone sufficient to make that claim. However, we will see that the mid-nineteenth century was an extraordinarily tumultuous period in giving birth to neuroscience, beyond what anyone realized at that time. Most of these advances are fading from memory. I've asked many of my contemporary colleagues in recent years if they attach any special significance to advances in the 1950s. It is usually only after I begin to recite some of the advances recorded in this book that they nod in agreement.

Some of the milestones in this revolution are indicated in the graph in Table 1.7. It is presented in terms of the main levels of organization of the nervous system. This begins at the most fundamental with molecules: the genes that carry the information for building the body and the molecules involved in signaling between cells to build the brain during development and to process information. Above this come basic cellular structures and physiological properties. On this are built the circuits that carry out the functional

Table 1.7 Timetable of Discoveries at Different Organizational Levels

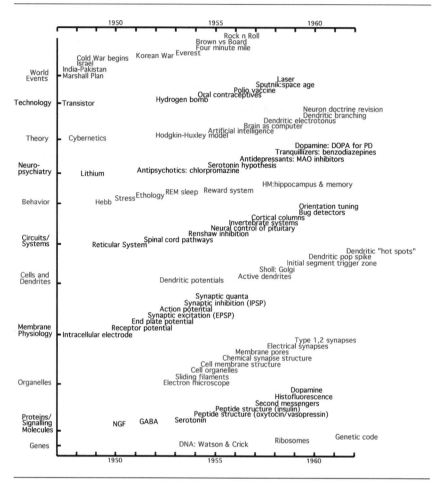

operations which constitute the neural basis of behavior. We end with the clinical disciplines that deliver the basic science to the bedside. Table 1.7 will serve as an overview and reference for the reader that situates the discoveries in relation to their level in the hierarchy of organization and to the other discoveries within that level and in comparison with the other levels.

The density of discoveries during those brief years is evidenced in Table 1.7. This tremendous, one may dare to say unparalleled, burst of creative activity not only laid the foundations for most of the levels of biological organization, from the gene to behavior, but also defined problems within those levels that are still the driving forces for much of modern neuroscience. If you, the reader, gain a deeper understanding of how this has come about, it will be well worth the effort!

Those origins have their own origins, many of which go back to the remarkable period of the late nineteenth and early twentieth centuries when the foundations of biology and all the other sciences were being built. I've therefore relaxed the focus enough to give sufficient acknowledgment of those accomplishments, which go back to the founding of the neuron doctrine in the nineteenth century, a subject covered in a previous book, *Foundations of the Neuron Doctrine* (Shepherd, 1991). On the other hand, I've included consideration of how the concepts arising from the pioneering studies in the 1950s have themselves provided the foundations for much of the research being carried out on the nervous system today and will likely continue to be relevant well into the future. Those developments from the 1960s to the present are to be covered in a subsequent volume.

Rationale for the Book

The challenge to write a definitive history of a subject is characteristically, and rightly, the province of the professionally trained historian of science. This account is by a person active in research in that field. It thus has the character of the introductory chapter of a doctoral thesis, where the student absorbs everything about the history of the subject relevant to his or her research interests. In addition, it includes the lore of the field, told by mentors and colleagues or dug out of obscure papers and monographs. Thus, I hope that the lack of the skills of the professional historian is at least partially balanced by the gains in the judgment by an active participant of what is relevant to the subject at hand. It is for that reason that I regard these as essays rather than definitive historical accounts. What is recorded here is written to acknowledge the peers who were there when the events occurred. Those times are fading, and those peers are becoming fewer. I hope that this account will help to keep those contributions fresh and relevant for the modern investigator.

Plan of the Book

The present account attempts to knit together all of these strands into a contribution to the history of modern neuroscience. Each chapter deals with the main discoveries made at one of the hierarchical levels of organization. Excerpts from the classical papers are provided. An appendix lists Web sites where the classical papers are available online. In fact, the course I teach at Yale on this subject is taught mainly through these online resources. Some references to the older literature are indicated in secondary more accessible sources, particularly online, a proven effective aid in stimulating an interest in history in the busy modern student and providing a context from a modern perspective.

The attempt has been made to give a systematic review of the main discoveries that laid the foundations for modern neuroscience. No account can, of course, be complete from all points of view, and I apologize for omissions of work that some may well believe should have been included. The aim has been to cover the main discoveries, both those that are well known and those that are often overlooked but nonetheless have been seminal in forming new fields that have been critical in creating modern neuroscience.

Summing Up

From our modern perspective, the 1950s may be seen to have been, paraphrasing Shakespeare, a "brave new world that had such people [and such science] in it." (The Tempest, v, i). The value of learning more about these people is expressed well by Andrew Huxley in his reflections on the history of research in muscle:

> It is common enough to mention the most outstanding of the discoveries that have led up to present-day opinions, but this sort of cursory glimpse is actively misleading in at least two ways. First, it gives the... false impression...that Science always moves forward, that is to say progresses. Secondly, it suggests that any scientist who put forward opinions which have not been upheld was either stupid or perverse, and that no intelligent person at the present day is in danger of falling into equivalent errors. The more I read the works of late nineteenth-century biologists, the more I am impressed by their ability, by their range and versatility, and by the modernity of their outlook. Biologists of all kinds owe a tremendous debt to their predecessors of around a century ago.
>
> (A. Huxley, Reflections on Muscle, 1980, 1–2)

As we shall see, the same sentiments can be applied to our predecessors of a half-century ago.

Chapter 2

Genes: Starting with DNA

The discovery of the molecular structure of DNA in 1953 was sufficient to claim the 1950s as the greatest decade in the history of modern biology. Although the discovery did not have an immediate impact on neuroscience, its importance for all organ systems was manifest, particularly as it became clear that a majority of the genes are expressed in the nervous system. The race to DNA also became a new paradigm for the conduct of investigations in modern biology, in which issues regarding the ethics of competition between laboratories and of the adequate recognition of contributions by women were brought to light. The subsequent characterization during the 1950s and early 1960s of the different types of RNA; the identification of the enzymes involved in mitosis, meiosis, transcription, and translation; the formulation of the "central dogma" of molecular biology; and the race for the genetic code are all part of the lore of modern biology, in general, and molecular neuroscience, in particular.

The Historical Depth of Molecular Biology

We take for granted that understanding a biological system begins with knowledge of the genes that are expressed by the cells in that system and of the RNAs and proteins that the genes encode in the form of structural molecules, enzymes, and receptors. In the middle of the nineteenth century, when modern biology began, this idea arose only as a distant vision in the minds of the first anatomists to use the microscope to describe the cells of the body and the first physiologists to use electrical instruments to record nerve activity.

It may have been distant, but when we consult the texts of the time, we find that the vision was formulated with deep passion and amazing clarity. (For modern readers, citations of this older literature may be found in "Foundations of the Neuron Doctrine" (Shepherd, 1991) and other more accessible sources which include commentaries from modern perspectives). The passion was especially true of the pioneers of electrophysiology, as related by Cranefield (1957). Emil Du Bois-Reymond was one of them. The first book on the electrical activity of nerve fibers (Du Bois-Reymond, 1848) set out the new principles that were needed:

> The true method ... lies ... in the effort to determine the basic connections of the natural phenomena beneath the mathematical structure of their relationships.... It cannot fail that ... physiology ... will dissolve into organic physics and chemistry.
>
> (Shepherd, 1991, 31)

In a similar fashion, the first textbook of histology (Kolliker, 1852), describing the cells of the body for the first time, predicted that when "the molecules which constitute cell membranes, muscular fibers, axial fibers of nerves, etc., should be discovered ... a new era will commence for Histology" based on a "molecular theory" and a "law of cell genesis" (in Shepherd, 1991, 31).

To read these texts is to realize that the molecular biology we now take for granted had been a goal of biologists for a very long time. The steps toward knowledge of genes are an exciting part of the struggle toward that goal. The story leading up to the discovery of the gene is rapidly becoming a part of the lore of that struggle (e.g., see Passarge, 1995). Although it mostly concerns the body in general, it also contains the first clues to the roles of genes in the nervous system. We provide a brief review of the rise of concepts beginning in the nineteenth century, before focusing on those aspects that are most relevant to the nervous system.

Genes and Their Terminology

It will be useful at the start to have some background on how our modern terms and concepts were derived.

To begin with, the reader may have noticed the use of "cell genesis" in the previous quotation, reflecting its definition referring to "origin" (from the Greek *gen*, "produce"), as in the book of Genesis. The adjectival form is "genetic." These terms had no scientific relevance but were used in the general literature in the early nineteenth century to refer to "genetic histories" of poetry or "genetic development" of the parts of speech. A "genetic fallacy" was one "supposing that an opinion is discredited when its causal origins are revealed."(Oxford English Dictionary, 1901) In science, Foster's *A Text-book of Physiology* (1897) stated that "Regarded in its genetic aspect, the spinal cord is a series of cemented segments," where we would now probably refer to its "developmental" aspect.

Darwin, in *Origin of Species* (1859), referred to "genetic connexions" (common origins) occurring between separated geological formations.

The first steps toward knowledge of the genes as we understand them occurred in the late nineteenth century (references to the background literature covered in this section may be found in textbooks of genetics (see Passarge, 1995) and online in Wikipedia (History of Genetics) and Wikipedia under the author's name). Colorful strands were described in stained tissue within the cytoplasm of dividing cells by Walther Flemming in 1879. These were named "chromosomes" (from the Greek *chrom*, "color," and *som*, "body") by Wilhelm von Waldeyer in Germany in 1888. Cell division into two daughter cells as occurs in somatic cells was termed "mitosis" by Flemming. The stages of cell division were termed "prophase," "metaphase," and "anaphase" by Eduard Strasburger, who also introduced the term "meiosis" for cell division that leads to daughter cells that contain only one of the chromosomal pair, as occurs in germ cells (summarized in Strasburger et al., 1894). These studies were part of the rise of cytology in the late nineteenth century and took place without any knowledge of, or connection to, Gregor Mendel's studies of the characteristics of inheritance in garden peas in the 1870s.

In 1900 Mendel's "laws of hereditary recombination" were rediscovered by Correns, Tschermak, and DeVries (Passarge, 1995). Mendel's proposal that heredity is the outcome of "independent factors" led William Bateson in England in 1906 to suggest the term "genetics" as a specific biological term for the study of the rules of heredity. Following Bateson, Wilhelm Johannsen in Denmark in 1909 proposed the term "gene" for the "independent factors", as well as "genotype" for the combination of genes in an individual and "phenotype" (from the Greek *phainen*, "to show") for the combination of features due to the genes and their interaction with the environment (see Ryan et al., 2000).

That chromosomes are the carriers of the genes became recognized by studies of the fruit fly *Drosophila melanogaster*, introduced by Thomas Hunt Morgan in the United States. The rapid reproductive cycles of *Drosophila* were a critical factor in the ability to analyze genetic mechanisms. In 1915 Morgan and colleagues suggested the "chromosome theory of inheritance," which slowly became accepted.

Mendelian laws governing the inheritance of human metabolic diseases were first discovered by Garrod and reported in his book *Inborn Errors of Metabolism* in 1909. This work was the first to implicate genetic mechanisms in diseases affecting the nervous system and to recognize that there are differences in genes and biochemical constituents among normal individuals.

Changes in genes were called "mutations" (from the Latin *mutatio*, "change"). It was shown that mutations could be induced by X-rays, by H.J Muller in 1927, During the Second World War it was found that mutations could be induced by chemicals: mustard gas by Lotte Auerbach and Rab Robson in England, and urethane by Friedrich Oehlkers in Germany (summarized in Beale (1993). This provided powerful tools for investigating genetic mechanisms.

Just as Mendel's garden peas opened one era and Morgan's fruit fly another, so the introduction of microorganisms, with their single-cell composition and rapid reproductive cycles, gave genetics a powerful thrust. Although studies of bacteria started in the 1920s, studies of the fungus *Neurospora* by Beadle and Tatum in the United States were the first to gain wide recognition and led to the concept of "one gene one enzyme." In 1946 Tatum and Lederberg showed that genetic information can be exchanged between different strains of mutant bacteria. This was the first evidence for genetic recombination.

Although these studies set genetics on the right track, there was still no idea of what stuff genes were made of. Physicists were attracted by this challenge. Niels Bohr, the central figure in the revolution of quantum physics in the 1920s, used his concept of "complementarity" to speculate on the physical nature of biological material (see Shepherd, 2000). Another quantum physicist, Erwin Schrödinger, of the wave equations as well as the cat, published a small book in 1945 entitled *What Is Life?*, which stimulated much interest across scientific disciplines and the lay public in the problem of the hereditary material. Many physicists have mentioned how this account of the problem of the biological basis of heredity was phrased in a way that, though containing errors about the biology, was accessible and stimulated their move to molecular biology. I well remember the impact on a young student of these cogent musings on the possible biochemical and physical nature of the genes.

The road to Schrodinger started with the discovery in the early 20th century of viruses that infect bacteria, Frederick Twort in the U.K. and the French-Canadian scientist Felix d"Herelle, who named them "bacteriophage" ("bacteria eaters"). There was great interest in developing bacteriophage as a means to combat infections, until antibiotics proved more effective in the 1940s. However, bacteriophages were to have a greater impact on science. Summers (1999), in his biography of d'Herelle, dates the origins of molecular biology to the discovery of bacteriophage. The path then led to Max Delbrück. As a young physics student, Delbrück was stimulated by a lecture by Bohr on his concept of complementarity in physics to pursue evidence for this concept in biology. In 1939 Ellis and Delbruck introduced phage as a means to further genetic research, which led to the formation of the phage group and the beginnings of modern molecular biology – and stimulated Schrodinger to write his book.

Clues to DNA

Experimental evidence for the nature of the gene came first in 1928 when Frederick Griffith in England reported a genetic transformation between two strains of pneumococcus. This remained in doubtful status until Oswald Avery, Colin MacLeod, and Maclyn McCarty (1943) in the United States demonstrated that the "transforming principle" was a long-chained nucleic acid, called "deoxyribonucleic acid" (DNA). It is often said that this now famous study went relatively unnoticed for several years. However, there is plenty of testimony from contemporaries that those interested in the nature of the hereditary material were well aware of the experiments. There was also continuing concern about the possibility of protein contaminants in the preparations. Supporting evidence was adduced by Hershey and Chase in 1952 that genes are indeed DNA. It was recognized that the chemical structure of DNA would reveal the long-sought mechanisms of the hereditary material.

The New Research Environment of the 1950s

This "holy grail" galvanized biochemists in many laboratories on both sides of the Atlantic. It was a propitious time. The Second World War (1939–1945) had recently ended. The effective large-scale organization of scientific research in the United States and Great Britain had been crucial to the Allied Nations' success, most notably in the development of radar and the atomic bomb. In the United States, under the leadership of Vannevar Bush and other enlightened scientists and politicians, this concept of large-scale scientific organization was converted in peacetime to a tremendous rise in investment by the federal government in basic research, not only in the physical sciences but also in the health sciences through a rapid expansion of the National Institutes of Health (NIH). In the United Kingdom, this led to increased support for both traditional and new laboratories in atomic physics and to the creation of the Medical Research Council for supporting basic research in the different health disciplines.

In the United States, the key funding strategy was to make research grants available on a competitive basis, directly to the "principal investigator" applying for the funds rather than to the chair of the department or only to senior professors. This maximized the creative potential of young investigators and left them free to decide for themselves on a particular research strategy. In addition, fellowship funds were made available to graduate students and postdoctoral fellows to pursue their research with mentors of their own choosing, with few strings attached.

This increased support provided funding that, by current standards, would be considered modest; but it created a research environment in which the best laboratories had what they needed in terms of facilities and, more importantly, the freedom to pursue projects, many of which today would be considered high-risk and therefore unfundable.

The Race to DNA

We have taken this digression to describe the upsurge of funding for freely pursued basic research in the aftermath of the Second World War because it provided the critical basis for the race to DNA (as well as biomedical research in general in the United States).

Although many established biochemical laboratories joined in the race, the prize went to two postdoctoral fellows, James Watson from the United States and Francis Crick from the United Kingdom. Watson was born in 1928 and, as a precocious child, was one of the "whiz kids" on the radio program of that name in the late 1930s. He then became a precocious postdoctoral fellow in his early twenties, who got a fellowship to study biochemistry and wandered through several European laboratories looking for something stimulating to work on. Crick, on the other hand, born in 1919, was trained in physics and became an "ageing" postdoctoral fellow, hanging around the famous Cavendish physics laboratory under Lawrence Bragg at Cambridge University, also looking for something stimulating to do. The two got together and decided they would try to win the race to discover the structure of DNA.

The story is now legendary. Drawing on data obtained from several collaborators, including most notably very early crystallographic data on DNA structure by another young investigator, Rosalind Franklin, in the laboratory of Maurice Wilkins in London, Watson and Crick constructed a physical model which showed that DNA consisted of two complementary intertwining helices of matching base pairs, a purine and a pyrimidine (the nucleic part), attached to outer sugars (the deoxyribose part) and a monophosphate (Fig. 2.1).

They made their report in a short article in the April 25, 1953, edition of the journal *Nature*; it was accompanied by a report by Franklin and Wilkins on the crystallography. Some books and articles are famous for their first sentences; theirs became famous for the last sentence (p 737): "It has not escaped our notice that the specific pairing we have postulated immediately suggests a possible copying mechanism for the genetic material." (See Appendix 2.1.)

Given the high level of publicity that attends even quite modest advances today, it is amusing to note how this momentous paper reached the general public. The customers at the Eagle Pub in Cambridge heard about it the same day the model was finished, for at the end of the day Watson and Crick walked over with their laboratory colleagues to raise a pint in celebration and declare to all the patrons that they had "discovered the secret to life." However, the news did not reach the U.S. public until 6 weeks later, when the *New York Times* ran a single-column story on an inside page stating that two scientists in England had reported on the chemical nature of the gene (see New York Times, 1953 Appendix 2.2).

> It was a momentous spring: Everest climbed, Elizabeth crowned, Stalin dead, *Playboy* born. The biggest event of all—life solved—caused barely a ripple (Ridley, 2006, 73).

On the personal level, the story of this race was first recounted in Watson's *The Double Helix* (1968), followed by Crick's *What Mad Pursuit* (1988), Ridley's *Francis Crick: Discoverer of the Genetic Code* (2006), and many other books and accounts, the most complete being by Horace Freeland Judson, *The Eighth Day of Creation: Makers of the Revolution in Biology* (1996).

The early reports of the discovery of DNA, and particularly Watson's book, had a large impact on the way biological science, including neuroscience, has been conducted since that time (though the book came after the decade of the

1950s). This was partly because it gave a new perspective on doing science, making it out to be an exhilarating race between the gifted and their plodding, or clueless, contemporaries, rather than a modest account of the steps toward the truth. The move away from the laboratory uniform of white coats, suits, and ties toward tee shirts and sneakers dates from that time.

The book also raised questions about the ethics of using other people's data. Watson and Crick did no experiments themselves but gathered hints, experimental insights, and critical data from others. Rosalind Franklin's pioneering crystallographic data, essential to building the structural model, was made available to them without her knowledge. For her part, Franklin generously acknowledged the correctness and beauty of the final structure and became friends with both of them in the years before her early death.

Finally, the book's description of the interactions with Franklin highlighted the injustices done to women in their struggle for equality of opportunity and recognition in laboratory research. She has become a totemic example for this struggle, which is still being waged (see Maddox, 2002). The fact that she was not allowed into the lunchroom at King's College where she worked to be with her male colleagues indicates the distance between those days and our own. Will our own time be looked back on from a similar distance in 50 years?

It is also worth noting that the discovery of DNA was a result of both experiment and theory. The experimental data were essential, but so was the model, proving that the molecule could exist in the postulated entwined double helices. To those who hold to the belief that progress in biology depends solely on data obtained by experiment, the DNA story is a strong refutation. It was the intellectual stimulation of solving the structure with a model that enabled the goal to be reached.

(I heard Crick give a talk on the work in Oxford in 1962. Someone asked what kind of a future he saw for modeling. He thought that perhaps it had served its main purpose. By then his colleague Max Perutz had solved the structure of hemoglobin, also demonstrated with a model. However, in the future, beyond those laboriously assembled physical models, lay molecular models assembled by computer, now an integral part of molecular biology. Someone also asked Crick the secret to teamwork in the laboratory, and he replied "Success depends on not being courteous to each other—though the Japanese might be an exception"!

The rush of biology into the molecular age was dramatized for me at the time by a talk given by Peter Medawar at Oxford around 1961 in which, reviewing recent developments in the cellular and molecular bases of tissue transplantation, he made the offhand remark "Of course, no one uses the term 'protoplasm' anymore." There was an audible gasp from the audience. In the question period a timid soul raised his hand and wondered whether protoplasm still had some utility. It was obvious that the term was still part of the vocabulary at Oxford! Medawar said in reply that he hadn't meant to offend anyone, but it was probably time to change.)

How Does DNA Work?

Although many biologists accepted the structure of DNA as potentially the most important discovery in biology since Darwin, there was little immediate practical effect on either biologists or the public because, although the principle of replication by pairing of the bases was obvious, how it actually occurs was a complete mystery. The first report was therefore a beginning, not an end, which is true of most great discoveries in science. Many years of hard work lay ahead. In fact, the double helix structure of oppositely oriented sequences was not finally confirmed until the early 1980s (Crick, 1988).

The developments in the 1950s involved the blurring and reinvention of traditional disciplines, another mark of the revolution taking place that has repeated itself ever since. One of these changes involved the new fusion of the study of nucleic acids with enzymology and biochemistry. This led to a big step forward in 1951, when Sanger and Tuppy in the United Kingdom combined these methods to determine the amino acid sequence of insulin. (This was the first sequencing of a protein acting as a body hormone which was shown subsequently to be a neuroactive compound acting in the brain; see Chapters 3 and 11. The peptide hormone antidiuretic hormone was sequenced in 1953; see Chapter 11.) This showed that a protein consists of a simple sequence of amino acids (also called amino acid "residues," i.e., what is left after parts of the molecules are used for the bonds between them). It implied a correlation between the sequence of base pairs in DNA and the sequence of amino acids in the protein. Furthermore, it was known by then that DNA resides in the cell nucleus and proteins are synthesized in the cytoplasm. So the problems were as follows: How does DNA undergo replication within the nucleus? What is the form of the information in the DNA sequence? How is this information transferred to the cytoplasm? How is it read out to produce the proteins?

Discovering RNA

Long before the structure of DNA was revealed, several lines of investigation began to lead toward the identification of ribonucleic acid (RNA) in the functions of the cell (see the summary and early references in Gall et al., 1981).

Beginning with the work of Garnier in France around 1900, a series of studies from various laboratories demonstrated a basophilic substance in the cytoplasm of glandular cells that was implicated in producing the secretory products of the cells. In the 1930s this substance was shown to be RNA. By the early 1940s it was postulated that RNA is important for protein synthesis. A variety of methods were used to isolate it and characterize its functions. These methods played a large role in the development of cellular biochemistry.

With high-speed centrifugation of cell contents, RNA was found in the "microsome" fraction (Claude, 1943). Early studies of cell fine structure with the electron microscope (EM) showed that the cytoplasm contains a network of membranes, termed by Keith Porter (1953) the "endoplasmic reticulum

(ER)", and that there is smooth ER and rough ER, the latter with attached small particles (Palade, 1955a,b). Much work, using radioactively labeled RNA, finally brought the two lines of work together, showing that the microsomes contain particles rich in RNA and that these are equivalent to the particles seen with the EM.

This work dramatized the impact of electron microscopy in opening up the new era in the biology of the cell and the way that fine structure could be correlated with classical biochemical methods such as subcellular fractionation.

The new methods enabled a direct attack on the question, how does the rough ER synthesize protein?

The RNAs and Protein Synthesis

Among the technological fruits for biology of the Second World War was the advent of radioactively labeled isotopes, especially ^{14}C. This approach has had wide application in biology, including neuroscience, as we shall see (e.g., the work on cerebral circulation, Chapter 13).

An obvious early target was to trace how radioactively labeled amino acids are assembled into proteins. It was soon realized that for the most effective application of this approach, cell-free protein-synthesizing systems were needed. These were developed around 1950. By 1954, just after the double-helical structure of DNA was discovered, it was possible "to dissect the protein-synthesizing system into four constituents: amino acid, an ATP-donating component, a soluble enzyme function, and a microsomal fraction" (Siekevitz and Zamecnik, 1981, 54s). It appeared that a separate enzyme in the soluble fraction was needed for activating each amino acid, and the site of amino acid polymerization into protein was shown to occur in the microsomes. This led to the identification in 1958 by several groups of transfer RNA (tRNA). It was recognized that tRNAs function as the "adapter" molecules carrying a triplet code for each amino acid, as postulated in the same year by Crick. Where does protein synthesis take place? Further study of the microsome particles by ultracentrifugation indicated that the particles that contain both RNA and protein are identical with the particles seen with the EM and appeared to be involved in protein synthesis. The term "ribosome," reflecting their content of RNA, was proposed for the particles; and RNA in the ribosome came to be called ribosomal RNA ("rRNA.") However, an understanding of the relation between rRNA and protein synthesis required identification of yet another actor in the production line.

Whereas rRNA is biochemically stable (i.e., has a slow turnover), evidence was obtained for a different, labile RNA (with a rapid turnover) involved somehow in protein synthesis(Astrachan and Volkin,1958). A convergence of work from the laboratories of Jacob and Monod in France, Brenner and Meselson in the United Kingdom, and Watson and Gilbert in the United States provided evidence for an RNA species that has a rapid turnover as it associates and dissociates from a ribosome particle. This came to be known as "messenger RNA" (mRNA). Converting the information in DNA into mRNA came to be called "transcription." Converting the information in mRNA into protein, through the interactions of tRNA and mRNA, came to be called "translation."

At a meeting in 1957, in his talk "On Protein Synthesis" to the Society of Experimental Biology, meeting in Canterbury, England, Crick reviewed the evidence for the unidirectional flow of information from DNA to RNA to protein. On theoretical grounds, he made two fundamental predictions. The "sequence hypothesis" was that the sequence of bases in the DNA specifies the sequence of amino acids in the protein, which is all the information needed for the protein to fold into its three-dimensional structure. The "central dogma" hypothesis was that "once 'information' has passed into protein, it cannot get out again" (Ridley, 2006, 333). As expressed eloquently by Judson (1996, 332–333),

> if there is one statement from the new science that deserves the general currency of that equation [$E = mc^2$] of Einstein's, it is this assertion of Crick's [DNA to RNA to protein].... [it] was the restatement—radical, absolute—of why characteristics acquired by the organism in its life but not from its genes cannot be inherited by its offspring.

Ridley (2006) states that "On Protein Synthesis" defined the field and compared it to Newton's *Principia* and Wittgenstein's *Tractatus*. Crick's predictions provided the guideposts toward breaking the genetic code. It was another example of how important theory can be in guiding experiments.

Breaking the Code

In Crick's talk on protein synthesis, the "sequence hypothesis," that "the specificity of a piece of nucleic acid is expressed solely by the sequence of its bases, and that this sequence is a (simple) code for the amino acid sequence of a particular protein" (Judson, 1996, 332), was a bold claim, a belief held by many of his audience but still without any evidence. The information must be converted from being contained in sequences of four different purine and pyrimidine bases—adenine, cytosine, guanine and thymine—to sequences of amino acids. But how?

Up to that time biochemists had identified a large number of different amino acids in proteins, but no one had asked which were the essential ones. It started with a physicist. Crick (1988) describes how, soon after the published description of the double helix, he and Watson received a letter from the cosmologist George Gamow with the proposal that DNA was the direct template for protein synthesis and that all proteins were made of just 20 amino acids. This stimulated Watson and Crick to carry out an exhaustive review and generate their own list. They came up with a somewhat different set of precisely 20, which have remained the commonly occurring essential amino acids since then.

Crick; Gamow; ex-physicists such as Seymour Benzer; another leading cosmologist, Fred Hoyle; and others were attracted to the problem like moths to a flame, speculating on how combinations of the four nucleic acids could encode 20 amino acids and how this could be built into an "adaptor" molecule to convert the information contained in DNA into protein. These theoretical endeavors suggested that a triplet code was likely, that is, combinations of three adjacent nucleotides in nucleic acids encode one amino acid. Since four types of nucleotides (adenylate, cytidylate, guanylate and thmidylate) give 64 possible triplet combinations, it was also likely that the code was degenerate (i.e. redundant), that is, an amino acid could be encoded by more than one combination of three nucleotides.

The discovery that protein synthesis occurs on ribosomes and that the sequence of the protein synthesized by a ribosome was determined by the nucleotide sequence of the messenger RNA attached to the ribosome opened an approach to the experimental study of the genetic code. This approach required generating synthetic RNA (more precisely, synthetic polyribonucleotides). An enzyme capable of doing this, polynucleotide phosphorylase, had been discovered in 1955 by Ochoa and his colleagues (Grunberg-Manago et al., 1956); this enzyme could generate homopolyribonucleotides (e.g. polyadenylic acid: poly A) or random co-polynucleotides.

A biochemist at NIH, Marshall Nirenberg, used a cell-free protein-synthesizing system, whose synthetic activity could be enhanced, e.g. by tobacco mosaic virus. As a control he also tested polyuridylic acide (Poly U). Remarkably, this turned out to promote the formation of polyphenylalanine (Nirenberg and Matthei, 1961). This experiment was the first to identify the nucleotide code for an amino acid, which was most likely to be a triplet. Such a triplet of nucleotides was called a "codon" by Crick and Brenner (Crick et al., 1961).

Progress after that was rapid, and by 1966 all 64 triplet codes were known for all the essential amino acids and, therefore, the universal DNA code for making all proteins in all species. During this time, DNA was very much in the public eye and ear. I was at the NIH in the early 1960s and well remember the excitement that went through the audience when we gathered in the main auditorium of Building 10 in 1964 to hear Nirenberg explain the code and how it worked. Friends at dinner parties would say proudly that they had read about DNA and RNA and asked what it was going to mean for them. It was obviously a great achievement, but the practical significance lay in the future.

Replication, but Not in the Adult Human Brain

While the code breakers were attacking the problem of how DNA makes proteins, others were attacking the equally fundamental problem of how DNA replicates itself. The Watson-Crick model implied that genes do this by reproducing the same sequence during cell division (mitosis) and cell reproduction (meiosis). But how?

Biochemists soon isolated an enzyme from the bacterium *Escherichia coli* that catalyzes the synthesis of DNA. Since the synthesis involves adding nucleotides together in a sequence to make a polymer of nucleotides, the enzyme was called "DNA polymerase." This came to be called "polymerase I," acting in concert with many other enzymes to open the double helix and add nucleotides one at a time to form new complete DNA molecules. The mechanisms of DNA replication are covered in textbooks of biochemistry and cell biology.

It was realized that some organs, such as the liver, can regenerate most of their substance; and it was known since the 1880s that cells undergo mitotic renewal in most organs of the body, including skin, gut, and blood. However, it was also known that the brain is different because it does not regenerate itself after injury, and when cytologists (microscopists studying the internal structure of the cell) were able to observe the chromosomes within the cell, they could see no evidence of mitosis in adult brain cells. Thus, the turning off of replication was special for adult brain cells.

Why replication is turned off in adult brain cells was one of the great mysteries about the brain and still is. How to overcome this, in order to allow injured parts of the brain to regenerate, was recognized as one of the greatest challenges in neuroscience. It was clear that the factors that control DNA replication must be involved.

Dynamic Genes

Far removed from the research centers working on DNA, an investigator in the tradition of Gregor Mendel was working on the inheritance of characteristics in Indian corn (maize). In 1951 Barbara McClintock gave a lecture at Cold Spring Harbor on her theory of mobile "controlling elements" in maize, a theory so controversial that she refrained from publishing her data, sharing it instead with trusted colleagues until her theory of *mobile genes* was ultimately confirmed. McClintock's studies in the 1950s indicated that the phenotype of a corn plant, reflecting mutations of specific genes, could be due to remote genes and that remotely related genes could move about within the chromosomes. She characterized these as mutable and unstable loci, acting as controlling genetic elements. It would take almost 30 years for the significance of this work to be merged with the traditional view of the molecular biology of gene structure, to give an understanding of the dynamic nature of the genome.

How Many Chromosomes?

Apart from the fundamental discoveries of the molecular mechanisms of the genes, advances in understanding other aspects of genes were being made. In the early part of the twentieth century it was found that the *karyotype* (the arrangement of the chromosomes; from the Greek *karyo*, "nucleus") of the fruit fly has only four chromosomes. They are huge and wax and wane in size in relation to the cell cycle; therefore, they became inviting targets for research. From that time it was believed that the human karyotype consisted of 23 pairs (called "autosomes") plus an additional two X chromosomes in females or an X and Y chromosome in males. In 1956 it was finally determined that the human karyotype consists of only 22 pairs of autosomes plus the sex chromosomes. The karyotype of the mouse is 19 autosomes plus the sex chromosomes.

Human Genes

A new opening in studies of human genes came with the discovery that certain clinical disorders are associated with chromosomal abnormalities. First were sickle cell anemia, due to a defect in the gene for hemoglobin (Pauling et al., 1949), and glycogen storage disease, caused by a defect in the gene for the enzyme glucose-6-phosphate, which normally phosphorylates glucose when it is taken up from the bloodstream into cells. Further genetically based disorders were reported in 1959, including Down syndrome, associated with trisomy 21 (an extra number 21 autosome) (Lejeune et al., 1959), and several other developmental disorders.

Several of these disorders were shown to be associated with changes in the structure of cells in the cerebral cortex, especially deformations of tiny structures called "spines" that cover the dendrites of the main output neurons, the pyramidal cells. Spines are the sites of synaptic connections, which will be described in Chapter 7. These studies began the study of the link between single-gene defects and the highest cognitive functions in the human. We will return to this study in Chapter 12.

From Physics to Molecular Biology to the Brain

The great advances of the 1950s, especially the discovery of the structure of DNA, marked the end of speculations that biology could be based purely on classical physics, showing instead that, at the molecular level, biology is based on principles of chemistry and biophysics. Pauling mentioned Bohr's concept of complementarity but never followed it up (see Pauling and Delbrück 1940). Crick told me that he and Watson never used Bohr's idea of complementarity in their work, even though the essence of the DNA model was the complementarity of the DNA strands. Delbrück spent his life attempting to find examples of complementarity in biology but finally gave it up (Delbrück, 1972). Henceforth, the hereditary material was firmly in the domain of biological structures operating by biological mechanisms.

The essence of those structures and mechanisms, however, was to be found in the information they contained and read out to provide the blueprint for the organs of the developing creature. The most complex information would obviously be found in the blueprint for the most complex organ, the brain. In the 1950s the distance between the gene and the brain seemed infinite. However, the essential steps to the present occurred relatively quickly: after the structure of DNA in 1953, the genetic code was obtained by 1963; recombinant DNA and rapid DNA sequencing ushered in the era of DNA engineering in the 1970s; the polymerase chain reaction in the late 1980s enabled identification of any arbitrary gene and protein in any cell, including in the brain; and the sequence of the full human genome was obtained in 2000, with half the genes expressed in the brain. It has brought us to the threshold of a new golden age.

In conclusion, the 1950s may truly be termed a "golden age" for biological research, the greatest in history. By itself, the discovery of the structure of DNA is enough to warrant that claim. Will we advance so strongly in our new, increasingly large-scale, industrialized era of big science? Will we go on collecting data, or will we emulate those pioneers in the 1950s by advancing with huge steps based on small groups of scientists interacting fruitfully between experiment and theory? Our review of the history indicates how high they set the bar.

Chapter 3

Signaling Molecules: The First Growth Factor

Like all organs of the body, the nervous system arises from a single fertilized egg. Classical histologists visualized this process through the cells of the changing embryo. The first great synthesis was the idea of an organizer that directed the formation of the organs. The crux for the nervous system was how connections are established between cells, which implied the presence of intercellular signals. The clearest evidence for such a signal, called "nerve growth factor", was reported in 1951. Subsequent experiments identified its molecular structure, which came to be known as NGF, the first of a growing number of neurotropic and neurotrophic factors involved in neural development and in the plasticity of connections that underlie learning, memory, and response to injury. The orderly arrangement of the connections was hypothesized to require chemoaffinity between axons and their targets. These dynamic processes require trafficking of appropriate molecules in the axons, by a process of axonal transport. The 1950s can therefore be regarded as laying the foundations for the molecular basis of development.

The Axonal Growth Cone

Early insights into how nerve cells develop came from Wilhelm His in Basel in the 1880s (summarized in Shepherd, 1991). He was the founder of neuroembryology, gathering his observations in a monumental tome (His, 1880–85). Here, we note his observations relevant to the outgrowth of the axon and dendrites.

Using microscopic observations of stained tissue in fetal animals of different ages, he observed the sequence of events in the emergence of neuronal branches. A developing motor neuron in the spinal cord first sent a single long axon toward a ventral root, followed by emergence of multiple short processes (His, 1886). This observation contained two rules that have stood the test of time: nerve cells that develop an axon produce only one and the axon develops before the short processes. The short processes had been termed "protoplasmic prolongations"—literally, extensions from the cell body. His introduced the term "dendrite" to refer to them, which was immediately adopted.

The outgrowing axon was examined more closely in brain cells by Ramón y Cajal (1892) in Madrid, who identified the axon tip as a distinct entity, calling it the "axonal growth cone." He imagined it as a kind of battering ram, forcing its way through intervening cells and fibers to make specific contacts with target cells.

His and Ramón y Cajal represented what has been called the "histological tradition" in developmental studies, that is, inferring mechanisms from observations of fixed and stained cell structures. At the time it was the only possible strategy because physiological methods were lacking.

The "experimental histological approach" began with Ross Harrison (1870–1959) (Purves and Lichtman, 1985). He studied at Johns Hopkins and Berlin, one of the early American biologists to receive training in Europe. Returning to Johns Hopkins, he addressed the problem of how the axon is formed.

Despite the evidence of His and Cajal, there were still holdouts who claimed that the axon was formed by coalescence of glial cells. To meet these objections, Harrison dissected out small pieces of the neural tube of an early frog embryo and kept them in a dish devoid of other cells, bathed only in frog lymph. His microscopic observations gave dramatic pictures of the individual outgrowing axons and their growth cones extending into the surrounding lymph (Harrison, 1910). This paper was an instant classic (Appendix 3.1). Harrison's images of the outgrowing axons and their growth cones are still reproduced in textbooks today.

These experiments proved that axons arise only from nerve cells and that nerve cells are separate entities in making connection by contact with other cells. This was a final brick in the edifice of the classical neuron doctrine (Shepherd, 1991). These experiments were also of great general significance in introducing in vitro ("in glass") tissue culture methods into biology.

The Organizer Principle

During the first half of the twentieth century the experimental methods for studying development were limited. Apart from tissue culture, the only means for observing and manipulating single cells was at the earliest stages of favorable models such as the large eggs of sea urchins. The methods were wonderfully inventive. At the four-cell stage, it became possible to separate the cells under a dissecting microscope by ligating (tying) them with a single human hair! Beyond the first few cell divisions, however, the embryo became a complicated organism that could be studied by only two main methods: *ablation* (destruction) of a part of the embryo and *transplantation* of one part onto another.

Transplantation experiments were critically important for generating ideas about the key mystery in development: How do undifferentiated cells give rise to differentiated cells and organs? A key experiment was carried out in the laboratory of Hans Spemann by a student, Hilde Proescholdt (who published under her married name of Mangold).

Spemann (1869–1941) had studied in Wurzburg, Germany, and became skilled in microsurgical techniques. In his early studies he showed that the dorsal part of the egg is essential for organizing the development of the embryo. He established a school in 1919 at Freiburg, which became a center for training developmental biologists; best known among the students were Viktor Hamburger and Johannes Holtfreter.

As a graduate student, Proescholdt carried out transplantation studies at very early stages of embryonic development, when the egg has developed by only a few cell divisions into a ball of cells called a "blastula." In the next stage the blastula develops a pore; the cells on the surface move to the pore and migrate through it into the interior of the embryo to begin to form the organs of the body. Using the strategy of a pigmented donor embryo and an unpigmented recipient (host) embryo, she transplanted the lip region of the blastopore of the donor into the belly region of the recipient and found that the transplanted tissue could induce a second neural plate in the host and, sometimes, an entire secondary embryo grafted onto the first. In their classic paper, Spemann and Mangold (1924) suggested that this region of the blastopore had special organizing properties. This special ability became known as the "organizer principle." Tragically, Hilde Mangold, after obtaining her degree, died soon after her marriage in an accidental domestic fire. Many believed that she should have shared in the recognition that came to Spemann as a pioneer in development for the work she did with him.

The idea that the dorsal lip of the blastopore has special "organizer" properties soon gave way to evidence that many regions of the embryo have this ability to a greater or lesser degree, as do a variety of biological tissues, hormones, and even foreign substances. Nonetheless, the concept that development is the outcome of organizer properties of antecedent cell populations was established, although the question of what organizes the organizer seemed to constrain the understanding of development to an infinite regression of organizers back to the egg.

The indeterminate character of the organizer concept was unavoidable given that experiments could be carried out only at the level of pieces of organs and tissues. In this respect, the situation was similar to that obtaining in other disciplines during this period; for example, in pharmacology the search for neurotransmitters was similarly limited to the organ level. As Viktor Hamburger (1996, 228) later observed, "In retrospect it seems remarkable how much information was obtained by these modest methods." The same can be said of experiments on the pharmacology of neurotransmitters, also limited to the organ level, as we shall see in Chapter 4.

Nerve Growth Factor

A major question in embryology that investigators grappled with through the 1930s and 1940s was the relation between developing neurons and their target cells. Ramon y Cajal believed that "the immense majority of the neuroblasts [primitive nerve cell precursors] survive to term and succeed in collaborating [i.e., connecting] with the normal structures of the adult nervous system" (see Purves and Lichtman, 1985, 137). This process, however, was shown to be a dynamic one by Margaret Shorey, a student of Frank Lillie, one of the pioneers in embryology in the United States. In 1909 Shorey showed that removal of the limb buds in early embryos of the chick and salamander produced severe losses of the sensory ganglion cells and motor cells in the spinal cord. This implied that a substance in the muscles normally sustains the nerve cells. In 1920 Sam Detwiler, a student of Harrison, repeated the experiments; rather than a loss of cells, he found in the salamander that grafting on a new limb bud produced an increase in the sensory cells.

At this point, Viktor Hamburger (1900–2001) enters the scene (Fig. 3.1A). A student of Spemann at Freiberg, he traveled in 1932 to Chicago to spend a year on a Rockefeller Fellowship with Frank Lillie to learn neuroembryology. Lillie was another of the pioneers in embryology in the United States. His book *Embryology of the Chick* was a classic in the field (see comment below). Lillie suggested to Hamburger to begin his studies in neuroembryology by repeating the Shorey–Detwiler experiments to see if he could resolve their differences.

Hamburger confirmed Shorey's finding of reduced numbers of sensory and motor neurons in the spinal cord. He found he could quantitatively relate the reduction in cell number with the amount of muscle and peripheral sense organs removed. He formulated the following hypothesis (Hamburger, 1996, 232):

> 1. The targets, that is, the musculature and the sense organs, generate two specific agents, one controlling the spinal ganglia and the other controlling the lateral motor columns.
> 2. The agents travel retrogradely in the nerves to their respective nerve centers, the lateral motor columns and the spinal ganglia.
> 3. The agents regulate the development of the nerve centers in a quantitative way.

As Hamburger noted, "two decades later, the discovery of nerve growth factor (NGF) identified one of the two agents postulated in the first point."

Hamburger sent a reprint of his 1934 article to a colleague, Giuseppe Levi, in Turin, Italy, who passed it along to his associate Rita Levi-Montalcini (Fig. 3.1B). Her subsequent experiments, carried out under the most difficult conditions imaginable during the war in Italy in the 1940s, led to somewhat different results from those of Hamburger. In a characteristically generous gesture, Hamburger invited Levi-Montalcini to join him in St. Louis to work together to resolve the differences in their results. In their first experiments (Hamburger and Levi-Montalcini, 1949), they showed that not only is there central cell death in the spinal cord near the site of an extirpated limb but it also occurs in other unaffected central areas. This was the first observation of naturally occurring nerve cell death during embryonic development (though incorrectly interpreted as due to a peripheral effect on cell proliferation: D. Purves, personal communication). Since that time, it has become increasingly recognized that development involves not only the generation of new neurons but also their pruning by cell death.

What was the chemical agent necessary for maintaining new cells in the face of dying ones? As they cast about for preparations to attack this question, Hamburger received a reprint from a former student, Elmer Bueker, at Georgetown University. Bueker had tested whether an implanted, rapidly growing tumor would more effectively stimulate a nerve center than a transplanted limb. In the chick he found that an implanted mouse sarcoma strongly stimulated ingrowth of sensory nerves from the spinal cord (Bueker, 1948).

This suggested a preparation that would produce large amounts of the sought-after chemical agent. With Bueker's consent (though with his later regret for not having followed up on his result himself [Purves and Lichtman, 1985]), Levi-Montalcini and Hamburger took up Bueker's approach, confirming the stimulating effect of a tumor on nearby dorsal root ganglia (Fig. 3.2). They obtained evidence that the effect must be due to a substance secreted by the tumor and called this hypothetical substance "nerve growth stimulating factor" (Levi-Montalcini and Hamburger, 1951; Levi-Montalcini et al., 1953; Purves and Lichtman, 1985) (Appendix 3.2).

Levi-Montalcini was determined to pursue the nature of this factor. To do this, she first traveled to the laboratory of a friend, H. Meyer, in Rio de Janeiro, Brazil, to develop a tissue culture assay in which the degree of outgrowth of fibers from an explanted chick sensory ganglion registered in a semiquantitative manner the amount of growth factor to which it was exposed. In the same period a postdoctoral biochemist, Stanley Cohen, joined the Hamburger laboratory, to work on identifying the biochemical nature of the growth factor. Chemical analyses showed that the tumor extract contained both nucleic acids and proteins. To remove the nucleic acid in order to purify the protein, they exposed the extract to snake venom, which contained a phosphodiesterase that would cleave it. However, control experiments showed that the venom itself stimulated the cells, which was subsequently shown to be due to high levels of growth factors within the venom (Levi-Montalcini and Cohen, 1956). Since the venom of the snake is secreted by the salivary gland, Cohen investigated the salivary (submaxillary) gland of the mouse and found that it contained large amounts of growth factor, which led to its purification (Cohen, 1960).

The sequence from Bueker's tumor to snake venom to mouse submaxillary gland is a classic illustration of how "chance favors the prepared mind". Using large numbers of submaxillary glands as a source, the growth factor was finally sequenced by Angeletti and Bradshaw (1971). Nerve growth factor became universally known as NGF.

Nerve growth factor (NGF) was the first of a large and growing family of trophic factors that control neuron targeting and survival during development and into adult life. This work has shown the difference between neurotropic and neurotrophic action. A *neurotropic* action is one that affects the direction of neuronal growth, whereas a *neurotrophic* action is one that is necessary for neuron survival (Gilbert, 1991). Many other growth factors as well as NGF have both actions.

As a footnote to this account of Viktor Hamburger, experimental embryology was my favorite course as an undergraduate at Iowa State College in the early 1950s. The teacher was Howard Hamilton, the lecture text was Weiss's *Principles of Development* [1939], and the laboratory text was the second edition of Lillie's *Embryology of the Chick*, revised by Howard Hamilton [1951]. Among our guest lecturers was Carroll Williams of Harvard, an outstanding insect developmental biologist who was a discoverer of insect developmental hormones. Hamilton was a meticulously prepared lecturer and laboratory instructor and an inspiration to a new biology student like myself. It must have been one of the best courses in the subject anywhere. It illustrates how quality is spread broadly across institutions of higher learning in the United States.

In preparing the revision of Lillie's classic book, Hamilton had invited Hamburger to join him in introducing a more precise staging of the chick's development, based on the appearances of clear morphological features rather than simple chronology, the early stages appearing at hourly intervals and the later daily. Their staging was published in Hamburger and Hamilton [1951]. Nearly a half-century later Hamburger [1996, 244] noted, "The Hamburger–Hamilton stage series is still one of the most frequently-quoted publications in developmental biology," reflecting the soundness of their staging concept and the rising numbers of investigators using the chick for developmental studies—another enduring contribution of the 1950s. The modern reader can confirm this by simply googling "hamburger hamilton".

Organizing the Connections

If growth factors are necessary for cell survival and the outgrowth of nerve processes to their targets, what are the factors that determine the specific connections that a given cell makes with a given target cell? This specificity is necessary for an orderly arrangement of cells in one region to interact with an orderly arrangement of cells in another. The modern reader can follow this history in Purves and Lichtman (1985).

Chemiotaxis. The background for this problem was Cajal's (1892) idea that when axons grow out to make connections some kind of chemical interactions are involved. The first experiments addressing the problem were in the 1890s by John Langley in Cambridge, England (this was at the time he purchased the *Journal of Physiology* in London to save it from bankruptcy and became its long-serving editor). He cut the preganglionic fibers to the superior cervical ganglion and found that reinnervation occurred in a precise manner: Electrical stimulation of the preganglionic motor fibers from different spinal segments activated the appropriate end organs innervated by the postganglionic fibers. Somehow the appropriate synaptic connections were made in the ganglion. Langley (1895; cited in Purves and Lichtman, 1985, 255) speculated that

> there is some special chemical relation between each class of nerve fibre and each class of nerve cell, which induces each fibre to grow towards a cell of its own class and there to form its terminal branches. At bottom then the [phenomenon] would be a chemiotactic [*sic*] one.

This observation in fact anticipated nerve growth factor as well as a mechanism for organizing the growing axons.

Resonance Theory. In the 1920s this problem was taken up by Paul Weiss, who trained in Vienna and was later at Chicago and Rockefeller Universities. In the frog Weiss studied the innervation of the muscles in a grafted limb and found that each muscle of the grafted limb contracted exactly together with the muscle of the corresponding host limb (Weiss, 1924). He speculated that the motor axons innervated the grafted muscle in random fashion, with specificity conferred by specific patterns of activity; each muscle was believed to be tuned to respond selectively to a specific activity pattern. In analogy with a violin string resonating to a particular tone, he termed the idea the "resonance hypothesis." In this hypothesis spatial patterning is of no importance; the pattern of impulses carries the code.

The resonance theory appeared to be disproved by the finding that during muscle movement impulses do not occur in all nerves but only in the nerves to the active muscles, *with little difference in their patterning* (Wiersma, 1931; Purves and Lichtman, 1985).

In retrospect, the resonance hypothesis appears as an early example of an idea that often occurs in brain theory, that spatial mapping specificity can be accounted for or replaced by temporal signal patterning. Another example was in the early theories on the neural basis of memory formation (see Chapter 12).

Contact Guidance Theory. Weiss (1934) then carried out experiments showing that in culture systems axons tend to follow physical features, such as scratches on the bottom of the culture dish. This gave rise to yet another theory, the "contact guidance theory," in which axons aimed at neighboring target cells tend to bundle together in order to arrive in appropriate alignment at their neighboring target cells. Weiss postulated that these neighborly relations could be maintained by physical contact throughout the trajectory of the axons to their targets without need for chemical signals between them (see Purves and Lichtman, 1985).

The Chemoaffinity Hypothesis. One of Weiss's graduate students at Chicago was Roger Sperry. He obtained his PhD in 1941 with Paul Weiss and did a postdoctoral fellowship with Karl Lashley at Harvard. Lashley was a behavioral psychologist who believed that the cerebral cortex mediated specific functions despite, in his view, being organized in a diffuse manner without discrete functional regions (see Chapter 12). Despite his training with these two opponents of the specificity of neuronal connections, Sperry set out to test for specificity using the pathway from the retina to the optic tectum, the region in the midbrain where the retinal ganglion cells project in an orderly manner to represent the visual field projected onto the retina. He used newts, goldfish and frogs, which have powerful regeneration abilities. The experiments involved cutting one optic nerve and rotating the eye 180°. When regeneration of the optic nerve was complete, he found that the axons grew back to their previous target sites; the map of the retina onto the tectum was preserved, despite the rotation of the eye and the disorganization and regrowth produced by the transection. The animals as a consequence behaved as if their visual world was upside down (Sperry, 1943, 1948).

Sperry therefore postulated that individual axons and their individual target cells have matching biochemical "identification tags" so that they establish synaptic connections by a chemical affinity between them. He suggested that this mutual affinity is responsible not only for the reestablishment of connections during regeneration but also for the establishment of connections during normal development (Sperry, 1959). The idea was therefore called the "chemoaffinity hypothesis" As pointed out by Purves and Lichtman (1985), it was the realization of the concept suggested by Langley over a half-century earlier (Appendix 3.3).

Sperry's results were therefore directly opposed to the notions of nonspecific neuronal connectivity of Weiss and Lashley. As Viktor Hamburger later observed, "I know of nobody else who has disposed of the cherished ideas of both his doctoral and postdoctoral sponsor, both at that time acknowledged leaders in their fields" (Hamburger, 1979, 5; also in Purves and Lichtman, 1985, 259).

The chemoaffinity hypothesis became the focus of much further testing and refinement, and the retinotectal pathway proved to be an excellent model for these studies. It is probably fair to say that most theories of the development of maps in the brain assume some variation on the chemoaffinity hypothesis (i.e., that the growth cones of the incoming axons and their target neurons must have some cell surface identification molecules that enable the two participants to recognize each other).

With regard to the *identity* of the molecular tags, these data had to await the development of the field of cell surface markers in the 1980s and 1990s. With regard to the *arrangement* of the molecular tags, Sperry (1963) envisaged that they are laid down in spatial gradients across the populations of projecting axons and target cells; two tags in gradients orthogonal to each other would define unique x and y coordinates within the tectum. The original hypothesis stressed rigid genetic mechanisms underlying the resulting patterns of synaptic connections in the nervous system. Subsequent research has focused on multiple signal molecules that are expressed in a position-dependent fashion at the sites where the axons originate in the retina and terminate in the tectum (reviewed in Purves and Lichtman, 1985). The interest in NGF has expanded to the multiple cell-signalling molecules that control cell-cell interactions, from development to learning, ageing and repair (Lichtman and Sanes, 2008).

For most systems, the main molecules identified thus far are growth factors and axon guidance molecules that affect all members in the cell assemblies; molecules that identify individual cells have been elusive. However, the best example of specific molecules that enable axons to differentiate between different cell targets are the olfactory receptors, which form families of up to 1000 or more different members. Their mRNAs are expressed at low levels in the axons and axonal growth cones of subsets of olfactory receptor cells and are involved in guiding the axons to different glomerular targets (Vassar et al., 1993; Ressler et al., 1993; Mombaerts et al., 1996a).

Axonal Transport

The work on growth factors and cell surface proteins implied transport through the axon to bring growth signals back to the cell body and to bring the growth factors and proteins produced in the cell body forward to the axon terminals to interact with the recognition molecules in the target cells. Although traffic in the axon belongs perhaps more logically in the chapter on the cell, we consider it here because the first evidence came from a laboratory in neural development, that of Paul Weiss.

Weiss and Hiscoe (1948) carried out the simple experiment of tying a fine thread (ligature) around a nerve bundle and observing the consequences. They found a swelling on the cell side of the ligature, implying that there was a net flow of material within the axon from the cell body to the periphery, in the centripetal (*centri*, "center"; *petal*, "away") direction. Recall that Weiss believed in physical contact controlling axonal outgrowth, so his attention was on these physical properties of what came to be called "axoplasmic transport" (Appendix 3.4).

At first, this evidence was tested with similar experiments, requiring interpretations of what aspects of the traffic (i.e., flow rate, intra-axonal pressure) accounted for the bulging of the axon. (I remember this kind of physical effect being reported in a seminar at Oxford around 1960.) By the early 1960s radioactive tracers were introduced, which soon showed that there were several types of transport. Fast transport of proteins, traced by radioactively labeled amino acids that were taken up and incorporated into protein, proceeded at a rate of up to 400 mm per day, equivalent to 15 mm per hour or, at the microscopic level, 4 μm per second. This occurred in large myelinated axons (Ochs et al., 1960; Grafstein, 1967, 1999) and in the finest unmyelinated axons (Land and Shepherd, 1974). Subsequent work showed the molecular basis of the transport along the microtubules (Schnapp et al., 1985). (I recall one of the exciting moments at the Society for Neuroscience annual meeting in the 1980s, when Tom Reese showed the first videos of vesicles scurrying along microtubules in the squid axon.)

This transport is the critical link for traffic related to the growth of the axon and the sensing properties of the growth cone, in delivering vesicles and other components of the presynaptic active zone, and in providing the maintenance and repair of the axon and all its synapses. Intracellular transport takes place not only in axons but also in dendrites, where it plays an equally critical role in the development and maintenance of postsynaptic (and in some cases presynaptic) elements.

Chapter 4

Signaling Molecules: The First Neurotransmitters in the Brain

In addition to the signal molecules between cells that mediate development are the signal molecules between nerve cells that mediate behavior. The key signal molecules for these functions are neurotransmitters, neuropeptides, internal second messengers, hormones, and pheromones. Apart from the sex hormones, most of these major types of components were first identified and their significance recognized in and around the 1950s. Before the 1950s, the biochemistry and pharmacology of the brain were essentially nonexistent. By the end of the decade, all the major categories of signaling agents had begun to emerge and the first textbook of brain biochemistry had appeared. However, it wasn't until the 1980s that a consensus began to emerge on the main neurotransmitters. Second messengers were discovered in 1957 and have been an essential motif in neurobiology since the 1970s. Neuropeptides were also first discovered in the 1950s and became a major theme in the 1970s, linked to second messengers. Pheromones were identified and named in the 1950s and are recognized to control the social behaviors of most animals, including significant roles in humans. These fields have expanded exponentially, and the mechanisms are the subject of intense investigation. Are current investigations opening the doors to new under-standing as widely as these initial discoveries?

We move from chemical signals between cells involved in the development of the nervous system to chemical signals between cells, to enable them to carry out the information processing that underlies the ability of animals to engage in the range of behavior characteristic of different species.

Early Experiments

To the histologists of the mid-nineteenth century, the idea that nerve cells need chemical signals to communicate with each other—what came to be called "chemical transmission"—was not apparent and took a long time to be established. Much of the history of neuroscience has been given to discovering and characterizing these signal molecules: what they are, how they are produced, how they act on their target cells, and how they are modulated by activity.

The concept of chemical transmission in the nervous system began with evidence that there might be junctions between excitable cells. The first clues emerged from the work of Claude Bernard in Paris on curare, the arrow-tip poison brought back to Europe by explorers in South America in the early nineteenth century (called also "tubocurare" after the tubes in which the curare was shipped) (Bowman, 1983, 109–110). A curare-tipped arrow caused instant paralysis and death. What was the cause? Bernard showed in 1856 that curare applied directly to the muscle had no effect but applied to the nerve and the muscle induced paralysis. He speculated that the curare was transported by the nerve back to the spinal cord to cause the death of the central end of the motor nerve (see Bowman, 1983, 110). His student, Vulpian, extended these studies in 1866, concluding correctly that the likely site of action of the poison was the junction between the muscle nerve and the muscle (Bowman, 1983, 110).

This was a classic experiment, introducing the motor nerve and its muscle as a subject for physiological study and providing a starting point for both the physiology (normal function) and pharmacology (effects of drugs) of the junction which came to be called the "synapse." The only idea of mechanism at the time was a brief comment by Emil du Bois-Reymond (1877) in Germany, that normal activation of the muscle could occur through "stimulatory secretion" of a "powerful stimulatory substance" by the nerve endings on the muscle.

In the early physiological laboratories of the time, the isolated beating heart of a frog or turtle became a standard preparation, in which a routine demonstration was the slowing of the heart produced by electrical stimulation of the vagus nerve. However, the fact that nerve impulses in the vagus nerve produced inhibition of the heart, in contrast to excitation by peripheral nerves to skeletal muscle, made it difficult to interpret the relation between nerve impulses and their actions on target cells (the explanation came only after the demonstration that the vagus nerves excite the parasympathetic ganglion cells in the sinoatrial node, which are inhibitory to the cardiac cells) (Bacq, 1983).

In the 1860s Schmiedeberg in Germany showed that an alkaloid substance called muscarine, from *Amanita muscaria*, mimicked the inhibitory action of vagal stimulation on the heart (see Bacq, 1975, 52). This may be regarded as one of the first pharmacological studies of synaptic transmission, long before any clear concept of this process.

"Chemical Mediators" and "Receptive Substances"

The first clear evidence came from Thomas Elliott, a student at Cambridge, England. His mentor, John Langley, had defined the autonomic nervous system in 1898 and by 1905 had further differentiated the autonomic nerves. Those associated with the cranial (head) and sacral (behind) parts of the autonomic nervous system he termed "parasympathetic" and those associated with the trunk were termed "sympathetic" (see Chapter 9). Elliott found that the compound adrenaline, obtained from the adrenal glands, mimicked the effects of sympathetic nerve stimulation. He tested the effects of adrenaline on several organs before and after denervation and presented a preliminary communication on his work to The Physiological Society (Elliott, 1904) entitled "On the action of adrenalin", which contained these lines (p 21):

> the point at which the stimulus of the chemical excitant [adrenaline] is received, and transformed into what may cause the change of tension of the muscle fibre, is perhaps a mechanism developed out of the muscle cell in response to its union with the synapsing sympathetic fibre. *Adrenalin might then be the chemical stimulant liberated on each occasion when the impulse arrives at the periphery.* (italics added)

The sentence in italics has been regarded as the first statement of the chemical theory of synaptic transmission (see O'Connor, 1991). We have already met Langley as credited with the first statement, at this same time, of the concept of chemotaxis in development (Chapter 3).

The studies of Elliott and Langley introduced the concepts that a "chemical mediator" is secreted by active nerve terminals and that it acts on "receptive substances" on the target cells. In addition, there was the idea that the junction forms during development due to some "trophic," growth-stimulating, effect of muscle on nerve. Finally, since all impulses are alike (see Chapter 6), it is the junction that determines the nature of the muscle response, whether it is excited or inhibited. This was the origin of the concepts of excitatory and inhibitory synapses. Given the fact that the experiments were carried out on the whole organ, the insights into cellular and even molecular mechanisms were remarkable.

The Concept of "Lock-and-Key"

At the time of these early pharmacological studies the best models for activation at the molecular level were for enzymes acting on their substrates. In the 1890s Emil Fischer in Germany published studies of sugar-converting enzymes in which he proposed that the interaction between an enzyme and its substrate has a specificity that can be likened to a "lock-and-key" mechanism. Based on this idea, Paul Ehrlich developed the concept of a molecular nucleus with "side chains" that bound distinct antitoxins to explain the specificity of interactions in the immune system. The "lock-and-key" model became a popular analogy for explaining chemical reactions in biology. However, the idea that interactions between enzymes and their substrate molecules would be similar to interactions between "receptive substances" and their receptive molecules was slow to penetrate the pharmacological literature. In fact, the explicit application of the methods developed for analysis of enzyme kinetics to the properties of receptors was to await the modern era.

Organ Pharmacology

The studies of Langley and his students early in the 1900s on identifying active substances at autonomic nerve endings in body organs provided a clear thrust forward. But proving the presence of a chemical mediator and its receptive substances was to consume the interest and ignite the passions of biochemists and pharmacologists for most of the first half of the twentieth century. The crucial obstacle was not lack of effort or insightful experiments but being confined to whole-organ preparations. The studies were limited to stimulating nerve trunks and observing effects on glands or muscles, collecting the perfusates, and testing them on biological assays. Although these studies allowed growing support for the existence of chemical transmission, they could not provide proof regarding the synaptic mechanism at the cellular level.

Important early advances were the characterization of acetylcholine as a potential chemical mediator by Walter Dixon (1907) and Henry Dale (1914a, 1914b) in England. Two kinds of actions were identified, a rapid one mimicked by nicotine (as at the neuromuscular junction) and a slower one mimicked by muscarine (as in the heart). The culmination of this line of work was the demonstration in 1921 by Otto Loewi in Germany that the vagus nerve inhibits the heart by liberating a substance, "vagusstoff," and the demonstration of its equivalence to acetylcholine (Feldberg and Krayer, 1933). The diagram of the two frog hearts, the one stimulated to release a substance (acetylcholine) into the perfusing fluid that acts to inhibit the beating of the other, is a classic in the history of both physiology and neuroscience. An inhibitory transmitter at synapses in the central nervous system was suggested by Edgar Adrian and Charles Sherrington in England.

Walter Bradford Cannon at Harvard made many contributions during this period. He extended Claude Bernard's idea of the constancy of the internal environment ("milieu interieur") to the broad concept of "homeostasis", and characterized the "fight or flight" emotions aroused during an animal's response to threats. This led to studies during the 1930s of adrenaline and noradrenaline as the transmitter substances for the sympathetic nerves to the viscera and for their roles in the behavioral actions related to aggression and fear (summarized in Cannon, 1945).

Dale and Feldberg and others showed that acetylcholine acts at all parasympathetic junctions. Dale (1935) introduced the distinction between "cholinergic" nerve fibers, which release acetylcholine, and "adrenergic" fibers, which release "adrenaline-like sympathin." He further suggested that these mediators act on "cholinoreceptive receptors" and "adrenoreceptive receptors," respectively;

however, the terms "cholinergic receptors" and "adrenergic receptors" have become universal instead. This set the precedent for terms characterizing other types of receptors for other types of chemical mediators at the synapses in the brain.

The "Soup vs. Sparks" Debate

During the 1930s the evidence built up for chemical transmission. Dale and his colleagues (1936) showed that acetylcholine is released from a stimulated muscle nerve and that, when injected into the bloodstream to an isolated muscle, causes it to twitch. However, while Dale and Loewi and others were laying the foundations for the view that synaptic transmission takes place through chemical messengers, many neurophysiologists continued to hold the opposite view, that synaptic transmission occurs by means of electrical current passing from one neuron to the next. They objected that many of the biochemical experiments involved collecting substances in perfusates of isolated organs that were stimulated at high rates so that the results were "pharmacological" rather than "physiological," a concern with all experiments involving application of drugs. It was also difficult to generalize from these peripheral organs to synapses in the central nervous system, where experimental methods, both physiological and biochemical, were at that time almost completely lacking (for an insightful review by a participant, see Bacq, 1975).

The controversy during the 1930s came to be known as the great "soup vs. sparks" debate (there are many accounts: see Cowan et al., 2000). The Australian neurophysiologist John Eccles, the last student trained by Sherrington in Oxford, was the most vociferous proponent of the "sparks" side. At meeting after meeting he challenged the pharmacologists defending the "soup" side. The pitched battles between the younger, aggressive Eccles and the older, pugnacious Dale are part of neuroscience lore. Bernard Katz, newly arrived in England in 1935, recorded his impressions (see Katz, 1996, p 373):

> To my great astonishment [at the meeting of the Physiological Society] I witnessed what seemed to be almost a stand-up fight between J. C. Eccles and H. H. Dale, with the chairman E. D. Adrian acting as a most uncomfortable and reluctant referee. Eccles had presented a paper in which he disputed the role of acetylcholine as a transmitter in the sympathetic ganglion. . . . When [he] had given his talk, he was counterattacked in succession by Brown, Feldberg, and Dale . . . [However] it did not take me long to discover that this form of banter led to no resentment between the contenders, it was in fact a prelude to much fruitful discussion over the years and indeed to growing mutual admiration between Dale and Eccles.

Others have, however, noted Dale's annoyance with Eccles' refusal to accept the chemical evidence. Eccles' pugnaciousness was met by the equally pugnacious Dale, whereas Eccles' attacks on others less able or willing to behave in this manner were regarded by many as excessive and unfair (see Chapter 7).

(It may also be observed that this kind of free-wheeling criticism was largely possible because it took place in an era of low budgets for research in which people functioned with largely independent support. As noted in Chapter 2, that era was replaced after World War II by government support of research, with larger budgets which, however, depended on "peer review" by colleagues that often included one's adversaries. For better or for worse, the intensity of open debate declined, while the intensity of anonymous reviews of manuscripts for publication and proposals for grant support rose.)

Some sense of soup vs. sparks controversy at the end of the 1930s can be gained from the remarks of Alexander Forbes (who was able to maintain his good humor) of Harvard, summing up the symposium on the synapse that was held in 1939, p 471:

> So goes the controversy. Dale in discussing it remarked that it was unreasonable to suppose that nature would provide for the liberation in the ganglion of acetylcholine, the most powerful known stimulant of ganglion cells, for the sole purpose of fooling physiologists. To this Monnier replied that it was likewise unreasonable to suppose action potentials would be delivered at the synapses with voltages apparently adequate for exciting the ganglion cells merely to fool physiologists.

The Intracellular Electrode Resolves the Controversy

At that moment, the introduction of the glass micropipette for electrical recording enabled observation of the electrical response at the synaptic junction for the first time. With these methods the electrophysiologists began to move the evidence for synaptic mechanisms from the organ to the cellular level. We take up that story in Chapter 7.

Neurotransmitters in the Brain

At this point the Second World War (1939–1945) intervened. After the war, studies of chemical mediators diversified. In one line, electrophysiologists, using the microelectrode, revealed the physiology and pharmacology of the synapse at the cellular level; we discuss this work further in Chapter 7. In a separate line, biochemists and pharmacologists attempted to obtain evidence for bioactive substances that could function as chemical mediators in the brain. We take up this part of the story next.

It will be difficult for the contemporary student of neuroscience to imagine the paucity of means at midcentury for studying chemical transmitters and their receptors in the brain. There was essentially no field of brain biochemistry or neurochemistry, no textbook or journal for either field, and few methods for biochemists or pharmacologists other than to grind up tissue and use rudimentary means to see what was there. In these, as in so many respects, the brain was the most refractory of the body organs.

Books on the chemistry of the brain had appeared from time to time, beginning with Thudichum's *Treatise on the Chemical Constitution of the Brain* (1884), largely concerned with documenting the presence of lipids. Himwich's *Brain Metabolism and Cerebral Disorders* (1951), contained early evidence on metabolism in brain tissue.

The new era began with the First International Neurochemical Symposium in Oxford in 1954 (published as *Biochemistry of the Developing Nervous System*; Waelsch, 1955) and the publication of *Biochemistry and the Central Nervous System* by Henry McIlwain (1955), a pioneer of the field, at the Maudsley Hospital in London. (I purchased both books as a medical student at the time.) There soon followed the publication of W. D. M. Paton's (1958) "Central and Synaptic Transmission in the Nervous System; Pharmacological Aspects," Gershenfeld and Tauc's (1961) "Pharmacological specificities of neurones in an elementary central nervous system", Hugh McLennan's (1963) *Synaptic Transmission*, and Eccles' (1964) *Physiology of Synapses*.

The contrast between the last of these books and the state of knowledge of brain neurotransmitters around 1950 can be gained from what was covered in the authoritative textbook entitled *The Pharmacological Basis of Therapeutics*, second edition, by Goodman and Gilman, published in 1955. (I used this text in the pharmacology course in medical school in 1957.) With regard to the substances we now know to be transmitters, the available information at the time can be summarized as follows:

Acetylcholine: Described mainly in relation to its parasympathetic autonomic actions on visceral organs. Studies of its possible central actions in the spinal cord were only beginning.

Norepinephrine: Mentioned only for its role in sympathetic autonomic actions at visceral organs.

Serotonin: Not mentioned

Dopamine: Not mentioned.

Glutamate: Glutamic acid (glutamate) was mentioned for its possible use in the symptomatic treatment of epilepsy.

γ-Aminobutyric acid (GABA): Not mentioned.

That was it.

Against this background, it is remarkable that in the course of the 1950s the first evidence was in fact obtained for most of the major neurotransmitters in the brain that we recognize today. We briefly discuss each in turn. The evidence came from several methods: biochemical studies, electrophysiological studies (see also Chapter 7), and histofluorescence studies (see Chapter 7).

Criteria for Transmitter Identification

The early studies of the physiology and pharmacology of synapses recognized that a set of strict criteria had to be met to establish the identity of a neurotransmitter substance (see Eccles, 1964):

1. appropriate enzymes for synthesizing the transmitter in the presynaptic terminal
2. sufficient quantities of the substance in the presynaptic terminal
3. sufficient release upon stimulation of the presynaptic axons
4. identical action of the substance when artificially applied
5. identical pharmacology of experimental and natural substances
6. an inactivating enzyme or other mechanism for substance removal

As we have seen, these criteria had been difficult enough to meet for accessible peripheral synapses and posed much greater challenges for the central, almost inaccessible synapses. Although initial progress was made in the 1950s, it took well into the 1980s and even 1990s before general agreement emerged on the neurotransmitters in the main pathways in the brain; and even now the hard evidence is patchy, with many of the criteria not met for many types of synaptic connections.

Dale's Law

A further criterion for identifying a transmitter was based on a suggestion of Dale. In a review of synaptic transmitters in the autonomic nervous system (Dale, 1934, 329), he wrote

the phenomena of regeneration appear to indicate that the nature of the chemical function, whether cholinergic or adrenergic, is characteristic for each particular neurone, and unchangeable. When we are dealing with two different endings of the same sensory neurone, the one peripheral and concerned with vasodilatation and the other at a central synapse, can we suppose that the discovery and identification of a chemical transmitter of axon-reflex dilation would furnish a hint as to the nature of the transmission process at a central synapse? The possibility has at least some value as a stimulus to further experiment.

This modest suggestion was later elevated by Eccles and others to Dale's law. It implied that during development some process of differentiation determines the particular secretory product a given neuron will manufacture, store, and release. The usefulness of the law in the analysis of synaptic circuits is explicit in Dale's statement, for if a substance can be established as the transmitter at one synapse, it can be inferred to be the transmitter at all other synapses made by that neuron. It was a corollary to the anatomical, physiological, metabolic, and genetic unity of the neuron as stated in the original neuron doctrine (Waldeyer, 1891; see Shepherd, 1991).

Dale's law applied only to the presynaptic unity of the neuron, not to the postsynaptic actions of the released transmitter. Subsequent studies, especially in invertebrates, were to show that these actions could be different depending on the types of neurotransmitter receptors in the target cells.

Early Evidence for Acetylcholine as an Excitatory Transmitter

The first evidence for the action of acetylcholine (ACh) at a central synapse was obtained by Eccles and co-workers (1954) for the Renshaw pathway in the spinal cord (see Chapter 9). In this pathway, ACh acts as an excitatory transmitter at the synapse from motoneuron axon collaterals to Renshaw interneurons, which then feed back inhibition onto the motoneurons. Its excitatory action is similar to its excitatory action at the neuromuscular junction, taken as an expression of Dale's law.

This early evidence stimulated a search for excitatory actions of ACh elsewhere in the brain. No clear evidence was found at the time. As a consequence, the search shifted to other substances.

Early Evidence for Glutamate as an Excitatory Transmitter

Little progress was made during the 1950s toward this goal until the end of the decade, when Curtis and co-workers (1960) reported that injection of acidic amino acids, including aspartic, glutamic, and cysteic acids, by a technique called microiontophoresis, near an electrode from which one is making recordings causes the neuron to discharge impulses repetitively. The similarity to the depolarization and repetitive discharges of Renshaw cells responding to ACh suggested that these amino acids could be specific excitatory transmitters. However, in an authoritative review, Eccles (1964, 71) noted that the authors

argue against identification with the synaptic transmitting agent, and suggest instead that they are non-specific excitants that act at receptor sites on the subsynaptic membrane other than the sites of action of the synaptic transmitters.

This excerpt indicates how cautious the initial investigators were about identifying a substance as a specific neurotransmitter in the absence of the ability to meet the proposed criteria. In follow-up studies the authors (Curtis and Watkins 1961) showed by topical application that these amino acids were powerful excitants of cells in the cat cerebral cortex. They also showed that a new substance, N-methyl-D-aspartic acid (NMDA), was the most powerful excitant, some 10 times more powerful than D-glutamic acid. Although aspartic acid subsequently faded from contention as the main excitatory neurotransmitter in the brain in favor of glutamic acid, in the form of NMDA it has been at the forefront of studies of plasticity of glutamic acid receptors and their role in learning and memory.

The best evidence for glutamate and other acidic amino acids as specific excitatory transmitters first emerged in studies of invertebrates. Takeuchi and Takeuchi (1963) demonstrated that receptor sites on crustacean muscle fibers, activated by local application of these substances, corresponded to synaptic sites on these fibers.

Despite this evidence, acceptance of glutamate as an excitatory neurotransmitter was slow in coming. As late as 1972, in the authoritative *Basic Neurochemistry*, edited by Albers, the main evidence noted was that of Van Harreveld and Mendelson (1959) (not cited by Eccles), who showed that brain extracts containing the acidic amino acids, when applied to the cerebral cortex, caused muscle contractions (through the descending motor pathways).

(I can attest to the difficulty we all had of accepting during the 1960s and 1970s the mounting evidence because of its piecemeal nature and the inability to satisfy all of the fundamental criteria for transmitter identification. It was not until the 1980s that glutamate began to be widely accepted as the main excitatory neurotransmitter in the brain.)

Early Evidence for GABA as an Inhibitory Transmitter

In contrast to glutamic acid, evidence that another acidic amino acid, GABA, might be an inhibitory transmitter at central synapses emerged early in the 1950s.

In 1950 GABA was first identified in extracts of mammalian brain, by the laboratories of Awapara, Udenfriend, and Roberts (summarized in Bennett and Balcar, 1999). It was initially assumed that GABA is involved in the metabolism of glutamate. Several investigators are credited with the first suggestion of GABA as an inhibitory neurotransmitter. T. Hayashi (1954) made this suggestion on the basis that GABA is found in the brain and has anticonvulsant activity (Koelle, 1955, 431). A key step was made by Ernst Florey (1954), who reported that brain extracts contain an inhibitory "substance I," as judged by inhibition of impulse firing of the crustacean stretch receptor in response to stretch (Koelle, 1955, 431). Substance I was then identified as GABA (Bazemore et al., 1957).

The upsurge of work on GABA led to a large interdisciplinary conference in 1959 to discuss its possible role as an inhibitory neurotransmitter in the brain. Despite the fact that the brain contains high concentrations of GABA and the early evidence for its inhibitory function, there was much skepticism. A primary concern was that the criteria for a transmitter had not been met, chiefly that no one had yet demonstrated its ability to produce an inhibitory postsynaptic potential. There were many reports against it; for example, it was reported that GABA was undetectable in the crustacean central nervous system, suggesting "All available evidence speaks... against it playing a role as inhibitory transmitter in vertebrates" (Florey, in Roberts, 1998, 371). These and other experiments giving negative results were all shown later to have been due to inadequate methods. Nonetheless, the outcome at the time was that "the curtain appeared to have been brought down on the candidacy of GABA as inhibitory transmitter" (Roberts, 1998, 373). A most discouraging prospect.

Resolution of this controversy occurred beyond our focus on the 1950s. Eccles (1964), for example, argued that intracellular recordings showed that inhibitory synaptic actions always produce a membrane hyperpolarization, which was not produced by GABA application. However, it was soon realized that the inhibitory action was due to an increase in Cl ion conductance, which could hold the membrane from being depolarized at its reversal potential without needing to cause hyperpolarization.

The definitive evidence was provided by a systematic study by Edward Kravitz and his colleagues, working in the new multidisciplinary Department of Neurobiology at Harvard Medical School under Stephen Kuffler. They showed in the lobster that GABA is synthesized by glutamic acid decarboxylase (GAD) in the motor nerves, is present there in high concentration, is released from inhibitory axons on stimulation, and when applied to the junction has the same inhibitory action as stimulating the nerves (Otsuka et al., 1966). In the mammalian brain the situation was otherwise; during the 1960s various studies suggested that GABA was not a transmitter there. As recalled by Bowery and Smart (2006), the first definitive evidence for GABA as an inhibitory transmitter in the mammalian brain was by Krnjevic and Schwartz (1967), who showed, using microelectrode recordings, that GABA mimics synaptic inhibition when iontophoresed onto cat cerebral cortical neurons. Subsequent studies rapidly showed that GABA is the major inhibitory neurotransmitter in most regions of the brain.

By the end of the 1970s the role of GABA as an inhibitory transmitter was established at several types of central synapses and thereafter at most such synapses. By modern definitions, the early studies were on fast-acting GABA-A synapses; later studies have identified different mechanisms related to different postsynaptic receptor types.

Early Evidence for Serotonin as a Neurotransmitter

It was known from the middle of the nineteenth century that when blood clots are formed they release a substance into the blood that causes the smooth muscle of the blood vessels to constrict, increasing vascular "tone." By the turn of the century blood platelets were identified as the source of this substance. In 1948, Rapport and colleagues isolated this substance, calling it "serotonin" (*sero*, "serum"; *tonin*, "tonic"), and showed that it was the chemical 5-hydroxytryptamine (5HT). It was synthesized in 1951. It was realized that 5HT was identical to a substance that had been shown to be widely distributed within the gut and other organs, with a variety of stimulating and depressing effects.

In 1953 5HT was found to be present in the brain, which suggested that it might have a role as a neurotransmitter there. Interest really perked up with the discovery that the extremely active hallucinogen lysergic acid diethylamide (LSD) has a similar chemical structure and that it antagonizes the stimulating actions of 5HT using a standard physiological preparation of smooth muscle, a strip of the guinea pig ileum (Gaddum, 1953; Woolley and Shaw, 1954). After the discovery of the tranquilizer reserpine (see Chapter 15), it was found in animal experiments that administration of LSD causes a deep fall in the 5HT content of the brain (Brodie and Shore, 1957)

This attracted enormous interest, among both research workers and, for better or worse, the public. The rumored powers of 5HT to expand consciousness attracted much attention, from young people wanting a wild ride to adults wanting to analyze their minds. The former were exemplified by the kids who gathered at Woodstock in 1969, the latter by the novelist Aldous Huxley. The effects were hallucinations, which were usually extremely disturbing and sometimes fatal. From that time, 5HT has been a leading candidate as a neurotransmitter for a wide range of normal and abnormal brain functions and as a target for a wide range of psychoactive drugs (Goodman and Gilman, 1955, 614; also Siegel et al., 1999, 264).

Subsequent research on 5HT split into several paths: the pharmacology of the receptors, metabolic pathways for synthesis and degradation, mechanisms of synaptic release, identification of serotonin transporters, and localization of 5HT brain pathways. Currently, 5HT is attracting considerable interest in the treatment of mood disorders through development of drugs to increase serotonin levels through selective serotonin reuptake inhibitors (SSRIs) (see Chapter 15).

Catecholamine Transmitters

A large family of neurotransmitters consists of molecules with aromatic rings and an amine side chain that are derived from dietary tyrosine. The biosynthetic pathway was worked out by Hugh Blaschko in the United Kingdom in 1939, passing from tyrosine to dihydroxyphenylalanine (DOPA) to dopamine to norepinephrine and finally epinephrine (Fig. 4.1). It was known at that time that epinephrine is an excitatory transmitter in the peripheral nervous system, but it was assumed that the others were not bioactive. This, however, changed rapidly in the 1950s when evidence came forward that they were widely present in the brain.

A breakthrough occurred in research on the actions of reserpine. This work will be considered in greater detail later (see Monoamine Histofluorescence) and in Chapter 15. Here, we note that work by Arvid Carlsson and his colleagues at

Lund showed that the behavioral effects of reserpine were due to depletion of catecholamines (Fig. 4.2). They found that dopamine is present in the brain and is released by reserpine along with noradrenaline and serotonin, suggesting that they are biologically active in the brain, possibly as neurotransmitters (Carlsson et al., 1959). It was shown that dopamine was present in high concentrations in the basal ganglia, which led to the hypothesis that the symptoms of parkinsonism (sedation and akinesia) produced by reserpine administration are due to depletion of dopamine in the basal ganglia. These symptoms could be relieved by administration of the dopamine precursor L-dopa (Carlsson, 36) (Appendix 4.1). During this time, Oleh Hornykiewicz in Vienna also carried out pioneering studies of dopamine in the human brain and its possible involvement in diseases of the extrapyramidal system (see Chapter 13).

These findings, together with those of other laboratories, led to an international meeting on adrenergic mechanisms in London in 1960 to discuss the status of these mechanisms in the brain. The meeting was dominated by British pharmacologists, led by H. H. Dale, who had figured so prominently in the soup vs. sparks debates with Eccles in the 1930s. The general attitude to the new findings from Carlsson and others was highly skeptical. Dopamine given in high doses was lethal; perhaps it was acting as a general poison in the experiments that were reported. These and other criticisms led to the general conclusion that "there was absolutely no evidence that the catecholamines in the brain act as synaptic transmitters" and "any of the theories on a relation between catecholamines or serotonin and behavior is 'a construction which some day will be amended'" (Vogt, in Carlsson, 38).

The outcome at this point for catecholamines was thus similar to that for GABA mentioned earlier: evidence for a role as neurotransmitter but skepticism, largely because the classical criteria for transmitter identification had not been met. Similar to the case of GABA, it took until well into the 1970s for the evidence regarding dopamine as a neurotransmitter to be convincing.

A patient step-by-step analysis of the pathways for degradation of the monoamines by Julius Axelrod and his colleagues was at the center of these efforts (Axelrod, 1958). In the mid-fifties Axelrod was invited by Ed Evarts to set up a Laboratory of Pharmacology in Evarts's Laboratory of Clinical Sciences in the National Institute for Mental Health (NIMH), under the intramural research director Seymour Kety. Kety had a wonderfully clear view of how to support basic research (Axelrod, 1996, 62):

> The philosophy of Seymour Kety . . . was to allow investigators working in the laboratories of the NIMH to do their research on whatever was potentially productive and important. Kety believed that without sufficient basic knowledge about the life processes, doing targeted research on mental illness would be a waste of time and money.

This emphasis on freedom in carrying out basic research in the life sciences is one of the main themes we will see that drove the revolution of the 1950s. We will meet Kety again in Chapter 3 where his leadership in research on brain metabolism will be further described.

For his part, Axelrod built up an enormously productive group. He trained many subsequent leaders in neurotransmitter pharmacology, including Solomon Snyder in the U.S., Leslie Iverson in the U.K., and Jacques Glowinski in France, among many others. His research methods were elegant in their simplicity:

> One of the most important qualities of doing research, I found, was to ask the right questions at the right time. I learned that it takes the same effort to work on an important problem as on a pedestrian or trivial one. When opportunities came I made the right choices.
>
> (Axelrod, 1996, 74)

Monoamine Histofluorescence

Evidence for noradrenaline, dopamine, and 5HT was gathered during the 1950s by several biochemical approaches; but confirmation of their presence in neurons at the cellular level was urgently needed. This required a histochemical approach, which had to be invented.

The first step was the discovery by Eino Eränkö (1956) in Finland that monoamines could be rendered fluorescent by exposure to formaldehyde. He reported that in frozen sections of brain tissue exposed to formaldehyde a yellow-green fluorescence is produced from cells containing norepinephrine. This method, however, had a low sensitivity. A concerted effort was then made by the laboratory of Nils-Åke Hillarp in Sweden to test different methods for intensifying the fluorescence while retaining the monoamines within their cells. This led to treating sections of freeze-dried tissue with gaseous reagents. The most effective was found to be formaldehyde vapor, which produced an intense fluorescence in the noradrenaline-containing cells of the adrenal medulla. This eventually led to a reliable fluorescence of both peripheral and central monoamine-containing cells; the first reports in the brain were by Carlsson et al. (1962). Although development of these methods lies beyond our focus on the 1950s, we note that this was the first evidence that dopamine, noradrenaline, and 5HT are contained in neurons of the brain and can therefore potentially function as neurotransmitters. It was immediately confirmed for both the vertebrate brain and invertebrate ganglia. This led to a new field of **transmitter-defined central systems** originating in the brainstem that appeared to parallel their peripheral autonomic nervous system counterparts. Included were the **noradrenergic** system arising in the locus ceruleus, the **dopaminergic** system in the substantia nigra and ventral tegmental area, and the **serotonergic** system in the raphe nucleus, later to be joined by the **cholinergic** forebrain system.

These advances showed that a stain for a molecule could reveal a whole system. The systems had far-reaching projections throughout the nervous system and were immediately implicated in behavioral and psychiatric disorders. Most dramatic in this respect was the discovery of **dopamine** in high concentrations in the brain, its critical loss underlying Parkinson disease, and restoration of function with the dopamine precursor dopa (Carlsson et al., 1958), the first evidence for the molecular basis of a neurodegenerative disease (see Chapter 15).

Second Messengers

As we will see in Chapter 7, the emerging concept of signaling by neurotransmitter actions involved the opening of ion channels in the cell membranes at the postsynaptic site, but a new concept was introduced by Ernest Sutherland in 1957. The signaling molecule instead activated an independent receptor in the membrane that, through activation of intermediates, ultimately produced a **second messenger** that activated an intracellular enzyme. First obtained for the role of cyclic adenosine monophosphate (**cyclic AMP**) in the liver (Berthet et al., 1957), this finding was immediately realized to have wide implications for cell signaling throughout the body. In the nervous system it led to the search for second-messenger actions controlling membrane channels as well as slower enzymatic effects.

Because of the paucity of biochemical and pharmacological methods for application to the brain, these experiments focused first on the autonomic nervous system, especially on the superior cervical ganglion, where small, intensely fluorescent cells had been identified and shown to contain dopamine. Paul Greengard and his colleagues initiated their studies of dopamine and second-messenger signaling in the nervous system on this ganglion in the 1960s and 1970s (see Kebabian and Greengard, 1973), which were then widened to regions in the brain. Second-messenger systems are at the core of current interest in the vast field of cell-signaling mechanisms.

Hormones

Hormones come into our account because of their actions on the hypothalamus and related parts of the brain. The 1930s was the golden age of identification of the **sex hormones**. With Adolph Butenandt in Germany playing a leading role, the female hormones estrone and progesterone, and male hormones androsterone and testosterone were isolated and identified during that period.

In 1951 the hormone **insulin** was sequenced (painfully slowly, one amino acid at a time!) by Fred Sanger and his colleagues in Cambridge, United Kingdom. As noted in Chapter 2, this opened the door to sequencing of peptides and eventually proteins as a fundamental basis of modern biology, including neuroscience. Insulin was the first of the peptides that have actions in the nervous system to be sequenced and was therefore in retrospect the first neuropeptide, along with the posterior pituitary hormones oxytocin and vasopressin (Chapters 2 and 11). Beyond our focus on mid-century, beginning in the 1960s and 1970s, **neuroactive peptides** were understood to constitute an essential signaling system with differential effects acting in parallel with the classical neurotransmitters. Through such peptides as the enkephalins, they have widespread and essential effects on behavior.

Pheromones

After his studies of hormones, Butenandt turned his attention to discovering the substance that the female moth *Bombyx mori* uses to attract males. In 1959, after nearly three decades and the accumulation of extracts from a half-million female moths, he identified a long-chain alcohol, which he named **bombykol** (Butenandt et al., 1959) (Fig. 4.3). Independently, Peter Karlson, a German biochemist, and Martin Luscher, a Swiss entomologist, working on substances used by termites, introduced the term "**pheromone**" (*phero*, "excitement"; *mone*, "carrier") for signals that elicit specific behavioral responses in *conspecifics* (members of the same species) (Karlson and Luscher, 1959) (Appendix 4.2). Bombykol was thus the first of many pheromones to be identified, in both invertebrates and vertebrates.

The ability to test physiologically for the action of a pheromone or other odorous substance in the insect was introduced by Dietrich Schneider in Germany in 1957 by the discovery of the electrical response of the cells in the antennae, called the "**electroantennogram**." Independently, David Ottoson in Sweden in 1955 discovered the summed electrical response of the olfactory organ in vertebrates, called the "**electro-olfactogram**" (see Chapter 7)

Pheromone Effects in Mammals. The decade of the 1950s was also rich in breakthroughs providing evidence for pheromone-like signaling in mammals (reviewed in Ottoson and Shepherd, 1967). In 1952 Paul Dell and his colleagues (David et al., 1952) in France showed that electrical stimulation of the olfactory bulb in female cats interrupted the estrous cycle. In 1956 Van der Lee and Boot in the Netherlands showed an effect on pseudopregnancies in female rats housed together compared with apart, which came to be known as the "Lee-Boot effect." Wes Whitten in Australia in 1957 showed that females housed together suppressed each other's cycles and that this effect was mediated by the olfactory pathway; in 1958 he showed that the presence of males made the cycles shorter and more regular. These "Whitten effects" indicated that olfactory signals affect female reproductive behavior to suppress the likelihood of pregnancy in the absence of males and enhance it in the presence of males.

Added to this evidence from laboratories around the world was a new factor by Hilda Bruce in England. After mating, a female normally rejects intercourse with all males prepartum. However, Bruce (1959) found that when recently mated females were placed with an alien male, they readily mated with the stranger; this terminated the pregnancy, and continued exposure led to mating with the strange male. Further studies showed that exposure to only the odor of the strange male was enough to terminate the pregnancy, which did not occur if the olfactory bulbs of the male were removed.

Subsequent studies have shown that the "Bruce effect" is indeed mediated by the olfactory pathway, involving memory mechanisms for the strange male odor already in the olfactory bulb, with transmission to the hypothalamus.

The 1950s thus provided the first insights into the potentially powerful effects of pheromonal signaling on mammalian behavior, forerunners of the evidence reported by Martha McClintock in 1971 for synchronizing cycles in human females and for the influence of pheromones on human mate choice, which are the subjects of continuing research and controversy today.

Chapter 5

Cell Biology and the Synapse

Before the 1950s, cell structure could be studied only under the light micro-scope and the organelles that do the work of the cell were seen only indis-tinctly. By the end of the 1950s, the electron microscope (EM) and other methods had opened up an entirely new field of cell biology, in which each organelle was recognized as contributing its particular set of functions to the overall mechanism of the cell. Most importantly for the nervous system, the synaptic contacts made by nerve cells could be clearly identified and char-acterized. The revolution promised by the cell theory over 100 years earlier had finally arrived, bringing with it evidence that both contact and continuity were the bases for the building of neural circuits. The molecular basis of the synapse became one of the central themes of modern neuroscience research. Many neurological disorders are due to pathological changes affecting synaptic function, and much of pharmaceutical research on drug discovery is aimed at the synapse, as will become apparent in Chapter 15. We focus here on the chemical synapse as the organelle most special for nerve cells, but it should not obscure the other organelles, which appeared most relevant for other body cells at the time but are seen to be increasingly critical for nervous function as well.

Cytology—the study of the structure of the cell—had its origins in the light microscopy of the nineteenth century. Although by the turn of the century a number of organelles inside the cell were identified—chromosomes, mitochon-dria, neurofilaments, the Golgi body—they could be seen only indistinctly due to the optical limitations of the microscopes, fixation methods, and illumination techniques available. The introduction of cell fractionation by differential centrifugation (Claude, 1946) opened the door to biochemical analysis of cell fractions (see Chapter 2). Yet so contentious were the issues that as late as midcentury an exhaustive review of the literature by the authorities in the field suggested that the Golgi body was likely an artifact (Palade and Claude, 1949)!

Cell Organelles

All of this uncertainty was swept away by the application of the electron microscope (EM) in biology. Within the space of several years in the early 1950s (roughly 1952–1956), the fine structure (in other words, the ultrastructure as seen by the EM at magnifications of up to 50,000 times or more compared with less than 1,000 times under the light microscope) of all of the main organelles of the cell was identified and characterized. This history belongs to cytology and the new field of cell biology, but it is also increasingly relevant to understanding the special features that are adapted for the nervous system. These fine structural features of the cell revealed by the EM are summarized in Table 5.1. They are the major fine structural features and organelles that we recognize today.

It was one of the most dramatic episodes in the history of biology, equivalent in its effect to that of the cell theory in the 1840s. It defined the new field of cell fine structure, the new discipline of cell biology, and the new agenda for the molecular investigation of cell functions ever since. Each organelle has become a field of its own within cell biology. As recalled by Porter and Bennett (1981, XI):

Table 5.1 Discoveries of the Fine Structure of Cell Organelles, Which Laid the Basis for the New Fields of Cell Biology and the Molecular Biology of the Cell

---

Cilia (with characteristic 9 + 2 mitrotubule array) (Fawcett and Porter, 1954)
Endoplasmic reticulum, rough and smooth (Palade and Porter, 1954; Palay and Palade, 1954; Fawcett, 1954)
Golgi body (Dalton and Felix, 1954)
Lysosomes (Novikoff et al., 1956)
Mitochondria (Palade, 1953; Sjöstrand, 1953)
Mitotic spindle (Mazia and Dan, 1952)
Muscle structure ("sliding filament hypothesis") (Huxley and Niedergerke, 1954a, 1954b; Huxley and Hanson, 1954)
Myelin (Geren, 1954; Robertson, 1955)
Nucleus and nucleolus (Porter, 1955)
Nucleoprotein particles (Palade, 1955), subsequently renamed "ribosomes" (Roberts 1958)
Plasma membrane (Robertson, 1957a, b)
  (summarized in Gall et al., 1981, and Fawcett, 1981, which contain these and other references)

A new world was opening for investigation; a new information gusher had been uncorked. Excitement of discovery and community of purpose brought us together. The friendships and mutual respect engendered in those exciting days have endured and have fortified the field of cell biology.

It is indeed this "excitement and community of purpose" that draws us to the 1950s, a time period that set the standard for assessing the significance of discoveries in modern biology and neuroscience.

Background on the Synapse

Of most interest for the nervous system was the fine structure of the synapse. First, I provide a brief background on this problem and its origins.

When in 1891 the concept of the neuron was formulated (see Chapter 8), Ramón y Cajal's idea was accepted that neurons interact by means of "contacts" between their axons and dendrites. At the time there was no evidence for the nature of the action at such contacts. The best analogy with devices of that era seemed to be nervous actions in a manner like the electric currents in an inductor coil (Ramón y Cajal, 1911); that is, the electric currents in what we now call the presynaptic process electrically induce currents in the postsynaptic process, but there was little insight into how this might come about.

A New Term: "Synapse." The critical insight into the problem of interactions between nerve cells and their targets came from a young English physiologist, Charles Sherrington of London. Around 1890 Sherrington was just beginning his study of the reflex functions of the spinal cord. His work involved a painstaking analysis of the anatomy and physiology of the spinal nerves and spinal cord. The results provided the foundation for concepts of the reflex as a basic unit of function in the spinal cord and elsewhere in the nervous system, as will be discussed later.

Sherrington's results set him to thinking about how impulses entering the nerve endings in the spinal cord are transferred to the motor neurons that innervate the muscles. It seemed that the transfer from the endings must involve properties different from those involved in impulse conduction. If Ramón y Cajal and his colleagues were right and the sensory nerves arborize and terminate in free endings, these different properties must be associated with some kind of special contact between the endings and the motor cells. And so it was that, when Michael Foster, a leading physiologist of the day, came in 1897 to revise his standard physiology textbook of the day and asked Sherrington to contribute the chapters on the spinal cord, Sherrington (1897, 929) advanced a simple proposal:

> So far as our present knowledge goes, we are led to think that the tip of a twig of the arborescence is not continuous with but merely in contact with the substance of the dendrite or cell body on which it impinges. Such a special connection of one nerve cell with another might be called a *synapse*.

Forty years later, John Fulton, a former student, asked Sherrington how he arrived at the term. (The letter is in the Medical Historical Library at Yale.) His answer shows the careful reasoning that lies behind the selection of Greek terms for application to biology (Sherrington, 1940; reproduced in Shepherd and Erulkar, 1997, p 387; Appendix 5.1):

> You enquire about the introduction of the term "synapse"; it happened thus.—M. Foster had asked me to get on with the Nervous System part (Part iii) of a new Edition of his 'Textb. of Physiol.' for him. I had begun it, and had not got far with it before I felt the need of some name to call the junction between nerve-cell & nerve-cell [because that place of junction now entered physiology as carrying functional importance]. I wrote him of my difficulty, & my wish to introduce a specific name. I suggested using syndesm. He consulted his Trinity friend Verrall, the Euripidean scholar, about it, & Verrall suggested 'synapse', & as that yields a better adjectival form, it was adopted for the book.
>
> The concept at root of the need for a specific term was that, as was becoming clear, 'conduction' which transmitted the 'impulse' *along* the nerve-fibre could not—as such—obtain at the junction, a 'membrane' *there* lay across the path, & 'conduction' per se was not competent to negotiate a 'cross-wise' membrane ... 'synapsis' strictly means 'a *process* of contact' *i.e.* a proceeding or *act* of contact, rather than a *thing* which enables contact i.e. an *instrument* of contact. 'Syndesm' would not have had that defect, i.e. it would have meant a '*bond.*'

This proposal thus brought together the neuroanatomical and the physiological evidence into one term, wherein lies so much of the power it has had to stimulate virtually the entire range of studies of nervous organization.

Neuronism vs. Reticularism

At the time there were no anatomical methods to demonstrate the synapse. Ramón y Cajal and most of the classical histologists provided strong evidence with their Golgi stains for discontinuity at the site of termination of an axon on the cell body or dendrites of another cell, which became the basis of the "neuron doctrine." We will discuss this central concept for the rise of modern neuroscience in Chapter 8. Others insisted they could see continuity between these processes, which gave rise to the so-called reticular theory.

The inability to provide a clear morphological demonstration of a synapse hung like a dark cloud over concepts of how neurons interact. It was a situation in which a simple model could play a critical role in providing needed insight. Such a model was the junction made by a motor nerve fiber terminal onto its muscle, the so-called neuromuscular junction (NMJ).

The Neuromuscular Junction. The NMJ, also called the "muscle end plate," had in fact been studied for many decades by then. It was first described by several authors in the 1860s and 1870s. Willy Kuhne in Germany was one of the best known of these investigators. Even with the limited stains available, his diagrams of the microscopic views of the NMJ were not unlike the views and diagrams produced by later improved optics and stains (Kuhne, 1869).

Kuhne described the junction in great detail. It was assumed that an impulse spread from the axon into the terminal and that this led to the activation of muscle contraction by some unknown mechanism. Kuhne suggested that this could be a model for connections made between nerve cells in the nervous system. As noted elsewhere (Chapters 4, 7), Du Bois-Reymond (1877) suggested that muscle activation might involve "stimulatory secretion" of a "powerful stimulatory substance" by the nerve endings on the muscle, but this was ignored as a model by the authors who later were associated with the founding of the neuron doctrine.

Rene Couteaux. After Ramón y Cajal's final say on "neuron or reticulum" (1933), the field was left in need of investigators with new methods to resolve the issue. One of the first was Rene Couteaux in France. As Tsuji (2006, p503) observes, "Although it is of great importance, the historical contribution of Couteaux to the knowledge of the synapse has scarcely been reported in the textbooks of histology." This problem was the more unfortunate for those who, like Couteaux, published their results in a language other than English.

He was born in 1909, studied medicine, became interested in research, and in Paris started a thesis project on the structure of the NMJ. This confronted him with the issue of "neuron or reticulum." To resolve this question at the NMJ, the methods available at that time were impregnation of the tissue with gold or silver or vital staining (staining of the tissue without any embedding or fixation) with methylene blue. Neither method gave clear visualization, given the limited resolution of the light microscope, of the membranes of both the neural terminals and the muscle membrane, to allow determination of whether they were separate (as proposed in the neuron doctrine) or whether there was fusion or continuity by means of neurofilaments from one side to the other (as proposed by the reticular theory).

By the mid-1930s chemical transmission by means of acetylcholine (ACh) and adrenaline (epinephrine) had become established in the autonomic nervous system (see Chapter 4). Evidence was also beginning to accumulate for ACh as the neurotransmitter from nerves to skeletal muscles at the NMJ. This role implied a mechanism for inactivating ACh after it had acted on the postsynaptic membrane. It was proposed that this could be brought about by an enzyme, acetylcholinesterase (AChE), to hydrolyze (break it apart) and inactivate it.

Couteaux focused his research on demonstrating the presence and localization of this enzyme. With David Nachmansohn, who along with many other

Jews had to flee Germany during the 1930s, he showed using biochemical methods that AChE is localized at the sites where the nerves innervate the muscles and that it persists after the nerves have been allowed to degenerate (Couteaux and Nachmansohn, 1940), implying that it is present in the junctional membranes themselves. He carried on his thesis work during the Nazi occupation and found that staining with a dye, Janus green B, revealed a space, a "synaptic gutter," at the junction, with a "subneural apparatus" on the muscle side. This separation between nerve terminal and muscle provided the strongest support then available for the neuron doctrine at this model synapse (Couteaux, 1944, 1946; see Tsuji, 2006).

George Koelle. The localization of AChE was still not sufficiently precise to convince the doubters. At this stage George Koelle enters the picture. He was born in 1918, attended Swarthmore, and received his PhD after World War II at the University of Pennsylvania in 1946. He developed a histochemical method for localizing AChE by staining for a closely related molecule (acetylthiocholine) that was more easily visualized (Koelle and Friedenwald, 1949). This became known as the "Koelle method" and was widely used for demonstrating cholinergic systems throughout the nervous system. It earned Koelle a full professorship in 1952, at the age of 34, and subsequently double chairs at Penn. (As a frequent visitor to the Penn pharmacology department, I can attest to his continuing devotion well beyond retirement to tracking down every evidence of AChE activity; he enthusiastically insisted on showing me his latest experiments into the 1990s.)

Couteaux and Taxi (1952a, 1952b) made a basic improvement to the Koelle method, which gave further confirmation of Couteaux's previous results with Janus green B. Thus, according to Tsuji (2006, 503),

"Couteaux's work provided, for the first time in histology, a clearly defined morphological basis to the synapse."

The Chemical Synapse

For most neuroscientists, definitive demonstration of synapses could be achieved only with the high resolution of the EM. The first EM images of the structure of a synapse were reported in 1954, by Sanford Palay and George Palade in the United States and by Eduardo De Robertis and Bennett in Uruguay.

Sanford Palay. Sanford Palay was born in 1918 in Cleveland, grew up there, and trained in medicine at Western Reserve University. He began his scientific career working with Ernst Scharrer on secretory granules in nerve cells of the fish. We will encounter Ernst and Berta Scharrer as pioneers in the new field of neurosecretion in Chapter 11. It was a fruitful beginning for the young student. His memoir (Palay, 1992, 192) gives the flavor of being a graduate student with those mentors, a training in both science and life that shaped one of the outstanding scholars of modern neuroscience. It also gives a sense of loss due to the cataclysm that was destroying European and German science and culture:

> ...the Scharrers represented the life of the mind in an extraordinarily attractive manner. Their teachers had been the leading lights in biology of the first part of the twentieth century, and they continued the line of excellence that European and especially German science had achieved since the beginning of the nineteenth century. To a midwestern youth who had been outside northern Ohio only twice in his life, they represented the cultivated world of travel, literature, the arts, and renown. They could speak easily in English, French, and German, and they knew Italian and other languages as well. They knew the authors of the papers we read and the textbooks we studied. We discussed all sorts of subjects from the scientific questions we were studying to the state of the world, from the progress of the war in Europe and the Pacific to the dangers ahead in the postwar settlement. I spent every evening in the laboratory either studying or carrying on research.

When the war ended in 1945, Palay accompanied the Scharrers as they resumed their summers in Woods Hole, Massachusetts, where he had the opportunity that Woods Hole affords for young students to meet the leaders in biology from around the country. After a medical stint in the army, he joined Albert Claude for a postdoctoral fellowship in 1948. Claude, a refugee from the Nazis in the 1930s, was soon joined by George Palade, a refugee from Romania after it came under the Soviet Union in 1947, to begin their studies using the EM.

After Claude returned to Belgium in 1949, Palay became an instructor at Yale. In addition to a heavy teaching load, he was drawn to the EM as the methods for tissue preservation and sectioning improved. On leave from Yale in 1953, he joined Palade to apply the new methods to nervous tissue. Despite the difficulties, they obtained images of the fine structure of the neuron, including Nissl substance, endoplasmic reticulum, neurofilaments, and the Golgi apparatus, which was published in 1955 (Palay and Palade, 1955). Palay in parallel focused on a search for the synapse and found it by studying the motor cells of the abducens nucleus, which were known to be covered with axon terminals. It was these findings that he first reported in 1954.

Eduardo De Robertis. The other main pioneer in the discovery of the fine structure of the synapse was Eduardo De Robertis, who by now is almost forgotten. He was born in 1913 of Italian immigrant parents in Buenos Aires, Argentina. After training in medicine, he studied endocrine function on a fellowship to the United States in 1939–1941 and returned to Argentina during the war to continue his research. When Perón came to power in 1946, De Robertis exiled himself to the United States. At the Massachusetts Institute of Technology (MIT) he carried out one of the first EM studies of the axon with Frank Schmitt, in which they demonstrated neurotubules.

He was then recruited by one of Ramón y Cajal's former students, C. Estable, to the Biological Research Institute in Uruguay, where he set up the first EM in South America and carried out studies of the fine structure of the retina and began his interest in synaptic membranes and exocytosis of granules in cells of the adrenal medulla. Building on this work, he joined Bennett in Seattle in 1953 to study the synapse, which led to their first reports in 1954. (In 1957 he returned to Buenos Aires to head the Cell Biology Department, including a unit for electron microscopy.)

Discovering the Synapse. The assignation of priority has been contentious because the story came out first in short communications given virtually simultaneously at meetings in 1954. It is useful therefore to identify the relevant communications in some detail (Appendices 5.2–5.5).

At the American Association of Anatomists meeting in 1954, an abstract by George Palade ("assisted by Sanford Palay") was entitled "Electron Microscopic Observations of Interneuronal and Neuromuscular Synapses."

> In the central nervous system (cerebellar cortex and . . . medulla oblongata) typical end-foot or "bouton terminal" appearances were occasionally encountered with dendrites. In the axon ending an agglomeration of mitochondria and small vesicles (300–500A) was found, whereas the dendrite showed fewer mitochondria and vesicles in a rather fibrillar cytoplasm. The axon and dendrite appeared to be separated by their respective plasma membranes, which at the level of closer contact were denser and thicker. The space between the synaptolemmae was ~200A. . . .
>
> The neuromuscular synapses were studied in rat skeletal muscles. The axon endings had the same cytoplasmic appearance as central synapses. The sarcoplasmic sole showed large accumulations of mitochondria and small granules. The axon and the muscle fiber were separate. The membrane of the latter showed a number of deep narrow infoldings ~700A thick and 0.2–0.4 µ apart, within which thin, dense lamellae were sometimes encountered (subneural apparatus of Couteau).
>
> (Palade and Palay, 1954, 336)

This abstract was immediately followed by one by Palay ("assisted by George Palade") entitled "Electron Microscopic Study of the Cytoplasm of Neurons." Nerve cells were reported to have conspicuous masses of Nissl substance, composed of thin membranes and punctate granules. A second system of membranes without granules is described (likely the Golgi body, still an uncertain structure). The Nissl substance could be seen to extend into dendrites for a short distance, but beyond that dendrites and axons appeared similar (due to the poor fixation possible at that time). This study was important in showing that nerve cells have a fine structure similar to most cells of the body.

At the same meeting, Eduardo De Robertis from Montevideo, Uruguay, presented "Changes in the 'Synaptic Vesicles' of the Ventral Acoustic Ganglion After Nerve Section (an Electron Microscope Study)," having chosen this region (in the guinea pig) so that he could examine the effects on synapses there after destroying the cochlea.

> In normal presynaptic endings the most conspicuous component is represented by the submicroscopic "synaptic vesicles" previously described by De Robertis and Bennett (Fed. Proc., 13, No. 1, 1954) in synapses of the frog and earthworm. Besides a limiting double membrane, mitochondria, endoplasmic reticulum and an amorphous matrix may be observed in the terminal. At the synaptic membrane there is a direct contact with the postsynaptic cytoplasm. Degenerative alterations of the terminal are conspicuous at 22 hours and very marked at 44 hours. Early changes consist of swelling of the matrix and agglutination and lysis of the synaptic vesicles. Then there is lysis of the mitochondria, complete disappearance of synaptic vesicles and finally detachment of the membrane of the terminal from the synaptic junction. No changes in the postsynaptic cytoplasm were observed. . . .
>
> (De Robertis, 1954, 284–285)

This may be regarded as the confirmation at the fine structural level of the insight of Forel in his contribution in the 1880s to the classical "neuron doctrine": that degeneration is specific to the affected cell and does not pass as through a reticulum from cell to cell (see Shepherd, 1991). (This view has been modified by subsequent research showing the transneuronal degenerative changes that can be demonstrated in many cells.)

These early communications were followed by full papers (De Robertis and Bennett, 1955; Palay, 1956; Appendices 5.6, 5.7).

In his 1956 paper, Palay (p198) published the first full characterization of the synapse as seen in the medulla, cerebellum, and cerebrum of the adult rat. He defined it thusly (Fig. 5.1):

> Three essential structural features characterize the synapses studied in this paper: (a) the closely apposed limiting membranes of the presynaptic ending and the postsynaptic cell or dendrite; (b) the cluster of mitochondria; and (c) the collections of fine vesicles filling the presynaptic terminal. The absence of protoplasmic continuity across the contact surface between the two members of the synaptic apparatus is impressive confirmation of the neuron doctrine enunciated and defended by Ramon y Cajal during the early part of this century . . .

The morphological definition of the synapse soon came down to the accumulation of small vesicles on the presynaptic side and densifications of the apposed membranes. The vesicles were immediately postulated to contain and release neurotransmitter molecules that act on the postsynaptic membrane, to account for chemical transmission at the NMJ and at other synapses. The early work was reviewed by Palay (1958), and a clear representation of the synapse at different scales of magnification was provided by De Robertis in a review in 1959, including a diagram of the theory that the vesicle fuses with the plasma membrane to release its neurotransmitter contents (Fig. 5.2). This united the anatomical and physiological study of the synapse and set the agenda for the analysis of synaptic mechanisms that has continued to this day.

Who Discovered the Synapse? The foregoing account indicates that with the appropriate methodology (the EM) the synapse was there to be discovered. The judgment of posterity on who was the discoverer is divided.

Palay (1992) has since described his feelings at being, certainly for him, the first to observe synaptic vesicles. In 1988 he gave the History of Neuroscience lecture at the annual meeting of the Society for Neuroscience, sponsored by the Committee on the History of Neuroscience, of which I was the chair. During the talk and at dinner afterward, he was obviously moved when he came to discussing his contributions and did not mention the parallel work of De Robertis and Bennett. In his memoir, Palay (1992, 209) wrote "I well remember the moment when I discovered synaptic terminals [including vesicles] in my preparations." He placed a high value on the quality of the images on which priority was based.

On the other hand, according to Porter and Bennett (1981, p 10), De Robertis and Bennett (1955) provided the first "full description of synaptic vesicles and the inter-membranous synaptic spacing."

Both Palay and De Robertis were widely recognized in their lifetimes for their achievements. Both were outstanding examples of innovation and scholarship in spreading the word about the new fields of cell biology and the synapse. De Robertis had already published a textbook of cell biology in Spanish in 1946, which went through multiple editions also in Japanese, Russian, Italian, Polish, Hungarian, and finally English in 1970. Palay, together with Peters and Webster, published the *Fine Structure of the Neuron*, which went through several editions. To his friends and colleagues "Sandy" was a wonderful mix of the sweet and the prickly, a gentle human being as well as a scholar swift to criticize any lapse in scientific rigor.

Different Kinds of Synapses

Types I and II. In 1959, George Gray in London (with appropriate fixation methods) differentiated between **type I** synapses, with round vesicles and asymmetric membrane densities, and **type II** synapses, with pleomorphic (many differently shaped) vesicles and symmetric membrane densities (Appendix 5.8). Type I was suggested to be excitatory and type II inhibitory. This distinction has proven invaluable in identifying presumed excitatory and inhibitory synapses (Chapter 8) and their roles in specific brain circuits (Chapter 10). Thus, by the end of the 1950s, the agenda for analyzing the synaptic organization of neural circuits in the different regions of the brain was set.

Tight Junctions. Other types of junctions made up of closely apposed membranes were seen between cells, with different patterns of connection and modifications of the apposed membranes. These were eventually classified as **tight junctions**, with the function of physically holding cells together and forming barriers to extracellular substances, including the blood-brain barrier.

Neuromuscular Junction. Finally, let us return to the model with which we began, the NMJ. In parallel with the studies of synapse fine structure in the central nervous system, investigators were including the NMJ. J. D. Robertson, an early pioneer of the fine structure of the nerve membrane, carried out a study of the muscle membrane and NMJ in the reptile. Muscle membrane appeared to have a double-leaflet structure similar to that of other cells (Robertson, 1956). The NMJ consisted of the neural membrane on one side and, across a space, a convoluted membrane on the muscle side. On the neural side were multiple clusters of vesicles opposing the folds of the muscle membrane. These clusters subsequently became known as "active zones" (Couteaux, in Eccles 1964; Heuser et al., 1974). Release of individual vesicles was correlated with miniature end-plate potentials by del Castillo and Katz (1954a, 1954b, 1954c; see also Chapter 7). Within the space was a line of increased density, the "basal lamina," a structure special for the NMJ and not found in the synaptic cleft of central synapses. Soon, AChE was localized to the postsynaptic folds and eventually the ACh receptors themselves.

These components defined the classical structure of the NMJ. The structure was largely consistent with the simplified structure of central synapses, supposedly reflecting the more mechanically dynamic environment of the moving muscle fiber. Thus, in the mid-1950s, the concept of the morphological synapse as the basis of the neuron doctrine seemed established.

The Electrical Synapse

As happens so often in biology, a concept which seems universal soon is found to have exceptions. No sooner had the chemical synapse become accepted as the mode for neuronal communication than an electrical interaction between nerve cells was demonstrated. Although this was a physiological action demonstrated by physiological experiments, it is discussed here because of its immediate implications for a direct anatomical pathway between nerve cells.

The first report came from the laboratory of Bernard Katz, who, as discussed in Chapter 7, was the pioneer in analyzing chemical transmission at the NMJ. It occurred during the peak of the transatlantic flow of young American scientists seeking training in the foremost laboratories of the United Kingdom, in recognition of the breakthroughs there with the new microelectrode techniques.

Among them were Edward Furshpan and David Potter, postdoctoral fellows of the U.S. Public Health Service and the National Science Foundation, respectively.

For their project on extending the model of the physiology of the chemical synapse (see Chapter 7), they pursued the strategy then gaining favor of using a "simple" model in an invertebrate and selected the nerve cord of the crayfish. In this preparation, a giant axon extends the length of the abdominal nerve cord and was known to activate a large motor axon to the muscle. This was, therefore, an axoaxonic synapse.

But what were its properties? Furshpan and Potter (1957) inserted an electrode into the presynaptic and postsynaptic fibers, delivered a brief current pulse to elicit an action potential (see Chapter 6) into the former, and recorded the response in the latter. If the activation worked by a chemical synapse, there would have been a significant "synaptic delay" for the response to occur; but instead the postsynaptic action potential arose almost simultaneously. Even small currents, too weak to activate an action potential, nonetheless induced an equivalent weak response. This could not happen at a chemical synapse, and the authors inferred from this and other evidence that current was passing directly between the axons. Current did not pass in the opposite direction, a property known as "rectification" (one-way) (Appendix 5.9).

The authors concluded (Furshpan and Potter, 1957, 343):

> There is, then, good evidence that a one-way transmission process can take place by means of an "electrical" mechanism, namely, one in which the local currents can cross the synaptic membrane in only one direction. This conclusion, however, probably does not apply to some other junctions in the crayfish cord; for there are indications that even this same post-fibre has other synapses on it which rely on a chemical mediator.

These electrical connections soon came to be called "electrical synapses." At first, it was assumed that this type of transmission, involving a stereotyped action between two impulse-transmitting axons, might be limited to the simpler functional demands of invertebrate nervous systems. However, other examples soon followed in the brainstem of vertebrates (Bennett et al., 1963). It was assumed that this would be characteristic of the simpler types of synchronous integration that occur in brainstem nuclei and would not occur higher in the brain.

Meanwhile, the search was on among cells in the body for the structural basis of the electrical synapse, which led to the discovery of gap junctions (Revel and Karnovsky, 1967), pores across the membrane that not only conduct electricity but are large enough to allow the diffusion of molecules between the cytoplasm of two cells. It was soon found that gap junctions were widely distributed in the body and involved in a variety of functions, such as exchange of nutrient molecules and exchange of molecules involved in cell differentiation and growth (gap junctions are especially present during early development), as well as transfer of second messengers and passage of electrical signals in one direction or another. They were also shown to be modulated in a variety of ways, by Ca ions, pH, phosphorylation, and transmembrane potential changes.

In the nervous system, we now know that gap junctions and electrical interactions may be found between cells in many regions, carrying out a variety of functions such as those enumerated above.

New Perspectives on the Neuron Doctrine

If direct continuity through gap junctions is so widespread, does this disprove the neuron doctrine? Is the nervous system composed of a reticulum, as Golgi maintained? The answer may be found in the fact that the presence of gap junctions has not disproved the cell theory; we still regard cells with their nuclei as the basic building blocks of the body, even though there may be direct channels of continuity and communication between them. Since the neuron doctrine was an extension of the cell theory to the nervous system, we can draw the same conclusion for nerve cells. They are still the basic building blocks of the nervous system. However, the patterns of both electrical and chemical synapses produce neural circuits that have a complexity that goes far beyond that imagined in the original theory of the neuron. We will discuss the neuron doctrine in more detail in Chapter 8.

Myelin

A cellular structure unique to nerve was myelin, a fatty substance surrounding large nerve fibers. It had been recognized by myelin stains in the nineteenth century but not visualized at the fine structural level until the advent of the EM in the 1950s. The classical description came from the discovery by Betty Geren at Harvard in 1954 that peripheral myelin is formed during development by the plasma membrane of an enveloping Schwann cell wrapping around the axon multiple times to form a compressed multilayer structure like a jelly-roll (Appendix 5.10).

This fundamental report was quickly confirmed (Geren and Schmitt, 1954; Robertson, 1955) and became an instant classic in establishing the nature of the myelin sheath around nerve axons. It was soon shown that this multiple membranous wrapping was associated with a high-resistance, low-capacitance structure which facilitated the rapid conduction of the action potential, with boosting of the current at the nodes of Ranvier. This became the basis for understanding normal axonal function and abnormal function as in multiple sclerosis.

Chapter 6

Physiology: The Action Potential

Different parts of the nervous system are interconnected by long fibers called "axons," which enable them to function together to mediate the coordinated spontaneous activity, reflexes, perceptions, memory, and willed movements that constitute behavior. The key property of an axon, that is special for the nervous system, is to be "excitable," capable of supporting self-regenerating waves of electrical potential that can propagate rapidly over long distances. These waves are called "impulses," or "action potentials." Understanding excitability is therefore central to understanding the nature of nervous activity. By 1900 it was postulated that the action potential is due to a transient movement of electrical charge in the form of ions across the cell membrane. Because of the rapid nature of the action potential, this hypothesis could not be tested until the advent of electronic amplifiers in the 1920s. A large axon in the squid was discovered in the 1930s that provided an ideal preparation for this study. This led to intracellular recordings and the experimentally based model of Hodgkin and Huxley in 1952, showing the role of sodium ions in generating the action potential, which ushered in the new era of intracellular electrophysiological study of the neuronal membrane. The HH action potential immediately took its place among the great discoveries of modern science, as important for biology and neuroscience as the Bohr atom had been for physics.

The nerve impulse, also called the "action potential," is at the center of the essence of the nervous system. Without it, there would be no "nervous" action, no nervous system, no sensation, movement, or feeling. The nerve impulse was unknown until the advent of the first slow electrical recording devices in the nineteenth century, its true rapid time course unrecorded until the first electronic vacuum tubes in the early 1920s, and its mechanism not understood until the 1950s. The discovery of this mechanism is therefore as essential for understanding the neural basis of behavior as was DNA for understanding the gene and heredity.

Background

The earliest ideas about the nature of the signals in the nervous system, beginning with the Greeks, involved notions that the brain secretes fluids, or "spirits," that flow through the nerves to the muscles. A new era opened in 1791 when Luigi Galvani of Bologna showed that frog muscles can be stimulated by electricity. His postulate of the existence of "animal electricity" in nerves and muscles soon led to a focus of attention on electrical mechanisms in nerve signaling.

At first, there were no methods for studying these mechanisms. The discovery of the electromagnetic effect of the current by the physicist Hans Christian Oersted in Denmark in 1819 gave birth to the industrial development of electricity. The galvanometer was soon developed for measuring electrical current. In the 1840s, Galvani's countryman Carlo Matteucci used the galvanometer to obtain evidence in peripheral nerves for animal electricity as a brief wave of electric current. He was the first to use the term "electrophysiology" (Geison, 1987). Emil Du Bois-Reymond of Berlin then carried out an extensive series of studies of the electrical properties of nerves. Du Bois-Reymond was one of the famous quartet of young German physiologists (Du Bois-Reymond, Herman von Helmholtz, Carl Ludwig, and Ernst von Brucke) who took an oath to put physiology on a mechanistic basis of physics and chemistry (Cranefield, 1957; see Chapter 2), a theme which has dominated experimental studies in biology and in the nervous system ever since.

Studies around 1900 provided the theoretical foundation for the pioneering work at mid-century (summarized by Huxley, 1999). Walther Nernst in 1888 derived an equation, now called the *Nernst equation*, to describe the potential (*equilibrium potential, diffusion potential*) across a semipermeable membrane due to differences in the concentrations of charged ions between the internal and external solutions. Julius Bernstein in 1902 suggested that the resting membrane potential is inside negative due to an excess inside the cell of negatively charged ions (anions) associated with positively charged K ions. He postulated that the action potential is due to a transient increase in permeability to all ions, acting like a short circuit to reduce the membrane potential to zero. This became the accepted explanation of the ionic basis of the action potential for the next 40 years. Neglected was the prescient suggestion of William Overton, in the same year, that the change could involve specific increases in Na and K ion permeabilities.

The impulse came to be called the *action potential*. As early as 1874, Hermann (see Byrne and Shepherd, 2008) suggested that the action potential propagates through "local circuits" of current spreading forward along the axon membrane. The small perturbations of the resting potential spreading passively along the membrane in a decaying fashion, below threshold for eliciting an action potential, were called *electrotonic potentials*. Lord Kelvin had pointed out the similarity to the spread of electrical current through an electrical cable. Passive properties therefore came to be called the *cable properties* of nerve.

The ability of a nerve to respond to an electrical shock with an impulse was referred to as *excitation*, and nervous tissue was recognized as excitable. However, it was soon recognized that the action potential is not limited to nerves or, indeed, to animal tissue. Bowditch showed that an action potential could be recorded from the Venus flytrap when its petals snapped shut on its prey.

Importance of the Nerve Impulse for Psychology

In 1850, Du Bois-Reymond's colleague, von Helmholtz, later a famous physicist, measured the speed of conduction of the nerve impulse and showed for the first time that, although fast, it is not all *that* fast. In the large nerves of the frog, it is about 40 meters per second, or 140 kilometers per hour. This was another landmark finding (see Boring, 1950, for discussion of its significance), for it showed that the mechanism of the nerve impulse is more than the physical spread of electricity as through a wire; it has to involve an *active biological process* (ergo, the term "action potential").

The electrical nature of the nerve impulse and its finite speed of conduction were important discoveries for physiology in general, and indeed for all science, because they constituted the first direct evidence for the kind of activity present in the nervous system. Just as the heart pumps blood and the kidney makes urine, so one could now say that the nervous system makes signals in the form of impulses.

The fact that the impulse travels at only a moderate speed had tremendous implications for psychology, for it seemed to separate the mind from the actions that the mind wills—which could be interpreted as supporting the idea of dualism, dating back to Descartes, that the mind (our thoughts) is separate from the body (our impulse signals). But it was also the opening wedge for the materialistic view that the mind can be equated with the signals in the nerves. It was thus one of the steps toward the development of modern psychology and the study of behavior, as well as contributing to the debate on the nature of the mind and the body.

Recording the Impulse

During the nineteenth century there were no instruments with sufficient sensitivity and fast enough response time to record the impulse directly. It could be detected electrically as a change in the resting potential, otherwise only by the fact that if a nerve was stimulated while connected to its muscle, the shock was followed (after a brief period for conduction in the nerve) by a twitch of the muscle. The brief nature of the twitch indicated that an impulse must also occur in the muscle, so the muscle was also recognized as having the property of excitability.

In the early years of the twentieth century a refined type of galvanometer, called a "string galvanometer," was developed, which was sufficiently sensitive to register the impulse but still too slow to do so without considerable distortion. Its sensitivity made it susceptible to tiny vibrations, so investigators had to build heavy tables to hold the apparatus, a problem for electrophysiological recordings that has continued to this day. This reached extreme limits in the experiments of Keith Lucas in Cambridge, England, whose recording table weighed several tons. Lucas developed several basic types of physiological apparatus, including massive arcs of brass through which swung a pendulum to trigger shocks at specific times and intervals. Recordings of stimuli and muscle responses were made on smoked drums and electrical recordings on film. Lucas' apparatus represented the culmination of the *electromechanical era* of physiological instrumentation (see Shepherd and Braun, 1989).

Lucas carried out his experiments on the nerve–muscle preparation of the frog. Conceptually, he believed that this provided a model for properties of cells in the brain. This idea became one of the key strategies in driving modern neuroscience: the use of simple preparations to reveal general principles of structure and function. While valuable up to a point, this belief in its narrow form turned out, like so many biological rules, to be too restrictive. When the central nervous system could finally be studied on its own terms, from the 1950s on, it was shown to operate by a wider range of mechanisms than is present in any one peripheral preparation.

Recording Single Action Potentials of Myelinated Nerves

Although the extracellularly recorded action potential cannot give insight into the membrane mechanisms that generate it, as intracellular recordings can, it was the mainstay for electrophysiologists in the first part of the twentieth century. Keith Lucas at Cambridge was the leader, but he died accidentally in 1917 while working in a factory during the World War I (1914–18). His work was carried on by his student, Edgar Adrian. During the 1920s, Adrian and his students used the string galvanometer combined with recordings from single fibers to show the all-or-nothing character of the nerve impulse in sensory axons (Adrian and Zotterman, 1926a, 1926b), and motor axons (Adrian and Bronk, 1928). (Adrian's name always came before his students because The Journal of Physiology allowed only alphabetical order for authors.) The study with Zotterman was the first to involve dissecting out single axons from a peripheral nerve, putting them on fine recording wires connected to an amplifier, and obtaining the first extracellular recordings of *single action potentials in nerve fibers* (Appendix 6.1). On a slow time base, the action potentials looked like single lines and came to be called *spikes*.

In these axons leading from muscle spindles it was shown that stretching the muscle gives rise to a train of action potentials that varies in frequency with the duration and amount of excitation from the sensory receptor. These studies inaugurated the study of encoding of information in impulse trains in the nervous system, as summarized by Adrian in *The Basis of Sensation* (1928).

We will return to encoding of neural information in spike trains in discussing studies of sensory systems later (Chapter 9).

Recordings from Nerve Fibers

The modern *electronic era* of biological instrumentation began with the introduction of the cathode ray oscilloscope for recording the nerve impulse by Herbert Gasser and Joseph Erlanger in 1922 in St. Louis. It can be regarded as the first major discovery in neurophysiology coming from the New World. With a peripheral nerve resting on two wire electrodes connected to an amplifier, the extracellular currents associated with the impulse could be recorded and displayed on a trace moving swiftly across the face of the oscilloscope. This showed that the impulse is indeed very brief, lasting for only a few milliseconds. In a series of studies Erlanger and Gasser and their colleagues showed that in fact the action potential recorded from the whole nerve consisted of several components, of differing amplitude, duration, and conducting rate, followed by brief refractory periods and longer periods of recovery of excitability. These recordings were thus termed the *compound action potential*.

Because these recordings were of extracellular currents, they gave little insight into the mechanisms that generated them. They and a number of their colleagues called themselves "axonologists." In their view the action potential could be explained in various ways other than as a change in membrane potential. One line of experimental work was to describe the purely physical properties involved in electrically exciting the nerves. The action potential required a threshold cathodal current, which depended on the strength ("rheobase") and the duration ("chronaxie") of the current. Henri Lapicque of Paris tried to develop these into universal laws of nerve excitation.

This evidence led to attempts to explain the electrical excitation of nerve in physical terms, which produced formal theories by Rashevsky (1933), Monnier and Lapicque (1934), Hill (1936), and Rushton (1937). Lillie (1935) showed that a transient traveling wave of electrical charge could be induced in an iron wire model that had properties similar to the action potential, which suggested that the action potential in nerve could be an entirely physical phenomenon. O.H. Schmitt (1937) suggested a physical model in which the action potential is due to a transient change in membrane capacitance. These early studies are summarized in a monograph by Bernard Katz (1939), *Electrical Excitation of Nerve*, which covered his doctoral work and subsequent studies with Hill. When I told Katz that I had acquired a copy of his book, he smiled and encouraged me not to take it seriously, being the work of a young student in Germany before he joined A. V. Hill (see Chapter 7).

Recording the Membrane Action Potential in Plant Cells

In order to test the theory of Bernstein that the action potential is a transient breakdown of a membrane potential, physiologists needed to be able to insert an electrode tip inside a single axon to record directly the change in membrane potential. Most axons have diameters of only a few microns (a few thousandths of a millimeter, about the thickness of a human hair), too small for the methods of the time. But a few physiologists were also interested in the generation of membrane potentials in plant cells, and they had an advantage in that some plants have very large cells. A sponge, *Nitella*, was found to be composed of such large cells; furthermore, these cells conducted a transient change in membrane potential resembling that of an action potential, albeit a very slow one.

To record from this preparation, micropipettes were made by taking an ordinary glass capillary pipette of a few millimeters in diameter, heating it, pulling it out to a small diameter, and then cutting it off to form a fine tip. This soon led to the *microforge*, an apparatus likened to a delicate smithy's forge, for automating the process. In the late 1960s I visited the laboratory at Swarthmore College near Philadelphia where these micropipettes were first made and acquired one of the rotary pipette pullers based on the original model. With such micropipettes filled with a conducting salt solution, the first intracellular recordings were made by W. J. V. Osterhout and his colleagues, showing the action potential in *Nitella* (see, e.g., Osterhout and Hill, 1938). While these studies attracted great interest at the time, their insight into the mechanism of the action potential in axons was still limited.

Recording Local Circuits and Graded Potentials

The discovery of the mechanism of the nerve action potential was the result of the efforts of many scientists in the 1930s and 1940s. Two investigators played central roles: Alan Hodgkin (Fig. 6.1) and Andrew Huxley (Fig. 6.2). We focus on Hodgkin first partly because he was senior in the team of Hodgkin and Huxley and because he was a role model in stimulating the new generation of young scientists who were subsequently inspired to work on the molecular mechanisms implied by the Hodgkin–Huxley action potential model.

Alan Hodgkin. As a role model, Hodgkin was very much in the traditional mold, a shy person who inspired others by his quiet manner and thoughtful approach. In this he was a sharp contrast with the new kinds of role models that we have seen came forth in the 1950s: brash youngsters like Jim Watson, sharp-witted theorizers like Francis Crick, or superaggressive personalities like Jack Eccles.

Hodgkin was born in 1914 in Banbury, England, not far from Oxford. His father was a banker and a Quaker. As a Quaker he was a conscientious objector in the First World War and was sent on a mercy mission to the Middle East, where he died in 1918. His mother raised the three children with modest means but a supportive larger family, and Hodgkin had a generally happy childhood, loving bird-watching and eventually choosing natural history over history when he went up to Trinity College at Cambridge in 1932. His tutor advised him to read physiology while learning as much chemistry and mathematics as possible. Trinity was an exhilarating place for a young scientist, where students rubbed elbows with the likes of J. J. Thomson (discoverer of the electron), Ernest Rutherford (of atom fame), G. H. Hardy (the mathematician), and Edgar Adrian (the physiologist), to name just a few. In his early studies Hodgkin read all the papers of Keith Lucas, stimulated in part by the fact that Lucas had been a friend of his father when they were both students at Cambridge (an example of the closeness of British society at the time).

He soon decided to study cell membranes. In his memoir *Chance and Design* (1992, 63) he recalls the following:

> I had also read the excellent review by Osterhout (1931) on "Physiological studies of large plant cells" and was impressed with the evidence obtained by Blinks (1930) for an increase of membrane conductivity during the action potential of *Nitella*. It seemed to me this crucial piece of evidence was lacking in nerve...

This early interest in membrane conductivity during the action potential was to remain at the core of his contributions to neuroscience, not the only instance of graduate work setting the course for a career.

He started his research by testing for "this crucial piece of evidence in nerve" by testing for the excitability of the nerve at a block of the action potential. His description indicates the distance between how one went about research then and now:

> In those days laboratory life was rather informal, at any rate in Cambridge. I never worked for a PhD and didn't have a research supervisor. You might easily start in a bare room and have to build most of your equipment yourself, apart from smoked drums...and kymographs...all that mattered was that I should have enough equipment to do something new.
>
> (pp 66–67)

(Kymographs and smoked drums for making physiological recordings were also in use when I started my studies in 1955 at Harvard Medical School, but the new era was dawning with newly arrived Tektronix 502A oscilloscopes. In Oxford in 1962 I helped teach the physiology course also using smoked drums, plus Daniel cells as electrical supplies and Lucas pendulums to time the shocks to the nerves, soon to be replaced by the new electronic gear.)

In addition to the simple equipment noted above, Hodgkin notes he was lucky to inherit a Matthews oscilloscope and other electrical equipment from Grey Walter, though "it wasn't considered proper to use an amplifier built by someone else." His basic approach was to lay a nerve across two stimulating electrodes and test the effect of a cold block on the excitability of the nerve (elegant in its simplicity!). The results gave evidence of heightened excitability spreading beyond the block. This was of great interest because a series of studies on axonal electrotonus associated with the names of Bernstein, Herrmann, and Cremer (Cremer, 1929) had suggested that the action potential gives rise to *local circuits* of current that flow down the "core conductor" within the axon, cross the membrane, and return to the site of the action potential. It was predicted that the outward current across the membrane would raise the excitability to keep the action potential propagating along the nerve. Hodgkin's results supported this theory (Hodgkin 1937a, 1937b) (Fig. 6.2).

Hodgkin's experience in carrying out these experiments and writing them up entirely on his own is in sharp contrast with today, when graduate students are closely mentored and their results subjected to continual criticism by co-workers:

> When I finished writing my first paper in 1937 I took the manu-script to Barcroft [the head of department] and asked if it needed his approval before I sent it to a journal. He was quite taken aback and explained first that we did not do anything like that in Cambridge, and, second, that anything I wrote was entirely my own affair. (p. 68)

Hodgkin next immersed himself in cable theory (putting to good use the advice from his college tutor), to set up experiments to determine the length of nerve that needs to be excited in order to initiate an action potential. (Nowadays, young neuroscientists regard passive cable properties as a boring subject compared with active properties, but the lesson here is that a thorough understanding of the one is necessary for understanding the other. We will see evidence of the value of this approach in discussing the Rall model of dendrites in Chapter 8).

For these experiments, Hodgkin teased out single axons from crab nerves, as Zotterman and Adrian had first done in the same department a decade earlier (see "Recording Single Action Potentials of Myelinated Nerves" and Chapter 9), and was able to show that a shock that was just below threshold sometimes gave a small potential graded in amplitude that, when sufficiently large, gave rise to the full-blown action potential. This gave further evidence of subthreshold heightened excitability due to local circuits associated with the action potential. Furthermore, he obtained preliminary evidence that a graded potential elicited during the peak of an action potential is reduced in amplitude, as predicted if the action potential is associated with an increase in membrane conductance. Similar experiments and results were found by Bernard Katz in his first studies in A. V. Hill's laboratory (Katz, 1939).

(In a talk on the history of neuroscience in the late 1980s, Andrew Huxley [see also Huxley, 2004] noted this early work on local circuits of the axon as the key starting point for their work together on the action potential mechanism.)

Andrew Huxley. A junior but powerful collaborator with Hodgkin, Huxley has been an extraordinarily productive scientist in his own right, as we shall see. Like Hodgkin, he is also in the traditional mold, with a quiet manner but more outgoing, more at ease in conversation. He has one of those dense family connections that characterize the Cambridge academic world. In conversation he enjoys referring in a casual way to "my grandfather," Thomas Huxley (1825–95), the biologist and comparative invertebrate anatomist who gained renown and controversy as "Darwin's bulldog" after his 1859 defense of the new ideas of evolution. Thomas Huxley had eight children, of whom the fourth, Leonard (1860–1933), a writer and editor, had five children by his first wife, Julia Arnold (granddaughter of Matthew Arnold), including the biologist Julian and the writer Aldous, the latter of whom gain notoriety for experimenting with LSD in the 1950s (see Chapter 15). With his second wife (a Wedgwood) he had two sons, the youngest, Andrew, born in 1917.

Andrew Huxley (Fig. 6.1B) came up to Trinity College, Cambridge, in 1935 intending to become a physicist. As an undergraduate he began to show his extraordinary strengths as a scholar in mathematics and physics, as well as in his medical courses, but soon found himself attracted to physiology, stimulated also by the inspiring faculty such as Adrian and other students such as Hodgkin. In 1939, while still only 21 years old, he joined Hodgkin to begin his research career with their groundbreaking study of the action potential.

Discovering the Squid Axon

After Hodgkin's first papers, he realized that simple, elegant experiments needed a boost from modern instrumentation and accepted an invitation by Herbert Gasser to spend a year (1937–38) at the Rockefeller Institute in New York. Here, he found himself surrounded by the latest electronic amplifiers and cathode-ray oscilloscopes and the technical experts who were developing them, especially Jan Friedrich Toennies, from Germany, whose expertise enriched the research of many of the electrophysiologists of that era (see Chapter 7). He also visited Erlanger in St. Louis, who "expressed total disbelief in subthreshold activity in myelinated axons and was also very skeptical about the local circuit theory" (Hodgkin, 1992, 8).

In the meantime, the problem of finding a suitably large axon for studying the action potential had been solved when the anatomist J. Z. Young of London reported in 1936 that a fiber in the squid, previously thought to be a connective tissue sinew, was actually a giant nerve fiber, about 1 mm in diameter. He recommended that physiologists use it as a model system for studying the action potential. "J Zed" always thought he deserved the highest recognition for thus starting the revolution in nerve membrane excitability. A movie clip of Young dissecting his squid axon is at the link to Appendix 6.2.

K. C. Cole and H. J. Curtis at Columbia University had the instrumentation to do this and took up the challenge in experiments during the summer at

Woods Hole, Massachusetts. This was to give Cole a critical role in the action potential story.

Kenneth Cole was born in Ithaca, New York, in 1900. At first intending to become an electrical engineer, he was stimulated by the work of W. J. V. Osterhout on the electrical properties of seaweed in Hugo Fricke's laboratory. In the early 1920s, in response to an advertisement for biophysicists at the Cleveland Clinic, he sought advice from his advisor, who told him, "Darned if I know what a biophysicist is . . . [but] it looks like darned good fun" (Cole, 1975, 143).

After finishing his PhD in physics, he began research in biology by measuring the membrane capacity of the sea urchin egg. An interest in cell membranes became his controlling passion. He pursued this interest with the eminent Dutch physical chemist Peter Debye, until Debye, exasperated in trying unsuccessfully to move Cole's interest to other phenomena, told him, "You and your damned membranes!" He wrote to Cole's former advisor, "I've enjoyed having Cole here—but please don't send me more like him." Cole relates this in his memoir in his modest good-humored way (Cole, 1975, 145). In fact, he benefitted greatly from that year, and it led directly to his first academic job. Creative friction can be better than a pleasant interlude in one's career.

The key event for Cole took place in the 1930s, when J. Z. Young, proselytizing for physiologists to use his newly discovered squid axon, got his ear. The first summer (1937) at Woods Hole, Cole and Curtis measured the baseline passive transverse impedance of the axon. In the summer of 1938 Cole generously invited Hodgkin, during his stay at Rockefeller, to join them to study the action potential. Hodgkin thus observed the first experiments in which the impedance (the combination of electrical resistance and capacitance) across the membrane during an action potential was recorded. The oscilloscope trace of the impedance decrease associated with the action potential (Cole and Curtis, 1939) is one of the classic images in the history of neuroscience (Appendix 6.3).

Last Experiments Before the War

Cole and Curtis's result could be explained by either a decrease in capacitance or conductance of the membrane, and Hodgkin was eager to test his prediction that it would be the conductance. He first upgraded his equipment, with help from colleagues at Cambridge and the Rockefeller Institute, to new d.c. amplifiers, cathode followers, multivibrators, and cameras. He and Andrew Huxley, his new young student colleague at Cambridge, first carried out extracellular recordings from single crab axons, immersed in paraffin oil, which causes a very high external resistance and enables one to estimate the membrane potential relative to the cut end of the nerve. This showed that the action potential was much larger than the resting potential. (A similar result was reported in frog muscle fibers by H. Schaefer in 1936.) These were the first clues that Bernstein's and Overton's theories would have to be revised.

Hodgkin and Huxley pursued this approach on the giant axon of the squid at the Marine Biological Laboratory in Plymouth, England, in the summer of 1939. Their preparation consisted of the axon mounted vertically, with a micropipette inserted into one end to record the intracellular potential. In early August they achieved the result they were seeking: The resting potential was about 50 mV negative and the action potential was almost 100 mV positive, overshooting 0 to a value of almost 50 mV positive.

In early September the Second World War broke out in Europe. Hodgkin and Huxley wrote up their result as a note in *Nature* (1939). Within a short time they and all other physiologists, on all sides of the conflict, had plunged into scientific projects supporting the war efforts, and all physiological research was suspended. It was only as the war began to move toward its close that the two got together again to write the full paper on the squid axon (Hodgkin and Huxley, 1945). This paper left unexplained the overshoot because the recent literature contained reports that the action potential could not be due to ion flows, a result later shown to be incorrect.

Gearing Up After the War

The war in Europe ended April 5, 1945. Adrian gained Hodgkin's early release from the armed forces on the grounds he was needed for teaching. By August Hodgkin and Huxley had begun experiments again on crayfish axons, scrounging equipment and eventually benefitting by the flood of war-surplus equipment.

The return to research was greatly aided by the Rockefeller Foundation. In a review of those years, Adrian, then head of the Department of Physiology at the University of Cambridge, in some of his remarks gives insight into the importance of the foundation in helping recovery in Europe, functioning as a kind of Marshall Plan of its own:

> At the end of the war, the return to the Department of several research workers of great promise encouraged me to apply to the Rockefeller Foundation, who agreed to a grant of £3,000 per annum for five years. The Unit has been in charge of A. L. Hodgkin . . . the other members were A. F. Huxley . . . and D. K. Hill . . . joined [recently] by R. D. Keynes and P. R. Lewis . . . a number of scientists from various countries have come for periods ranging from a few months to two years.
>
> The Rockefeller grant has been used for apparatus and equipment, for paying salaries (whole or in part), and for maintenance grants to various workers who have been invited here. [The] . . . Foundation made the grant to encourage a new development and did not contemplate financing it after the initial five year period, but the Unit has already justified its existence and the research programme of the

Physiological Laboratory would suffer very seriously if the work in biophysics had to be curtailed.

(Hodgkin, 1992, 265)

Despite the evidence against the roles of ions in the action potential, Hodgkin and Huxley favored this view. They decided to look more closely at the amount of K+ that flowed out during the impulse (Hodgkin and Huxley, 1947). The calculations gave startling insight into the extremely small amounts of ions that were involved: One impulse releases 10,000 K ions through 1 cm^2, which is only 1/100,000 of the total internal K+, which translated into 1 K ion through an area of some 500 fatty acid molecules in the membrane (Hodgkin, 1992, 268). Richard Keynes then took up this project and pursued a valuable line of research on ion fluxes related to the action potential using the newly available radioactive labeling (see below).

During this time Hodgkin and Huxley began to think about possible models to explain an initial inward flow of Na ions followed by outward flow of K ions that could generate the action potential. They initially hypothesized a "carrier" molecule to transport the ions across the membrane. This model was disproved by subsequent experiments, but Hodgkin (p268) observes, "In spite of this defect, I feel that these early theoretical studies were important in helping us to decide on the right experimental approach." This is a useful reminder of how important theory has been for guiding experiments in many of the areas we are reviewing.

Initial experiments examining more closely the effects of Na ion removal from crab axons gave clear evidence that Na ions were involved in the action potential peak. From there, the path to the ultimate model ensued.

The story is a part of the lore of neuroscience. The analysis of the initial results took place during the bitter cold of the winter of 1947 in Britain, with Huxley "cranking a Brunsviga calculating machine with mitten-covered hands" (Hodgkin, 1992, 271). The definitive experiments to test the Na theory on squid axons in Plymouth were done by Hodgkin in collaboration with Katz because Huxley was getting married that summer (Hodgkin, 1992) (a collegiality unusual in any age).

The Goldman-Hodgkin-Katz Equation

In this work it was necessary to account for the reversal of the potential during the action potential in rigorous terms.

> ... it became increasingly clear we needed a theory which would predict the potential difference that would arise across a thin membrane, permeable to K+, Na+ and Cl−, and separating different concentrations of these ions. For this purpose we used a simple equation derived by Goldman (1943) who assumed that the voltage gradient through the

membrane was constant, that ions move under the influence of diffusion and the electric field, and that the concentration at the edges of the membrane are directly proportional to those in the aqueous solution.

(Hodgkin, 1992, 275)

This became known as the Goldman-Hodgkin-Katz constant field equation, containing in a quantitative form the ionic theory of the membrane potential. It was the basis for all subsequent investigations of membrane potentials in living cells by the intracellular recording method.

The Path to the HH Action Potential Model

An extended trip by Hodgkin to the United States in 1948 included a visit with Gerard in Chicago, where he heard about the first microelectrode experiments of Ling and Gerard (1947), and a visit with Cole and Marmont, where he learned about their development of the voltage-clamp method for observing transmembrane currents. Back in Cambridge, Hodgkin and Nastuk (1950) used the intracellular electrode to report the first recordings of the muscle action potential and evidence that this was due to Na current; this included, according to Hodgkin (1992), the concept of the equilibrium potential for an ion at which there is no net flow of current. (For these experiments Hodgkin filled the electrodes with a solution of 3 mM KCl, a value he recalls was a "pure guess" but became set in stone for much intracellular recording thereafter, including my own experiments in the Phillips laboratory; see Chapter 9.)

By the summer of 1948 a voltage-clamp amplifier had been built and the squid axon experiments to test the Na hypothesis were under way, with Katz helping out. (See Appendix 6.4 for the setup of the squid axon for intracellular recording.) The next summer brought the definitive experiments, which included both activation and inactivation of Na conductance as well as activation of a delayed K conductance.

The analysis of the results took the next 2 years. First, they rigorously disproved the carrier hypothesis. Then, they developed a kinetic model based on the idea of the movement of electrically charged particles across the membrane (Hodgkin, 1992, 291), with the time courses of the conductance changes described by m3h and n4. They then took their equations to the university computer, the early EDVAC, to be solved, but found that it was down for 6 months. Huxley returned to his hand-cranked Brunsviga calculating machine and solved the differential equations in 3 weeks (Hodgkin, 1992). The time courses of the membrane currents of Na^+ and K^+ in the model matched closely the experimental traces (Fig. 6.3). The experimental results were published in a set of three papers in the *Journal of Physiology* in 1952, followed by the paper comparing the results with the theoretical model (Hodgkin and Huxley, 1952a-d). A link to the final paper is included in Appendix 6.5.

The significance of modeling the action potential was assessed later by Hodgkin (1992, 297):

Fitting theoretical equations to biological processes is not always particularly helpful, but in this case Huxley and I had a strong reason for carrying out such an analysis. A nerve fibre undergoes all sorts of complicated electrical changes under different experimental conditions and it is not obvious that these can be explained by relatively simple permeability changes of the kind [we found]. To answer such questions we needed a theory and preferably one that could be given a physical basis of some kind. [He could have added, preferably one that could be tested experimentally.]

The model became the gold standard for understanding the mechanisms underlying nerve activity. It is no exaggeration to say that the Hodgkin–Huxley model of the action potential played a role in biology equivalent to that played by the Bohr atom in physics. With these studies we find ourselves at the heart of the events that made this period of a few years in the 1950s the golden age of neuroscience.

It remains to note that another young colleague of Hodgkin's, Richard Keynes, joined the project to obtain evidence for the postulated ion movements. (To continue the theme of genealogical connectedness in Cambridge physiology, Richard Darwin Keynes, born in 1919, is the nephew of the economist John Maynard Keynes; his mother was a granddaughter of Charles Darwin; his wife was the elder daughter of Edgar Adrian.) After the war Hodgkin suggested that Keynes use radioisotopes to track the movements of the ions across the axon membrane. Keynes was the first in Britain to make isotopes for this purpose. He carried out a series of experiments (see Keynes, 1951) proving the redistribution of Na and K ions in relation to the action potential as determined by experiment and predicted by theory.

Impact of the Hodgkin–Huxley Action Potential Model

In contrast to the delayed recognition of the Watson–Crick model for DNA, the Hodgkin–Huxley model for the action potential had immediate impact. This probably reflected the fact that the action potential belonged to electrophysiologists, and most of what we now call "neuroscience" at that time was "electrophysiology." The new model was immediately taught around the world, as I can attest from the course I took in physiology in 1954 at Iowa State College and from the strong impression it made on a young student, that the most explosive event in the nervous system could be due to the movement of common salt ions.

The physical basis provided by the HH model meant that it could be tested experimentally. This made the model the foundation of all future work on the mechanism of excitability in the nervous system. It was soon realized that calcium ions could also carry charge into the cell, and calcium action potentials were identified, particularly in cell bodies and dendrites. Beginning in the 1970s, a variety of different K currents were identified. Beginning in the

1980s, several distinct types of Ca currents were found that mediated other functions in the cell. With the advent of gene engineering, an array of channel subunits has been identified that are shuffled in different combinations to achieve different kinetic control over ion movements in different cells and parts of cells.

For all of these cases, an understanding of the mechanisms of ion selectivity, gating, and inactivation has been grounded in adaptations of the HH model approach. While this has been of great value, it nonetheless has not satisfied the need for a fundamental theory of excitability that builds on first principles. That goal is getting closer as structural analysis of membrane channel proteins is developing.

Pumping the Ions Back

Ions that cross the membrane down their electrochemical gradient have to be returned in order to maintain the normal concentration differences across the membrane. This requires a molecular mechanism called a "membrane pump," which pumps out the Na ions that have come in during the action potential and the K ions in. It must run on energy supplied by high-energy phosphates in the form of adenosine triphosphate (ATP).

In the 1950s the hunt was on for the identification of this pump. It was won by Jens Christian Skou, working in Aarhus, Denmark. His paper in 1957 reported the biochemical identification of the "Na/K ATP pump." It was a discovery fundamental for all biological membranes. With the development of genetic engineering, the molecular structure of the pump has been revealed, and a family of pumps critical to the maintenance of differing ion distributions in body cells, including neurons and glia, has been identified.

Chapter 7

Physiology: Synaptic Potentials and Receptor Potentials

After excitability, the second key property of nerve cells is the action that occurs at the synapses between cells. This is the crucial property that underlies the coordinated activity of neuronal populations. In analogy with the action potentials of the nerve fibers, the actions at synapses are called "synaptic potentials." The era of investigation of synaptic potentials was opened by the development of fine-tipped micropipettes that could record the membrane currents and potentials near the sites of synapses. A leading model for these mechanisms was the nerve–muscle junction, where Bernard Katz and colleagues showed that the invading action potential in the nerve activated an end-plate potential, shown to be due to the summed action of many miniature responses to transmitter quanta presumably corresponding to the release of vesicles from the presynaptic terminal. The other leading model was the spinal motoneuron, shown by John Eccles and collaborators to generate postsynaptic excitatory and inhibitory potentials due to presynaptic transmitter release. The universality of these mechanisms was confirmed in invertebrate preparations and in sensory receptors.

The Synapse as a Functional Concept

We have seen in Chapter 5 how the idea of neuronal interactions taking place by contact arose in the work of Ramón y Cajal and his colleagues in the 1890s and how the term "synapse" was introduced by Sherrington in 1897 to refer to this site of contact.

Sherrington, ever the precise thinker, was in fact in some doubt as to whether the synapse was primarily an anatomical or a physiological concept.

He initially seemed inclined toward the anatomical. But by the time he published his book *The Integrative Action of the Nervous System* (1906, 16) he was thinking primarily in functional terms. In a clear break with the traditional speculations, he outlined what some of the potential functions that a "surface of separation" at the nerve terminal might have:

> Such a surface might restrain diffusion, bank up osmotic pressure, restrict the movement of ions, accumulate electric charges, support a double electric layer, alter in shape and surface tension with changes in difference of potential ... or intervene as a membrane between dilute solutions of electrolytes of different concentration or colloidal suspensions with different sign of charge.

This passage shows how Sherrington, working at the systems level, was keenly aware of contemporary studies of membrane properties. He thought of synaptic interactions as possibly embracing a number of complex properties that were critical for understanding neural mechanisms underlying behavior. It is notable that he doesn't mention the "receptive substances" suggested by the pharmacologists several years before. Nor does he mention any kind of electrical induction mechanism as suggested by Ramón y Cajal. But he does speculate on "electrolytes of different concentrations," possibly indicating his awareness of the Bernstein-Overton theory of the membrane potential (see Chapter 6).

And there matters stood for almost four decades. It was not a question that could even be approached at the organ level, as the pharmacologists could do by collecting candidate neurotransmitter substances produced by stimulation of the nerves to an organ; the brain was too complex and seemingly impenetrable.

First Electrophysiological Evidence for Synaptic Transmission

The question eventually was attacked when microelectrodes were first introduced in the late 1930s (see Chapter 6), and recordings could be made from peripheral nerve preparations, the neuromuscular junction, and the sympathetic nerve ganglion. Several groups around the world—Gopfert and Schaefer (1938) in Germany, Feng (1941) in China, and Eccles and his collaborators (Eccles and O'Connor, 1939) in Australia—reported that the impulse invading the nerve terminal first leads to a local "end-plate potential" in the muscle at the end-plate region, which then triggers the muscle action potential. This end-plate potential was the first example of a synaptic response and the first direct recording of the physiological effect of a synapse. These results provided strong evidence that, at least at these peripheral synapses, chemical transmission takes place when acetylcholine (ACh) is released by the presynaptic terminal and acts on the postsynaptic terminal to cause, in the muscle cell, the end-plate potential and, in sympathetic ganglion cells, a postsynaptic potential. Even Eccles had to agree.

As noted in Chapter 4, this left open whether central synapses work in a similar fashion, and Eccles for one still clung to the idea that central synapses might involve passage of electric current from the presynaptic to the postsynaptic side.

The Impact of Intracellular Recordings

The evidence on this critical feature, to resolve once and for all the universality of the "soup vs. sparks" debate, required the development of reliable intracellular recordings.

Central neurons are small, their cell bodies ranging from only 5 to as much as 70 μm in diameter and their axons and dendrites from 0.1 to 20 μm; so the pipette tip must be very small, 1 μm or less. Furthermore, action potentials are extremely rapid, lasting only approximately 1 msec, which requires sophisticated electronic equipment, including high-impedance cathode followers, for accurate recordings. This equipment was not developed until after the war. One of the leaders in this effort was Jan Friedrich Toennies at the Rockefeller Institute in New York, who we have seen proved to be so helpful to Hodgkin in the work on the action potential (see Chapter 6).

As discussed in Chapter 6, intracellular recordings were essential for establishing the membrane mechanisms underlying the action potential. The recordings from the squid axon could be made by inserting a fine wire because of the unusually large diameter of the axon. The earlier recordings from peripheral nerves and ganglia were made with early methods for drawing and filling the micropipettes with conducting solution and with early electronic equipment for recording the potentials. However, for the technique to gain wider use it was necessary to devise a standard way to construct the pipettes on a microforge and improved electronic equipment for recordings. This was first accomplished by Gilbert Ling, in Chicago, working with Ralph Gerard, one of the leaders in neurophysiology at that time. The paper of Ling and Gerard (1947) showed the effectiveness of the method, using recordings of the membrane potential of muscle as the model system (Appendix 7.1) It took several more years for the method to be developed. Hodgkin and Nastuk (1950) made the first recordings of the muscle action potential. The race was on to develop the method in order to investigate all the preparations in which only extracellular recordings had been possible, in both the peripheral and the central nervous systems. Within a few years, the method had thrown open a new world of cell physiology, to complement cell structures revealed by the electronmicroscope. We begin with the first model synapse, the neuromuscular junction.

Bernard Katz and A. V. Hill

In the same way that the action potential is associated with Hodgkin and Huxley, the neuromuscular junction is associated with Bernard Katz. It will be useful to recount Katz's background, which he describes in a memoir (Katz, 1996), as an example of one of the key facts in the run-up to the breakthroughs at midcentury: the persecution of Jewish scientists by the Nazis, their escapes, and their enrichment of science in the democracies of the West.

Bernard Katz was born in Leipzig in 1911 but grew up without German citizenship because at that time Leipzig was under Russian hegemony. After the Russian Revolution he was therefore stateless. He was educated first in classics, then entered medical studies, and found himself attracted to the natural sciences, where he "realized the power and depth of scientific ideas and their continuous subjection to criticism and further trials by experiment" (p. 361). Among his teachers was Hans Held, the histologist who believed in continuity of nerve cells in opposition to Ramón y Cajal (see Chapter 5). Katz was drawn to neurophysiology, especially the subject as we have seen (Chapter 6) much debated at the time of the laws of electrical excitation of nerves, fascinated he wrote later "that one could make accurate and repeatable measurements of electrical excitability on living tissues and express the results by a simple mathematical equation" (p. 364). He carried out some simple experiments on muscle permeability and found an impedance response of muscle to stretching, which led to a couple of papers in *Pflügers Archiv*. This was significant for two reasons: It won him a research prize and the papers were noticed by A. V. Hill in London. Hill was one of the towering figures of British science and culture, an authority on nerve and muscle physiology, a leading critic of the rise of Hitler, and a central figure in trying to improve Britain's preparedness for the coming war during the 1930s.

During his student years Katz suffered along with other Jews the growing hostility of the Nazis and seriously considered emigrating to Palestine. However, after an interview with Chaim Weizmann, the well-known Zionist leader who knew Hill, and a letter of introduction to Hill by his professor, Martin Gildemeister, he was invited to join Hill in London. Without citizenship, the only way he could get a visa was with a "Nansenpass," "the green identification certificate that was issued to stateless persons by the League of Nations' Commissioner for Refugees" (p. 352). It is a pleasant irony that Katz, the neurophysiologist, was saved by Nansen, who began his career as a neuroanatomist, one of the founders of the neuron doctrine, before becoming the arctic explorer, world diplomat, and humanitarian (recounted in Shepherd, 1991).

Katz arrived in London in February 1935 and worked for four years with Hill on the electrical excitation of nerve. When in 1938 Hill was asked to write a review on this subject for *Ergebnisse der Physiologie*, he passed it along to Katz. In response to the submitted manuscript, the editor replied that the article could not be published without an Aryan coauthor. One of Hill's colleagues suggested Winston Churchill! The article was published as a monograph (see p. 73). Katz's background and this incident illustrate the extraordinarily vicious attitude toward Jews in general and academics in particular during the 1930s in Germany, relieved only by the successful attempts to emigrate or escape. The enrichment of scientific achievement in the West was incalculable, as the history of modern neuroscience well illustrates.

During his time in Hill's laboratory Katz became friends with the leaders of neurophysiology in Britain, including Alan Hodgkin and Jack Eccles. Eccles moved to Australia in 1937, where as we have seen he carried out the first recordings of the end-plate potential. He invited Katz to join him in keeping his research going in that rather isolated setting. Stephen Kuffler also joined him, and Katz spent two years with them; the photograph of the three of them walking down a street in Sydney is part of the lore of the field (Fig. 7.1). He then spent four years in the military, much of it in New Guinea. At the end of the war he got married and, as a wedding present from Hill, received a telegram inviting him back to London to be assistant director of research in Hill's biophysics unit. Hill's personal closeness to Katz and his wife is shown by the fact that for their first 2 two years back in London Hill put them up in his own house. How many of us could manage that for even our closest colleagues?

On Katz's return to the University College London laboratory, he scrounged for equipment, as we have seen Hodgkin and others did, to get his research going again in a badly damaged city that for many years endured continuing food rationing, coal shortages, and rebuilding. He picked up the threads of his former interest in nerve excitation and the properties of muscle membrane, including the observation of anomalous (inward) rectification. Several summers were spent working on the squid axon in collaboration with Hodgkin, as noted previously. The paper with Hodgkin on the sodium current in the action potential was his first to gain wider attention (Hodgkin and Katz, 1949). He then carried out his own first major study, on the muscle spindle of the frog, combining physiological recordings from the nerve in mineral oil with a very early electron microscopic study showing the thin nerve endings and bulbs in the spindle (Katz, 1950). I had many occasions to refer to this article in later work on the sensory response of the muscle spindle (Ottoson and Shepherd, 1971).

The End-Plate Potential and Synaptic Quanta

In 1948 an American, Paul Fatt, joined Katz and together they initiated an intracellular study of synaptic transmission at the frog neuromuscular junction. Fatt is a forgotten pioneer of that era, a brilliant experimentalist who collaborated in establishing two key advances: the muscle end-plate potential (EPP) with Katz and the nature of synaptic inhibition with Eccles.

The work with Katz identified the EPP as the postsynaptic response that elicits the muscle action potential (Fatt and Katz, 1951; Appendix 7.2). The role of ACh as the neurotransmitter was established by their work, as well as by the histological evidence of Couteaux in France (Chapter 5). The EPP became the leading model for understanding all chemical synapses and continues to play a valuable role today, even when current methods enable detailed analysis of central synapses. During this period other models for synaptic action were introduced, including the squid giant synapse (Young, 1938; Bullock, 1948; Bullock and Hagiwara, 1957). As we have seen, this was eventually shown to involve electrical as well as chemical transmission (see Chapter 5).

While recording the EPP at high gain, Fatt and Katz noticed very small unitary (all-or-nothing) potentials (Fig. 7.2). In later talks about these experiments, Katz joked that at first they checked the corridor outside to see if these might be due to A. V.'s heavy footsteps as he stalked down the hall. A thorough study by del Castillo and Katz (1954a–c) characterized these as miniature end-plate potentials (MEPPs) and showed that many of these "quanta" were released simultaneously by an action potential in the terminal to sum and produce the full EPP. The analysis of the quanta invoked an elegant mathematical and statistical approach that harkens back to what drew Katz to neurophysiology in the first place as a student, that "one could make accurate and repeatable measurements . . . on living tissues and express the results by a simple mathematical equation" (Appendix 7.3).

The approach is based on the statistics of random events, such as radioactive decay, as explained by del Castillo and Katz (1954a, 263-264):

> Suppose we have, at each nerve-muscle junction, a population of n units . . . capable of responding to a nerve impulse. Suppose, further, that the average probability of responding is p . . . then the mean number of units responding to one impulse is $m = np$. . . . when p is very small, the number of units x which make up the e.p.p. in a large series of observations should be distributed in the characteristic manner of Poisson's law (their relative frequencies being given by $\exp(-m)\, m^x/x!$).

These questions relate the amplitudes of quanta to the numbers available and their probability of release. The *frequency* of the miniature potentials is controlled by the properties of the *pre*synaptic membrane, while their *amplitude* is controlled by the properties of the *post*synaptic membrane. This formulation became as fundamental to understanding the synaptic potential as the HH equations were for understanding the action potential (Boyd and Martin, 1956). Additional studies showed that the release probability is controlled by the membrane potential (Liley, 1956), as predicted, and is affected by drugs (Nicholls and Quilliam, 1956). Later studies by Katz and his long-time colleague Ricardo Miledi (e.g. 1963) established the essential role of Ca^{2+} in the release mechanism.

These physiological quanta had not been predicted. It was immediately recognized that they could be correlated with the synaptic vesicles identified by the electron microscopists working independently at virtually the same time (see Chapter 5). A series of studies by Katz and others provided increasing evidence that a vesicle contains several thousand molecules of ACh, released simultaneously when the vesicle bursts open as it fuses with the plasma membrane.

The site of vesicle fusion came to be recognized as an *active zone* (see Chapter 5), and the release of a single synaptic vesicle and the action of its neurotransmitter on postsynaptic receptors has become recognized as the *fundamental unit of action* at chemical synapses, as essential to the functional organization of the brain as the chemical bond is to the organization and interactions of molecules. With the advent of recombinant DNA techniques, those mechanisms have come under unrelenting scrutiny, with many molecular players involved in each step of vesicle mobilization and fusion on the presynaptic side and activation of receptors on the postsynaptic side. Each of these steps is a potential site of action for a genetic disorder, for a toxin, or for a drug that can ameliorate a nervous system disorder.

Central Synapses: Eccles and the Spinal Motoneuron

The parallel revolution in understanding the mechanisms of synapses in the central nervous system was led by Eccles, Katz's mentor, friend, and colleague from Australia. Eccles was such a dominant personality in establishing the physiology of the neuron in the 1950s, publishing over his lifetime 500 articles and books and training over 200 students, that it will be appropriate to describe the trajectory of his career, especially since today memory of how our knowledge of central synapses was first wrested from the spinal cord as a model is fading. The following account is based on Shepherd (2008); see also the testimonial issue of Stuart and Pierce (2006).

Background. Eccles was born in Melbourne, New South Wales, Australia, in 1903. His parents were both schoolteachers and Catholics, a family background that shaped the future career. He received his undergraduate and medical training at the University of Melbourne, graduating in 1925 with first-class honors. He won a Rhodes Scholarship for study at Oxford University, where he joined the group of outstanding young investigators which included Derek Denny-Brown, John Farquhar Fulton, R. S. Creed, and E. G. T. Liddell, producing a series of studies under Charles Sherrington on spinal cord reflexes. This resulted in the landmark book *Reflex Activity in the Spinal Cord* (1932) by Creed et al. Liddell later told me that they put the manuscript together with some urgency to have it support the awarding of the Nobel Prize to Sherrington (together with Adrian) in that year.

During this time Eccles completed a BS at Oxford in 1927 and a DPhil in 1929 and then became a tutor at Magdalen College and a university demonstrator in 1934. Sherrington took him on as a research assistant for his last experiments on excitation and inhibition of spinal cord reflexes. Eccles then developed his own studies of synaptic transmission in sympathetic ganglia, in which he interpreted his findings in terms of electrical transmission between the stimulated nerves and the postsynaptic cells. This brought him into conflict with the emerging pharmacological evidence by H. H. Dale, Wilhelm Feldberg, Lindor Brown, and others for the release and action of chemical transmitters at the synaptic junctions between nerve cell fiber terminals and their target glands and muscles.

As described in Chapter 4, this engendered the "soup vs. sparks" debates, which often involved pitched battles between the participants at one meeting after the other throughout the 1930s. As mentioned in Chapter 4, Bernard Katz, as a refugee from Germany in the mid-1930s, was amazed at how violently the younger Eccles and the older Dale would attack each other during these meetings and was further amazed at how they would then retire to sherry and a convivial dinner together.

Isolation. Sherrington retired in 1935 (at the age of 75, having been granted a personal extension). Although Eccles was an obvious candidate to succeed him, his Australian brashness and pugnacity were a bit much for the Oxford scene, and John Mellanby was appointed. In 1937 Eccles left to return to Australia (a common career trajectory from training in England back to the colonies), to head a small medical research unit in the Kanematsu Institute of Pathology in Sydney. It was near oblivion for him, with no university connection, no access to students, and an unsympathetic administration. The onset of the war in Europe in September 1939 diverted most of his attention to the war effort. By great good fortune, he was joined by both Katz and another refugee, Stephen Kuffler, documented by the famous photograph of the three strolling down a street in Sydney (Fig. 7.1). As already noted, in 1939 Eccles reported electrophysiological recordings from the neuromuscular junction with evidence of chemical transmission, simultaneously with similar reports by Feng in China and Schaefer in Germany. Although this was a great breakthrough in the analysis of the physiology of the synapse, it also disproved his own electrical hypothesis, at least for peripheral synaptic transmission.

With prospects dim at the institute, in 1944 Eccles accepted the professorship of physiology at the University of Otago in Dunedin, New Zealand. Despite the remote location, it gave the opportunity to return to an academic setting for his research, though with a heavy teaching load. He describes how in his first year he gave all the physiology lectures, totaling some 500 contact hours. On the positive side, it gave him discipline in using his time and a broad grasp of physiological principles.

He was still depressed over the failure of his theoretical predictions in the 1930s, until meeting the philosopher Karl Popper in New Zealand. Popper was developing his philosophy of science, with the dictum that science can never prove a hypothesis correct but can only falsify it; the goal of the scientist is therefore to erect hypotheses that can be tested and disproven. According to this view, Eccles had been advancing science by proving himself wrong. This new concept of doing science rescued Eccles from his depression, and the two became lifelong friends. "I was urged by Popper to formulate the hypotheses of electrical excitation and inhibition in models that invited experimental testing and falsification" (Eccles, 1977, 6). Eccles added an implied corollary to this: Only Eccles would be allowed to disprove Eccles' hypotheses!

Despite the isolation of Dunedin, after the war he assembled a group of outstanding young students and colleagues from New Zealand and abroad, including on the faculty the electrophysiologist Archibald McIntyre and as a graduate student the American biophysicist Wilfrid Rall. For several years he pursued his hypothesis of electrical transmission at synapses in the spinal cord. This required convoluted reasoning to account for current flows that could cause postsynaptic inhibition. In his remote location, one less motivated might have lost out in the postwar era of gearing up for modern cellular research and drifted out of the mainstream.

However, around 1950 McIntyre returned from the Rockefeller Institute with the circuit for the new state-of-the-art amplifier built by Jan Friedrich Toennies, the outstanding German engineer (who before the war, as we have noted in Chapter 6, had trained Alan Hodgkin in cathode followers for his squid axon studies). Dexter Easton (personal communication) came with the news that J. Walter Woodbury and Harry Patton in Seattle were beginning to make intracellular recordings in the spinal cord. Easton related to me that this galvanized Eccles to a single-minded focus on this goal, with an intensity that could not be matched by the Seattle group.

The Drive for the Central Synaptic Potential. It was a singular moment for Eccles, "a crisis in my life." (p6) Spurred by fear of the competition, he resolved to get there first. He needed hands to do it. According to Rall (personal communication), Eccles asked John Coombs, a physicist, to help with the electronics for doing the microelectrode work. Coombs decided it was interesting and would do it himself, constructing the needed cathode follower amplifier with high-input impedance to reduce input capacitance and neutralize pipette capacitance by negative feedback.

Laurence Brock had just completed his medical course; he was good with his hands and pulled the micropipettes. This was done on a microforge, requiring (as I know from my own work a few years later on a similar apparatus) extreme concentration to pull the pipettes to a fine tip and luck to get them fully filled with the electrode solution. Rall had started earlier work with Eccles but decided he would do his own project under Archibald McIntyre for his PhD thesis. McIntyre was a mild-mannered person at an early stage in his career. Eccles at the time was using the classical mechanoelectric Lucas pendulum breaks for stimulators, recording the data on glass negatives that were developed as they went along. When he realized he needed McIntyre's state-of-the-art equipment, he simply took it over. The experiments in McIntyre's laboratory were done behind closed doors. All efforts were bent on beating the Americans. I once asked McIntyre if he would write a brief account of those times, but it was too difficult for him to countenance.

Eccles and colleagues plunged into making intracellular recordings from the motor neurons in the spinal cord in response to electrical shocks to the ventral roots, to activate the motor neurons backward (antidromically), and to the dorsal roots, to activate them by the normal forward route (orthodromically).

The recordings immediately showed that stimulation of the sensory nerves from an agonist muscle set up depolarizing, excitatory postsynaptic potentials (EPSPs) in a motoneuron. In analogy with the EPP recently demonstrated by Fatt and Katz, this was hypothesized to involve a nonspecific conductance increase to Na and K ions, depolarizing the membrane toward zero.

In contrast, stimulation of an antagonist muscle produced a hyperpolarizing potential that inhibited any activity by the cell; hence, it was termed the "inhibitory postsynaptic potential" (IPSP). Whereas the depolarization of an EPSP could possibly be construed as being due to current flowing from the presynaptic terminal, this could not explain the hyperpolarization of an IPSP. This and other arguments convinced Eccles finally that the electrical hypothesis of synaptic transmission was dead.

> ... an electrical explanation of inhibitory transmission seems most improbable. It would demand the postulate of special electrical properties qualitatively different from those revealed by exhaustive investigations of surface membranes.
>
> It may therefore be concluded that inhibitory synaptic action is probably mediated by a specific transmitter substance that is liberated from the inhibitory synaptic knobs, and causes an active hyperpolarization process in the subjacent membrane of the motoneurone.
>
> (Eccles 1953, 163)

The electrical hypothesis was triumphantly demolished by its own Popperian architect!

For a new mechanism, Eccles initially favored a sodium pump that would hyperpolarize the membrane by moving positively charged Na ions outward. As it happened, Fatt and Katz, as if their studies on the EPP were not enough, were also at this time carrying out a study of inhibitory fibers to the muscles of the crab. This took advantage of the fact that, whereas vertebrate muscles have only excitatory inputs (through the neuromuscular junction), invertebrates may have both excitatory and inhibitory fibers. This study (Fatt and Katz, 1952, 164) provided evidence that the inhibition is due to a hyperpolarization caused by an increase in conductance to K (similar to the hyperpolarization due to K following the action potential). In addition, experiments by Burgen and Terroux (1952) suggested that the inhibition that ACh produces in heart muscle (the classic preparation of Loewi, see Chapter 4) is most likely due to an increase in K^+ conductance. Further experiments showed clearly that this mechanism was the more likely, and eventually it was shown that it involves increases in Cl^- conductance as well.

Eccles' initial results were published in a series of articles in the *Journal of Physiology* beginning in 1951(Brock et al., 1952) (Fig. 7.3, Appendix 7.4).

In that year Eccles accepted the opportunity to move back to Australia, to be professor of physiology in the newly established Australian National University in Canberra. It took 15 months for the new laboratories to be ready, an interim that might have been fatal to the scientific career of a normal mortal at that critical juncture. However, Eccles typically used it to full advantage. He spent five months traveling in early 1952, first to a Cold Spring Harbor symposium on the neuron, where he learned about the Hodgkin-Huxley action potential model and the Katz neuromuscular junction work, then back to England to summarize the new results in the Waynflete Lectures, delivered at Magdalen College in Oxford in 1952 and published in *The Neurophysiological Basis of Mind: The Principles of Neurophysiology* in 1953.

In many ways this work and the book launched the modern cellular physiology of the central nervous system. It established the basic functions of chemical excitatory and inhibitory synapses, just before they were visualized morphologically for the first time with the electron microscope. They were furthermore developed firmly within the context of the emerging modern concepts of the properties of cell membranes, thanks to his rapid assimilation of the work of Hodgkin and Huxley in developing their model of the action potential in the squid axon and of Katz and Fatt in their model of the neuromuscular junction. It immediately laid out the future of cellular and circuit neuroscience, at a time when neurophysiology ruled studies of the nervous system, before the advent of the biochemical and pharmacological approaches which today we take for granted. For a young medical student in the 1950s determined to become a neurophysiologist, it was, if not the tablets of Moses, something close to them.

The air was suddenly cleared; chemical transmission was the way neurons communicate by means of synapses, which received strong support from the revelations of the electron microscope of the fine structure of the chemical synapse (see Chapter 5). Within a few years electrical synapses were described by Furshpan and Potter and their basis in gap junctions shown (Chapter 5), to give our present understanding of both chemical and electrical transmission in the central nervous system.

When the new laboratories were completed, Eccles, with a growing number of students from around the world and with a growing number of other laboratories joining the hunt, launched into studies of the synaptic organization of the neuron and the identification of the first synaptic pathways in the central nervous system. These studies are covered in Chapters 8 and 9, respectively, together with an assessment of Eccles' career and influence.

Extending the Model of Synaptic Action

The intracellular method was quickly taken up by other laboratories, testing the motoneuron model itself and extending it to other types of cells. These included the motoneuron in other species (Woodbury and Patton, 1952; Araki et al., 1953; Araki and Otani, 1955; Frank and Fuortes, 1955, 1956); cells of the fish electric organ (Albe-Fessard and Buser, 1954); and cerebral cortical pyramidal neurons, the first intracellular recordings of cells in the brain above the spinal cord (Phillips, 1955, 1956a, 1956b; Albe-Fessard and Buser, 1955). We will take up the studies in the brain in Chapter 9.

Invertebrate Simple Systems

A number of electrophysiologists pursued the study of synaptic properties in invertebrate animals. Of special importance among them was Ladislav Tauc (Fig. 7.4).

Ladislav Tauc. He was born in Czechoslovakia in 1926. In 1945, just after the war, he began his studies at Masaryk University, carrying out his first research on the electrical signals of plant cells. He then obtained a scholarship to pursue his studies in Paris, where he came under the wing of Alfred Fessard, the leading figure in the growth of electrophysiology in France in the 1950s, at the Institut Marey.(By the way, don't try to go on a pilgrimage to the Marey; it was razed to make way for Roland Garros, site of the French Open in tennis.) After pursuing further studies of the electrical activity of various cells in plants and nervous tissue, he decided to focus on the nervous system of the garden slug *Aplysia*.

The first use of *Aplysia* for electrophysiological studies was by Angelique Arvanitaki in Marseilles in 1941. According to Tauc's colleague Maurice Israel (2000, 47):

> The introduction of a "simplified" brain (the *Aplysia* nervous system) to study the cellular and molecular basis of organized neuronal interactions, is probably one of Tauc's essential contributions to neuroscience. When he introduced modern electrophysiology to study the nervous system of *Aplysia*, no one imagined that the simple brain of a mollusc would be so crucial to the understanding of more complex nervous systems. The very first microelectrode with which Tauc penetrated an *Aplysia* neurone was the breakthrough that started the modern studies of the biophysical properties of neurones. Because of its remarkable properties, this model has been used by hundreds of neurobiology researchers throughout the world. Indeed, each neurone has now been identified, and its ionic channels, transmitters and receptors characterized.

Just as the giant axon of the squid enabled Hodgkin and Huxley to reveal the nature of the nerve impulse and the motoneuron of the spinal cord revealed the nature of synaptic potentials in nerve cells, so the giant neurons of *Aplysia* allowed Tauc to take the next step and study membrane properties in identified neurons. In many cases these large cell bodies could be recognized across individuals; they could be given their own names! Beginning in 1954, soon after the reports of the Hodgkin-Huxley action potential (Chapter 6) and the synaptic potentials of the spinal motoneuron (see above), he initiated a series of studies, focusing on identified cells in the abdominal ganglion. These are summarized in Table 7.1.

Table 7.1 Early Investigations of the Electrophysiology of *Aplysia* by Ladislav Tauc

---

Synaptic responses (1955)
Basic types of induced (1955) and spontaneous (1955) electrical activity
Inhibitory postsynaptic potentials (1956)
Biophysical properties (1956)
Subthreshold oscillations (1956) (with A. Fessard)
Electrotonic potentials (1957) (with A. Fessard)
More about inhibitory potentials (1957)
Backfiring antidromic responses (1957)
Responses to injected substances (1958)
Repetitive synaptic responses (1958) (with A. Fessard)
Interneuronal actions (1958)
Effects of hyperpolarization (1958)
Proof of existence of interneurons (1959)
Long-lasting hyperpolarization (1959)

(See tauc l, in http://www.ncbi.nlm.nih.gov/pubmed/, for these references).

It was a remarkable pioneering series of studies. Unfortunately, the outside world was scarcely aware of it because every study was published in French. However, a few took note. As France began to recover from the war, its scientists reestablished contacts with colleagues outside. In the late 1950s Arvanitaki-Chalazonitis and Tauc visited the United States and gave lectures on their work on the electrophysiology of the giant neurons of *Aplysia*. Eric Kandel (2006) describes how, nearing the end of his training with Wade Marshall and Kay Frank at the National Institutes of Health, he was searching for a preparation that would enable him to pursue his aim of

> ... an animal with a simple reflex that could be modified by learning and that was controlled by a small number of large nerve cells whose pathway from input to output could be identified. In that way I could relate changes in the reflex to changes in the cells.
>
> (p 144)

He realized the advantages of *Aplysia* for this purpose and arranged to join Tauc for training after his psychiatry residency. During this interim Kay Frank himself spent time with Tauc, bringing the voltage-clamp method to bear on the membrane properties of *Aplysia* neurons. Kandel's first publication with Tauc was entitled "Mechanism of Prolonged Heterosynaptic Facilitation" (Kandel and Tauc, 1964) (in all, they published five studies together, three in English), which initiated the brilliant studies by Kandel of activity-dependent plasticity of synaptic actions that might underlie learning and memory. The rest, as they say, is history (see Kandel's memoir *In Search of Memory*, 2006).

Meanwhile, Hersch (Coco) Gerschenfeld, an Argentine neurophysiologist, joined Tauc in the late 1950s and initiated with him an analysis of neurotransmitters, starting with ACh. Although their studies extend beyond our primary focus on the 1950s, we note that their collaboration was significant for two reasons. First, it brought *Aplysia* into the mainstream of interest in the critical questions regarding neurotransmitters and their actions, leading to their breakthrough demonstration that a single transmitter could be liberated by a given identified neuron and have both excitatory and inhibitory effects on another identified neuron. Second, their publications (see Gerschenfeld and Tauc, 1961) were in English in the journal *Nature*, bringing *Aplysia* to the notice of the world outside France.

Tauc's influence also was important within France: Phillippe Ascher and JacSue Kehoe joined the laboratory later in the 1960s and, with Gerschenfeld, quickly became leaders in the field of electrophysiology of the nervous system in France, in particular making bridges to the Anglo-Saxon world.

Receptor Potentials of Sensory Receptors

The search for large and accessible cells for physiological analysis led J. S. Alexandrowicz (1953) to the stretch receptor cell of the crayfish. In this preparation, the dendrites of the cell end in branches that interdigitate within the muscle fibers. Stephen Kuffler and a postdoctoral fellow, Carlos Eyzaguirre, from Chile immediately took advantage of it for physiological study. Their recordings (Eyzaguirre and Kuffler, 1955a, 1955b) showed that stretch of the muscle sets up a depolarizing potential that spreads through the dendrites to the cell body to initiate the action potential, which sends the message on to the nervous ganglion of the crayfish. This was the clearest demonstration of the **receptor potential** of a sensory receptor cell to its stimulus.

They further showed that the stretch receptor cell also received synaptic inhibition from central nerve fibers and were able to study in detail how the interaction of the opposing depolarizing and hyperpolarizing potentials controls action potential initiation in the axon. Together with the work by the Eccles laboratory, this provided an elegant model for how postsynaptic potentials are integrated within the nerve cell. This integration involves the dendrites, which requires discussion of this next level of organization within the cell in Chapter 8.

Intracellular recordings from retinal cells were attempted by Gunnar Svaetichin in Stockholm in 1954, but successful results awaited the intracellular analysis of the mudpuppy retina by Frank Werblin and John Dowling in 1969 (Chapter 9).

Other Studies of Sensory Responses

Extracellular Single-Unit Recordings. As mentioned in Chapter 6, analysis of single sensory receptors began in 1926 with the study of Edgar Adrian and his student Yngve Zotterman of Sweden. They dissected a peripheral sensory nerve of the frog to a single fiber and showed with extracellular recordings that it responded with phasic and tonic firing to an applied stimulus, which increased in frequency with increasing strength. The extracellular unit recording method was used by Ragnar Granit in the late 1930s and was extended to the *Limulus* eye by Keffer Hartline and to the vertebrate retina by Kuffler and Barlow in the 1950s (see Chapter 9).

Some of the basic response properties of sensory receptors in the skin were evidenced by single-unit extracellular recordings from their axons during the 1950s. For example, recordings from the endings of pacinian corpuscles showed that they adapted extremely rapidly, responding with only one impulse to applied pressure when the surrounding capsule was removed (Loewenstein and Rathkamp, 1958).

Summed Field Potentials. In contrast to the recordings of single receptors, the responses of many receptors could be recorded as summed extracellular potentials due to the electric currents flowing outside the activated populations, similar to the electrocardiogram or the electroencephalogram. A summed field potential, the electroretinogram (ERG), was recorded from the retina, attributable to a succession of three responses: the responses to light of the photoreceptors, the synaptic activation of bipolar cells, and further activation of other cell types (Brown and Wiesel, 1961). The ERG is used in clinical settings to diagnose certain retinal disorders.

A summed field potential, the electro-olfactogram (EOG), was recorded from the frog olfactory epithelium in response to smell stimuli (Ottoson, 1955). This has been useful as a monitor of the overall stimulating effectiveness of different compounds used as odor stimuli.

These potentials had the advantage of ease of recording with large extracellular electrodes; they had the limitation of being of small amplitude, registering the combined activity of overlapping populations of cells and giving little insight into membrane properties and mechanisms.

Psychophysical Studies. Several important classical psychophysical studies were carried out during this time period. In the human exposed to light stimuli in total darkness, photoreceptors were found to respond to single photons (Hecht et al., 1941), leading to the estimate that the threshold of visual perception required the summation of approximately seven receptor responses. In hearing, the tympanic membrane was shown to respond to vibrations of the diameter of a single hydrogen atom. In smell, olfactory cells were estimated to be able to respond to single molecules (Stuiver, 1960). These studies thus combined to show that sensory receptors are able to respond to stimuli close to their theoretical limits (see review by Block, 1993).

Basilar Membrane of the Cochlea. A fundamental analysis of the mechanical response of the tectorial membrane to sound stimuli was carried out by Georg von Békésy (summarized in 1960). Although the experiments were limited by being carried out on cadaver material, the work nonetheless provided one of the foundations for modern study of the mechanical basis of the transduction of sound in the inner ear.

von Békésy worked in the basement of Sanders Theater at Harvard. In the summer of 1956, when I was working with Karl Pribram in Walter Rosenblith's laboratory at MIT, he arranged a visit during which von Békésy showed us with quiet pride his long model of a mechanical basilar membrane hanging across his basement room, where he could twitch the "oval window" end and demonstrate what must have been the world's largest standing waves.

Chapter 8

Functional Organization of Neurons and Dendrites

The "neuron doctrine" arose as an organizing principle for the nervous system in the late nineteenth century. The advances in the 1950s provided the first adequate tests of its validity, bringing about, in the words of Theodore Bullock, a "quiet but sweeping revolution" in the functional concept of the neuron, a revolution that continues to this day. Much of this revolution concerns the functional significance of the short processes, the dendrites, at the next higher level of organization of the neuron above the synapse. Neurons were seen to contain "complexity within unity." A new concept of the functional organization of vertebrate neurons emerged: Excitatory and inhibitory synaptic potentials combine to spread to the initial segment of the axon to activate the action potential, which then spreads backward into the cell body and dendrites. Wilfrid Rall built on the work of Hodgkin and Huxley to show the dominance of the dendrites in this integrative activity. The first studies of the physiological properties of dendrites and their spines were carried out. The expanded concept of the functional organization of the neuron is being greatly extended by current work. Nonetheless, a full appreciation of the importance of dendrites in the integrative action of the neuron continues to be one of the last frontiers of modern neuroscience.

The cell theory was introduced for plants by Matthias Schlieden in 1838 and for animals by Theodor Schwann in 1839. An outpouring of microscopic studies in the 1840s established the cell as the membrane-enclosed fundamental unit of organization of most tissues and organs of the body, but acceptance was delayed in the nervous system by the difficulty of visualizing under the light microscope how the branches of its processes end (reviewed in Shepherd, 1991).

The impregnation method discovered by Camillo Golgi in 1873 finally enabled visualization of individual cells in the central nervous system. With this method, Golgi established a number of firsts. He saw that the branching dendrites end freely, which disposed of previous theories of networks involving dendrites. He used the different dendritic branching patterns as the basis for classifying different types of nerve cells. He extended Deiters' observation of a single axon arising from a motoneuron to show that this was also true of central neurons in the brain. He classified cells on the basis of their axons into cells of long axon (projecting out of a region to other regions) and cells of short axon (which came to be recognized as interneurons). He showed that the axon has extensive branches, called "axon collaterals," the discovery of which he was most proud. In all these findings Golgi was the pioneer; all who followed him were building on his foundation, a fact probably not adequately recognized at the time and certainly not in our own time.

Beyond these fundamental findings, confirmed by Ramón y Cajal and later histologists, Golgi made a further observation and a fateful interpretation. In his stained preparations it appeared to him that the finest axon collaterals merged into a continuous network. His interpretation was that these widely branching collaterals, and only the collaterals, form a reticulum, which carries out the basic signaling functions of the nervous system.

The Golgi technique remained mostly ignored for over a decade until it was discovered by an obscure histologist in Spain, Santiago Ramón y Cajal. The story has been told many times, most vividly in Ramón y Cajal's own memoirs (Ramón y Cajal, 1937; Shepherd, 1991). In his first studies in the late 1880s, Ramón y Cajal confirmed Golgi's findings that the dendrites end freely, that their different patterns are the basis of different types of nerve cells, that the axon is usually single, and that it characteristically gives off collaterals in different branching patterns. However, he also found persuasive evidence that the axon collaterals, too, end freely. This implied that the collaterals do not form a reticulum but, rather, that communication between nerve cells is by contacts rather than by continuity.

Ramón y Cajal's findings and interpretations were supported by most of the other classical histologists who took up the Golgi method. Ramón y Cajal in particular worked furiously, producing an outpouring of papers on different cells throughout the nervous system during the 1890s. The consensus emerging from the early work was reviewed in 1891 by Wilhelm Waldeyer in Germany (see Shepherd, 1891, 183, for translation):

> . . . all those authors who do not accept a network formation of the nerve fibers inside the central organ (Ramon y Cajal, Kolliker, His, Nansen, Lenhossek, Retzius) can easily unite points I and II above into one common brief fundamental law of wider range. It would sound thus:
> *The nervous system consists of numerous nerve units (neurons), anatomically and genetically independent.*

This gave rise to the "neuron theory," which was soon elevated in status to the "neuron doctrine." As commonly understood, it states that each nerve cell is a separate individual, bounded, like all other cells in the body, by its plasma membrane. This conclusion was in line with the interpretation of the relations, by contact not continuity, between cells in other tissues and organs throughout the body. It is for this reason that the neuron doctrine was regarded as the extension of the cell theory to the nervous system. As we have seen, Sherrington suggested the term "synapse" for the contacts between the nerve cells (Chapter 5).

Dynamic Polarization of the Neuron

In addition to his insistence on the individuality of the entire nerve cell and its interactions through contact, Ramón y Cajal (1911) made two other conceptual contributions that were essential for understanding the functional significance of the neuron (summarized in Shepherd, 1991).

The first had to do with the flow of information through the nerve cell. Waldeyer had left this question uncertain. In further work in the early 1890s, Ramón y Cajal, together with Alfred van Gehuchten of Belgium, inferred that there was an overall direction of the flow of activity, from contacts on the dendrites and soma out to the axon and to the axon terminals (summarized in Shepherd, 1991). He termed this the "law of dynamic polarization." This gave a functional meaning to the nerve cell as an integrative entity, taking in inputs from different sources and distributing them to different target cells (Fig. 8.1).

The second concept built on the first. By applying his tremendous powers of imagination to the functional interpretation of the relations between his stained cells, he deduced the flow of information not only within each cell but also between the cells. He devised diagrams showing how these relations form pathways within a region to accomplish multineuronal functions, integrating inputs from different regional sources and distributing them to different target regions. This enabled him to represent the flow of activity through the cells of the olfactory bulb, for example, and compare it with an equivalent flow of activity through the retina. This approach provided persuasive evidence that the nervous system is built of interconnected nerve cells that form the circuits and pathways that carry out the functional operations of the different regions and systems.

Many authors have attested to the importance of the original neuron doctrine and these functional concepts for the rise of modern neuroscience. For example, David Hubel has observed that Ramón y Cajal's (1911) textbook of histology of the nervous system, replete with the evidence of nerve cells as separate entities, "is considered to be the most important work ever published in neurobiology" (Junquera, 1992, viii). On the physiological side, Sherrington made clear the central importance of the extension of the cell theory to the nervous system. In his great work *The Integrative Action of the Nervous System*, published in 1906 just after Ramón y Cajal's *Histologia* in Spanish, the first sentence reads, "Nowhere in physiology does the cell-theory reveal its presence more frequently in the very framework of the argument than at the present time in the study of nervous reactions."

In its simplified set of postulates the neuron doctrine thus provided the conceptual basis for the rise of modern neuroscience in understanding normal brain function and the rise of the clinical neurological disciplines in understanding neurological diseases. In this respect it can be said to have provided the fundamental organizing principle for modern cellular neuroscience, performing a role similar to that of the atom for modern physics, the chemical bond for chemistry, the cell for cell biology, and the gene for genetics and for molecular biology.

Modern Research First Confirmed, Then Challenged, the Classical Neuron Doctrine

Ramón y Cajal's last publication, in 1933, just before his death, was an exhaustive review of the evidence for the neuron theory against the reticular theory. We have seen that the advent of modern methods of cell biology in the 1950s, particularly the electron microscope for the fine structure of cells and the recording microelectrode for membrane and cell physiology, brought support for the fundamental validity of the classical doctrine. However, electrical synapses raised questions about the kinds of neuronal ensembles created by continuity for passage of electric current and small molecules in many cell populations, questions that continue to this day.

What about the functional concept of the neuron, the idea that there is a flow of activity from the dendrites to the soma and out the axon? If the function of the axon is to transmit impulses, what is the function of the cell body and its elaborate dendritic branches? Ramón y Cajal and the other histologists who established the neuron doctrine were unaware of any activity of nerve cells other than the impulse in axons, so they supposed that when the dendrites are excited they transmit impulses through their branches toward the soma to pass out into the axon.

Synaptic Integration and Action Potential Initiation

The discovery of synaptic potentials forced a rethinking of this idea because in the motoneuron model, with the graded activation of different numbers of synapses on the soma-dendritic membrane, a conversion took place between the summed synaptic potentials and the all-or-nothing impulse output. Where did this conversion take place within the neuron and how?

This question was addressed in the motoneuron by Kay Frank and Michael Fuortes (Fuortes et al., 1957) (Appendix 8.1) at the National Institutes of Health. They first examined how the motoneuron reacts to an action potential set up in the axon and invading backward (antidromically) into the cell body. They found that the large spike recorded from the cell body had a hesitation on its upstroke, which they attributed to the delay that occurred in the depolarizing ability of the local currents of the action potential as they spread from the high resistance of the small-diameter axon to the low resistance of the large expanse of the cell body and all the dendrites arising from it, an electrical difference called an "impedance mismatch."

Eccles and his laboratory soon joined in this work, building on their pioneering demonstration of excitatory and inhibitory postsynaptic potentials (EPSPs and IPSPs) (Chapter 7). The surprise was that this same spike sequence, from axon back to cell body and dendrites, also occurred when the cell was activated by synaptic excitation in the dendrites. The new concept, as summarized by Eccles in his widely read monograph *The Physiology of the Neuron* (1957), was that EPSPs and IPSPs spread through the passive soma-dendritic membrane to summate at the highly excitable initial segment to initiate the action potential, with subsequent propagation down the axon and spread back into the cell body and on back into the dendrites. Because of the mismatch in electrical impedance (the combined resistance and capacitance of the membrane) between the smaller initial segment and the larger soma-dendritic membrane, the spike recorded from the soma showed the same two successive components as in the antidromic case. These spike components were called "initial segment" (IS) followed by "soma-dendritic" (IS-SD) (Eccles, 1957) (Fig. 8.2) and "A" and "B" by Fuortes et al. (1957).

The evidence for this new concept in the motoneuron was indirect; what was needed was an isolated cell where recordings could be made directly from the different parts of the neuron. Carlos Eyzaguirre, working with Stephen Kuffler at Woods Hole, assessed this question in the crayfish stretch receptor (Eyzaguirre and Kuffler, 1955a, 1955b). As we have seen (Chapter 7), attention had been drawn to this cell by Alexandrowicz (1953). The cell can be easily visualized under the microscope. It is organized with its dendritic tips embedded in a muscle fiber so that when the muscle is stretched the terminals are depolarized, setting up what is called a "receptor potential." The potential spreads through the dendrites into the cell body to initiate an action potential output in the axon. Eyzaguirre and Kuffler analyzed the cell responses and showed how the stretch is converted into the receptor potential, which gives rise to the impulse output that faithfully encodes the rate of rise and degree of muscle stretch (Appendix 8.2). This use of a model cell to demonstrate a physiological principle in an elegant manner was Kuffler's trademark. We will encounter an even better-known example in discussing visual receptive fields (Chapter 9).

This still left the question of exactly where the action potentials arise from the receptor potential: in the dendritic terminals, dendrites, cell body, or where? Charles Edwards and David Ottoson in Kuffler's laboratory were given the project of probing with an extracellular recording electrode along the cell to determine where the inward current occurred, which would signal where the spike was initiated. As Ottoson later told me, they expected that it would be at the cell body. To their, and Kuffler's, surprise, the site turned out to be several hundred microns from the cell body out on the axon, equivalent to the axonal initial segment (Edwards and Ottoson, 1958) (Fig. 8.3). Thus, the depolarization of the receptor potential spreads through the dendrites and cell body and out the axon to initiate the action potential, which propagates further down the axon but also spreads back into the cell body and dendrites, analogous to the sequence indicated by the experiments in the motoneuron.

Although less well known than the motoneuron studies, the stretch receptor was the most elegant demonstration of a new concept of the integrative organization of the neuron. Rather than the simple progression of impulses through the cell toward the axon, the reception and integration of synaptic potentials in the cell body and dendrites could be seen as a first and separate step of integration before activation of the action potential in the initial segment of the axon. It could be conceived that a great deal of integration could take place below threshold for initiating an output, possibly changing the responsiveness of the cell in a way that could lead to mechanisms for learning and memory. In addition, the backward spread of the action potential informed the cell bodies and dendrites whether there had been an output or not, thus further affecting the future responsiveness.

This sequence became the classical concept of the **integrative organization** of the neuron for **action potential initiation** in a neuron, such as the motoneuron, with passive dendrites. It was confirmed by studies in the 1990s in which dual electrodes could be placed on both the soma and dendrites (Stuart and Sakmann, 1994).

Active Properties of Dendrites

These properties indicated that Ramón y Cajal's law of the dynamic polarization of the neuron required revision. There was also evidence in favor. Most of this evidence came not from intracellular recordings from a single neuron but from extracellular recordings. During this period it was becoming possible to deliver a single shock to a part of the brain and record responses with an extracellular micropipette. These recordings took generally two forms. One was a small spike indicating the action potential in a single nearby cell. Because the identification was unsure, these were usually referred to as "single-unit recordings." The other was the sequence of potential waves around a population of activated cells due to the summed flows of current around them. The evidence was not as definitive as that from the intracellular recordings, but the extracellular recordings were much easier to obtain.

Several groups investigated the active properties of the dendrites. In the first approach, Paul Fatt carried out recordings of single spike potentials around motoneurons and obtained evidence for active impulse invasion of the dendrites (Fatt, 1957a, 1957b). In the second approach, H.-T. Chang at Yale and George Bishop and Margaret Clare in St. Louis obtained evidence in cortical dendrites for "decremental conduction," that is, weakly active processes in the dendrites that decayed with distance from a site of local electrical stimulation. We will return to the studies of Chang later in this section.

The most persuasive evidence was obtained by a graduate student, Per Andersen, working in Oslo, Norway. He recorded the summed extracellular field potentials generated around activated neurons in the hippocampus.

These showed a sharp wave attributed to action potentials initiated in the distal apical dendrites of pyramidal cells by excitatory synapses; this wave propagated forward, through the dendrites toward the cell body and out the axon (Andersen, 1959) (Appendix 8.3). The study was one of the first to introduce the hippocampus as a model system for analyzing the functional organization of brain regions. The synaptically activated sharp wave, called a "**population spike**", became a valuable tool for this purpose, leading to the use of the hippocampus as a tissue slice for investigating the trisynaptic circuit (Skrede and Westgaard, 1971) and in the subsequent investigation of long-term potentiation as a candidate mechanism for the synaptic basis of Hebbian learning and memory; see Chapter 12. Forward propagation in dendrites was finally clearly demonstrated by the dual patch electrode method in olfactory mitral cells (Chen et al., 1997).

The first report of active dendritic properties using intracellular electrodes was by Eccles, Libet and Young (1958), who recorded small spikes indicative of dendritic "**hot spots**" in motoneurons undergoing chromatolytic degeneration after transection of their axons. The first report in normal cells of small "prepotentials" indicative of active "hot spots" at distant dendritic branch points in the apical dendrites was inferred from intracellular recordings from the cell bodies of hippocampal pyramidal cells in a classic paper by Alden Spencer and Eric Kandel in 1961. All of these studies were carried out in anesthetized animals.

These studies showed that dendrites were capable of generating active, impulse-like responses to excitatory synaptic inputs. However, in most recordings in the following decades, the dendrites appeared to lack these properties and were thus judged to have passive membranes, in contrast to the action potential–generating membranes of axons. It was only with the introduction of the patch electrode method for recording from central neurons in the 1990s that it began to be shown that most dendrites express voltage-dependent ion channels and that their ability to generate active responses depends on multiple factors, including the geometry of the dendritic branching trees, the density of the voltage-dependent channels, and the types of neighboring channels.

Dendritic Dominance and Wilfrid Rall

The early studies of dendritic properties could not make much headway in understanding the complex relations between these properties without a quantitative foundation built on the biophysical properties of the membranes. This had been the approach of Hodgkin and Huxley in producing their quantitative model of the action potential in the squid axon. The elaborate branching patterns of dendritic trees posed, however, a daunting obstacle to extending this approach to dendrites.

Wilfrid Rall. The solution to this problem was provided by Wilfrid Rall (Fig. 8.4), an American, born in 1922, who trained as a physicist at Yale during World

War II and on graduation moved to the University of Chicago to participate in the Manhattan Project, which built the first atomic bomb. During this time he met K. C. Cole, who had discovered the action potential in the squid axon (Chapter 6). Cole was setting up the first graduate program in biophysics, and Rall entered as one of the first students. After the war Cole prepared to return to Woods Hole to take up his experiments on the squid axon again (see Chapter 6) and invited Rall to join him.

Chicago had been a leading center in the application of mathematics to biology, through one of the pioneers in this effort, Nicholas Rashevsky. Typical of this approach were the equations to describe the electrical excitation of nerve, which as we have seen (Chapter 6) gave little insight into the biological mechanisms themselves. The new biophysics had the goal of understanding the physical basis of biological function but was determined that it should be based on a closer combination of experiment and theory. Thus, in Woods Hole, Rall learned to dissect the squid axon and take part in the experiments on the action potential, as well as assisting in the development of the electronic methods including the new voltage-clamp method and analyzing the electrical responses.

After completing his requirements for a master's degree, Rall decided to do his thesis work with Eccles in New Zealand, stimulated by Eccles' electrical theory of synaptic inhibition (Rall, 2006). He arrived there in 1949 and soon was engaged in an in-depth study of the synchronous responses of a pool of motoneurons to a synchronous activation of the sensory fibers to them. This required careful dissection of the spinal roots of the cat and long sessions recording the input–output relations. During this time, the news of the advent of intracellular recording techniques was brought to Dunedin, and Eccles threw himself into the experiments which led to his breakthrough in 1951–52, described in Chapter 7.

Rall, however, continued with his independent project under Archibald McIntyre. This resulted in a model of the input–output relations of a motoneuron pool which posited that either many synapses were equally distributed over the surfaces of the motoneurons or a small number were concentrated in a favorable region. While this result was somewhat indeterminate, it started him thinking about how synaptic potentials might spread in a cell and led him to the insight that in a cell body the potential would spread over its surface almost instantaneously. In contrast, it could be seen that the potential would spread more slowly and decrementally through the dendritic tree.

After a year's sabbatical, which he spent at the laboratories of Katz in London and Cuy Hunt at Rockefeller, he joined the biophysics group under Cole at the Naval Medical Research Center in 1956. However, the new executive officer made it clear that "Basic research is OK, a long as it is not too basic." This differed from the tradition that the Navy had built up during the war of supporting basic research, and to which it was to return in the future; but it was enough to stimulate an immediate exodus of the group. Rall moved across Wisconsin Avenue to the National Institutes of Health, where he spent the rest of his career in the Mathematical Research Branch, created by Dewitt Stetten in the

National Institute for Arthritis and Metabolic Diseases to receive the immigrant theorists.

In 1957 Eccles and several others published recordings from motoneurons showing the potentials produced by injection of current into the cell body (summarized in Eccles, 1957). The decaying phases of these responses were interpreted to follow a single exponential, as would be true of a simple circuit of resistance and capacitance representing the cell body membrane. From his previous analysis of transients in a cell body, Rall realized that the recorded transients were slower than expected and must be due to current flowing into the dendrites. He published a brief note in *Science* in 1957 showing that the transients could best be modeled by a cell body attached to a long cylinder representing the dendritic tree. Thus was born the concept of "dendritic dominance" in the integrative activity of a motoneuron. Since most other neurons have elaborate dendritic trees, the concept was generalized to most neurons.

Rall carried out a detailed study of branching patterns of motoneuron dendrites, which provided a rigorous basis for reducing a branching tree to a single cylinder. The papers were, however, rejected for publication, with Eccles clearly one of the referees, with the argument that the decaying transient in Eccles' recordings was due to a technical aspect of the instrumentation (subsequently shown to be irrelevant; see Jack and Redman, in Segev et al., 1995). This rejection was a setback not only for Rall, at this critical stage in his career, but also for the biophysics of dendrites, delaying its acceptance for over a decade. The study was published in 1959 and 1960 in *Experimental Neurology* (Rall, 1959, 1960) (Fig. 8.5). It was further noteworthy for showing that if successive branches in a tree satisfied the sum of the diameters raised to the 3/2 power, the tree could be modeled as an "equivalent cylinder". This provided a valuable tool for facilitating the electrophysiological analysis of dendritic properties.

These studies covered the steady-state spread of current and potential through a dendritic tree. Transient, time-varying spread was too complex to represent with analytical equations, so Rall introduced numerical methods, beginning by adapting a program developed by a colleague in the unit, Mones Berman, for describing the spread of radioactive substances through body compartments. Although these results fall in the next period in the historical development of modern neuroscience, we note that they were first presented at a conference in Ojai, California, in 1962 and published in 1964 (reprinted in Segev et al., 1995). This pioneering paper showed for the first time in a rigorous manner how electrical current spreads in a dendritic tree and how the conductances underlying synaptic potentials interact in a nonlinear manner (Appendix 8.4). The approach was applied to the motoneuron in a set of papers in 1967, which finally began the revolution in both dendritic function and computational neuroscience. However, the reluctance of many neurophysiologists, neuroanatomists, and computational neuroscientists to include the properties of dendrites in understanding neuronal and network functions continues to this day (see Chapter 16).

Revival of the Golgi Stain

After the death of Ramón y Cajal in 1934, there was little investigation of neuronal morphology, in general, or dendritic morphology, in particular. Revival of interest in **dendritic tree morphology** started with the biophysical studies of Rall and the anatomical studies of David Sholl, summarized in his widely read monograph *The Organization of the Cerebral Cortex* (1956). This not only focused anew on dendrites and their spines but also introduced statistical approaches to characterizing synaptic connectedness to dendritic trees. Sholl's work helped to stimulate new and more rapid modifications of the Golgi stain that brought many new investigators into the study of dendritic morphology.

Dendritic Spines

Some dendrites, such as those of motoneurons, have a smooth surface; but some, such as those of pyramidal cells in the cerebral cortex, are covered with small outcroppings called "spines." These were described by Ramón y Cajal and his contemporaries, but there was little insight into their function. The first physiological studies appear to have been by H.-T. Chang. Among all the young scientists who came to the United States because of World War II, his escape is one of the most dramatic, as he later described it (Chang, 1984).

Hsiang-Tung Chang was born in 1907 in a small village in Hopei Province in northern China. His circumstances were so impoverished that he was not able to start his primary education until the age of 14. His studies led to the National University of Peking, where he graduated with a BS degree in psychology in 1933. He then became an assistant to Ging-Hsi Wang in Nanjing (Nanking). Wang, head of the Institute of Psychology, was an outstanding investigator and teacher, training Chang in research in anatomy and electrophysiology, designing experiments, and writing research articles; Chang's first was on an auditory reflex of the hedgehog in the *Chinese Journal of Physiology*. At that time China was fortunate in receiving foreign visitors, such as Walter Cannon, of epinephrine fame, who were a vital link to science in the West and an inspiration to the young students aspiring to research careers. Among them were several who went on to make their mark, including T. P. Feng, who was among the first to record a synaptic potential in 1940 (Chapter 7); S.-C. Shen, who trained with Joseph Needham in Cambridge, United Kingdom; and, among the younger generation, Chang, who collaborated with Gaddum in neuropharmacology in the United Kingdom, and his son, Renji Chang, subsequently a leading neurophysiologist in China.

H.-T. Chang was in Nanking when the Japanese attacked in 1937 and carried out the brutal assault that was to become known as the "Rape of Nanking." Chang managed to get out on the last boat. For a while he helped with the desperate relief efforts, including salvaging the libraries and equipment of Chinese academies in front of the invading armies, and then found his way to a more protected part of China, where he was asked to take a job teaching physiology in the army medical school near Kuel-yang. While there, he found in the library a copy of John Fulton's *Physiology of the Nervous System* (1938). Fulton had studied under Sherrington in the 1920s; it was he who asked Sherrington about the origin of the word "synapse" (Chapter 5). He had become chair of physiology in 1930 at Yale at the age of 30. Through his association with Sherrington and Harvey Cushing, founding the *Journal of Neurophysiology* in 1938 and writing *Physiology of the Nervous System*, the first textbook on the nervous system, also in 1938, Fulton was one of the world's most famous neurophysiologists.

Inspired by the book, Chang told colleagues that he would like to work with Fulton, to which one of them replied, "If a poor man like you could ever go to the United States, the sun would rise in the west." Stung, Chang resolved to do just that and wrote a letter addressed simply to "John Fulton, Yale University, United States," inquiring about the possibility of studying in his laboratory. Three months later a telegram arrived with three words: "Yes letter follows." A month later the letter arrived, granting his application as a visiting fellow in physiology, with living expenses, if he could get to the United States.

Chang sold his belongings, made his way through endless bureaucratic red tape, and finally after 6 months received his passport, exit papers, and, with the Yale letter his only documentation, his visa to the United States. The only route out of wartime China was by military transport plane from Chungking to Calcutta, which he took on New Year's day 1943. Most travelers were stranded in the city, but Chang managed to find old friends from school, who helped him first book passage on a "liberty ship" (an old U.S. destroyer) leaving shortly for the United States, though he then shifted to another ship leaving from Bombay. Soon after, the first ship was sunk by the Japanese, with loss of nearly all on board. Chang's ship was grossly overloaded but managed to make its way south of Australia, past New Zealand into the south Pacific, and to arrive 30 days later in San Pedro, California. He made his way across the United States and, on March 24, walked into the rotunda at 333 Cedar Street in New Haven and presented himself to Professor Fulton as his new assistant at Yale!

It may be noted that this gesture of Fulton's was entirely consistent with his generous nature and magnetic personality. Through these qualities he had attracted a succession of outstanding faculty, students, postdoctoral trainees, and visiting scholars. It was a rich environment for anyone to be trained in, especially one who had begun with so little and had come so far.

Chang soaked up the new environment, plunging into a variety of projects, both at Yale and with colleagues who were part of the far-flung network around Fulton. Within 2 years he had obtained his PhD with a study of central pathways in the spinal cord, a 300-page opus that was turned into eight journal articles. He then collaborated on projects with Clinton Woolsey at Johns Hopkins and David Lloyd at Rockefeller, then returned to Yale to work on reverberating circuits between the thalamus and the cortex (see Chapter 10).

He soon became fascinated with dendrites in the cerebral cortex. In his contribution to the great gathering at Cold Spring Harbor in 1952 on the new physiology of the neuron he explained his pioneering approach (Chang, 1952, 160):

> Our investigation was an attempt to establish the existence of dendritic potentials in the cortex in response to weak electrical stimulation and to differentiate the dendritic potentials from the potentials accompanying the activity of intracortical neurons. We wanted to inquire about the properties of dendrites compared with those of axons....Our results [showed] that (i) the dendrites were excited by electrical stimulation, (ii) the dendrites were capable of transmitting impulses, and (iii) the dendritic potential differed from the axonal potential in that it was not an all-or-none response. It was suggested that the intensity of the stimulation induced graded responses.

He distinguished between synaptic actions on the cell body, which directly initiated a response of the cell, and those on the dendrites, which he suggested mediated "higher nervous activity, such as consciousness, perception, and thinking." The results were first published in 1951 and between then and 1955 led to eight more publications on dendritic potentials, a prodigious output considering how recently he had set out on his trip from China.

One of the most intriguing of Chang's findings related to dendritic spines, which he termed "gemmules." He discussed the distribution of gemmules on the apical dendrites of cortical pyramidal cells and made the following observations:

> Functionally, the gemmules on the dendrites constitute a mechanical barrier preventing the synaptic knobs from reaching the stem of dendrites directly, and hence they serve as a limiting factor for synaptic excitation. They also delay and attenuate the process of synaptic excitation because of the high ohmic resistance of the gemmules' extremely slender stalks.
>
> (Chang, 1952, 200)

This 1952 paper was widely read (Appendix 8.5) and helped to stimulate the revival of interest in dendrites, including the studies of Margaret Clare and George Bishop in the early 1950s. Chang's observation on the importance of the slender stem of the spine in attenuating the response spreading from the spine head to the parent dendrite was especially prescient. It was the first step toward subsequent functional analyses of spine properties and their contributions to the integrative actions of dendrites in work on the olfactory granule cell, cerebellar Purkinje cells, and ultimately cortical pyramidal cells.

Chang's subsequent career gives a window on the international politics of the 1950s. In 1955 he attended a congress in Scandinavia and suddenly vanished, returning home to China. Though cut off from the West, he became a central figure in developing neurophysiology in China, focusing on the physiology of pain. Doing this required a careful balance between meeting the rapidly rising technology of western science, while accommodating both the Chinese traditions of folk and medicinal acupuncture, as well as surviving the Cultural Revolution. He was most hospitable when I visited him in Shanghai in 1993, at the Shanghai Brain Institute he had founded there. With an impish smile he asked me to look under the cabinet in the second laboratory from the end of the corridor where he had inscribed his name before he left Yale in 1955. Unfortunately, the laboratories had long since been remodeled, but after all, the memory of his name scratched under that cabinet at Yale was all that mattered.

Rethinking the Neuron Doctrine

Putting together the studies during the 1950s on the synaptic actions on neurons together with the new evidence for the properties of dendrites, it began to be evident that the nerve cell was not the simple functional unit envisaged in the classical neuron doctrine. Given that Ramón y Cajal made all of his interpretations on the basis of only the histology of the neurons more than a half-century before any experiments could be carried out on cells in the brain, it is not surprising that the physiological evidence would give new insights. Theodore Bullock (1959, Appendix 8.6), in reviewing the electrophysiological studies of both invertebrate and vertebrate central neurons in the 1950s, argued that these results showed that, rather than functioning as a single element, the nerve cell has different properties in its dendrites and axons so that its function is characterized by "complexity-within-unity."

The impulse is not the only form of nerve cell activity; excitation of one part of the neuron does not necessarily involve the whole neuron; many dendrites may not propagate impulses at all; and the synapse is not the only locus of selection, evaluation, fatigue, and persistent change. Several forms of graded activity—for example, pacemaker, synaptic, and local potentials—each confined to a circumscribed region or repeating regions of the neuron, can separately or sequentially integrate arriving events, with the history and milieu, to determine output in the restricted region where the spikes are initiated.

In a well-known phrase, he characterized this as a "quiet but sweeping revolution" in our concept of the neuron. The evidence continued with discoveries of axoaxonal synapses (Dudel and Kuffler, 1960) and dendrodendritic synapses (Rall et al., 1966). This led eventually to suggestions to replace the functional concepts of the neuron doctrine, in which the neuron is the only functional unit, with a concept of functional units at different organizational levels. These can occur within a given neuron and within the multineuronal interactions that form the circuits and pathways of the nervous system (Shepherd, 1972, 1991). It is this concept of hierarchical levels that has been used in organizing the material in this book. The effort to incorporate the classical neuron doctrine into new concepts of multilevel, multineuronal functional units continues to the present (Bullock et al., 2005; Byrne and Shepherd, 2008).

Chapter 9

Neural Circuits: Spinal Cord, Retina, Invertebrate Systems

Armed with their new microelectrodes and electronic instrumentation for single-cell recording, electrophysiologists began the attack on how neurons are organized into pathways and systems. In the spinal cord, Eccles led the way to identifying the cellular basis of the reflex pathways and control of the muscles, key for understanding how we move normally and for effects of neurological disease. The discovery of "Renshaw" inhibition provided a model of recurrent and lateral inhibition that was tested in many parts of the nervous system. Of prime interest was visual processing in the retina; the studies by Keffer Hartline of the Limulus *eye and by Stephen Kuffler and Horace Barlow of the cat's eye provided models for the role of lateral inhibition in visual discrimination. Studies of both vertebrate and invertebrate systems began to enlarge the concept of the reflex, giving evidence of command neurons whose activation brings forth a coordinated output from a neuronal system, while other studies identified the neurons responsible for central pattern generation of coordinated motor activity. It became clear that interactions between excitatory and inhibitory circuits are key to how the nervous system generates and processes information.*

In the 1950s the microelectrode opened the door not only to understanding the properties of the individual nerve cell but also to how they are connected, how they "talk" to each other. Physiologists for the first time thus had the means to reveal the mechanisms of information processing in the brain at the cellular level. To the extent that this could be combined with knowledge of the cell properties involved in processing the inputs and outputs, properties we have covered in the foregoing chapters, one would have a complete description of the neural basis of behavior. It was an exciting prospect. But how to obtain it?

Intracellular recordings for this purpose were extremely difficult to obtain because methods for restraining the pulsing of the brain due to the beating of the heart and the heaving of respiration were inadequate. The spinal cord continued to be the best model system for working out circuit connections, while above, in the brain, the first attempts were being made. Faced with these difficulties, experimenters began using microelectrodes that could record extracellularly from single neurons. Since it was rarely possible to be sure whether one was recording from a cell body, axon, or dendrite, careful investigators referred to these as "single-unit" recordings (and with reason—mistakes were often made in confusing axon recordings with cell body recordings). These microelectrodes could be either the same micropipettes used for intracellular recordings (filled with extracellular salt solutions) or made of metal drawn out to fine tips, electrically insulated along their shafts up to the tips.

Two philosophies emerged. One was to aim at working out connections in order to build up the circuits responsible for the responses of the cells. This approach was exemplified by the work of Eccles in the spinal cord and set the standard for extension of the single-cell approach to other parts of the nervous system. However, another approach was to record and characterize the responses of the cells to physiological stimuli, to show what the brain does, and to leave to future work identifying the circuits involved.

Both philosophies arose in the 1950s and produced dramatic results that shaped all subsequent studies of the physiology of the central nervous system. We consider in this chapter the spinal cord, retina, and invertebrate systems and in the next chapter the work on systems in the brain.

Spinal Reflex Pathways and Renshaw Inhibition

In World War II Sweden avoided direct involvement in the fighting by maintaining its neutrality, and its science structure therefore remained intact, in contrast to its neighbors in Scandinavia and on the rest of the continent. During the war Lars Leksell, a young neurosurgeon at the Karolinska Hospital in Stockholm, took up a problem that had arisen from the experiments of Eccles and Sherrington. In 1930 they had reported that electrical stimulation of a large population of thin fibers in the motor nerves to the muscles did not actually cause detectable contraction of the muscle. What was their function? Leksell was able to show that in fact they are motor fibers to the muscle spindles, which are modified muscle fibers within long fusiform capsules within the muscles (Leksell, 1945). It was known that the muscle spindles have sensory axons innervating their central regions and that they sense the amount of stretch of the normal muscle fibers, thereby signaling to the spinal cord the state of shortening or lengthening of the muscles. This work completed the cast of actors involved in muscle reflexes and opened the door to physiological analysis of the relation between the muscles and the muscle spindles. Leksell went on to a distinguished career as a neurosurgeon, developing stereotaxic approaches to brain surgery and inventing the method known as radiosurgery (Chapter 14).

Anatomical studies began to reveal the beautifully complex nature of the sensory and motor innervation of the muscle spindle (Barker, 1948). Stephen Kuffler, Carlton Hunt, and colleagues then showed in a classic study that repetitive electrical shocks to the fine fibers elicited repetitive firing of the sensory axons from the muscle spindles (Kuffler and Hunt, 1949; Kuffler et al., 1951). Thus, the spindle was extremely sensitive both to the amount of stretch imposed by the surrounding muscle fibers as well as to its motor innervation from small motoneurons, so-called gamma motoneurons. The large muscles are controlled by the large alpha motoneurons, whereas the muscle spindle sensitivity is controlled by the small gamma motoneurons. Through this means, the spinal cord modulates the sensitivity of the muscle spindles in accord with the state of contraction of the muscles.

At this point we pick up Eccles' research as described in Chapter 7 (p. 90; Shepherd, 2008; see also Stuart and Pierce, 2006).

Eccles and Spinal Cord Pathways. With the ability to record intracellularly from the motoneuron and identify the properties of excitatory and inhibitory postsynaptic potentials (EPSPs and IPSPs), Eccles and his collaborators were in a position to use these responses to dissect the excitatory and inhibitory synaptic pathways that underlie the reflex activity of the spinal cord. This was the great problem presented by his mentor, Charles Sherrington, in his first landmark book *The Integrative Action of the Nervous System* (1906) and with Creed and other colleagues in *Reflex Activity in the Spinal Cord* in 1932. Eccles' first book, *The Neurophysiological Basis of Mind* (1953), summarized the first steps in this direction.

The cat spinal motoneuron was the first model in the early years not only for synaptic actions but also for identification of synaptic pathways. The most precise information was gained using the intracellular recording electrode. Recordings were made from a cell identified by observing whether its response to a peripheral nerve was antidromic, monosynaptic, or disynaptic and then looking up in Ramón y Cajal's great book *Histologie du Système Nerveux de l'Homme et des Vertébrés* (1911) to identify the likely neurons. Methodologically, this approach required the microforge for manual construction of the micro-pipettes; development of the cathode follower, amplifier, and oscilloscope for recording; and the Schmitt trigger for stimulating and synchronizing the shock with the start of the recording trace, the basic instrumentation for all subsequent electrophysiological recording studies. The standard preparation was the cat, as used in the classical studies of spinal reflexes beginning with Sherrington.

The spinal cord pathways attracted intense study, mainly from Eccles, Guy Hunt, Yves Laporte, and David Lloyd. Starting in his new laboratories in Canberra, Australia, in early 1953, Eccles led the way by virtue of his tremendous drive and focus on determining these pathways. The simplest synaptic pathway was the *monosynaptic excitatory pathway* from Ia muscle spindle afferents onto motoneurons, mediating the stretch reflex. A *disynaptic inhibitory pathway* was identified from Ib muscle spindle afferents to antagonistic muscles; these afferents made excitatory synapses onto interneurons, which in turn made inhibitory synapses onto the motoneurons. A third disynaptic pathway was identified from *Golgi tendon organs*. These circuits were directly correlated with the reflex activity that could be elicited not only from laboratory animals but also from human patients in the clinic. They were thus essential for understanding the neural basis for normal motor control involved in standing and walking and in the hyperreflex state (spasticity) that appears following strokes and other diseases of descending motor control from the brain.

A final type identified by Eccles in the 1950s was the pathway for *recurrent inhibition* of the motoneurons from their axon collaterals through an interneuron and back onto the motoneurons. This study was carried out with Paul Fatt (moving on from Katz's laboratory) and Kyozo Koketsu from Japan (Eccles et al., 1954) (Fig. 9.1, Appendix 9.1). The way this discovery came about was as follows. Single shocks were delivered to the motoneuron axons in the ventral root of the spinal cord. Each shock set up an action potential that traveled antidromically (in the reverse direction of normal) in the axons to invade synchronously the cell bodies in the spinal cord. The intracellular recording from the cell body showed the antidromic action potential followed by a long-lasting hyperpolarization. What caused the hyperpolarization? To test for this, the strength of the shock to the ventral root was successively reduced, stimulating fewer and fewer axons, until finally the impulse failed but a hyperpolarization still remained. This had the characteristics of an IPSP, presumably due to interneurons activated by collaterals of the motoneuron axons.

The inhibition of a motoneuron by an interneuron, presumably activated by recurrent collaterasl of motoneuron axons, had previously been predicted from recordings by a young investigator at Harvard, Birdsey Renshaw (1941, 1946). (Renshaw tragically died at an early age of polio in 1947. His mentor, Alexander Forbes, told me in 1959 that it was an incalculable loss to neurophysiology.) Further probing in the ventral horn by Eccles and his colleagues revealed cells that fired intense bursts of impulses in response to the ventral root volley, with an onset delay a millisecond before the onset of the motoneuron inhibition and a duration of discharge that was long-lasting, similar to the motoneuron IPSP. Eccles termed these "Renshaw cells" in Renshaw's honor, and they became the paradigmatic form of self- and lateral feedback inhibition, with examples being found subsequently in many different regions of the nervous system. (I found them using the same approach in my thesis work on the olfactory bulb beginning in 1959.) Paradoxically, in those other regions specific functions for the inhibition could be proposed, whereas the functions in the spinal cord remained elusive. A new synthesis of these results with intracellular recordings in other nerve cells was summarized in Eccles' widely read book *The Physiology of Nerve Cells* in 1957.

As we describe different styles of neuroscientists, it may be mentioned that during the 1950s Eccles engaged in several unduly harsh efforts to apply the Popper doctrine to falsifying the findings of colleagues. One was

David P. C. Lloyd, a former student at Oxford, over details of synaptic connectivity in the spinal cord. Another was his former student Rall, who brought forward evidence (Rall, 1959) from Eccles' own recordings for dendritic dominance of synaptic integration. As indicated in Chapter 8, Eccles would brook no opposition, claiming another explanation based on a postulated persistent current. Rall refuted this explanation, and Eccles eventually abandoned it. But as late as 1960 he was still defending the idea that dendrites had mostly nutritive roles, being too distant to affect synaptic integration, which he believed was focused at the cell body where his recordings were made.

Eccles' opposition greatly impeded recognition of the significance of Rall's work and the value of theory in neuroscience (see Chapter 8). Rall first adapted basic cable theory followed by his new methods of compartmental analysis to show that most synaptic integration takes place in the dendrites. However, as was typical of Eccles, harkening back to his interactions with Dale, when Rall and his colleagues came forward with evidence for novel interactions between dendrites in the olfactory bulb, it was Eccles who organized and invited Rall to co-chair with him a meeting in 1968 where these new findings were presented.

The reason for his harsh attacks, I believe, goes back to his training in England, where they could take place between colleagues within the clubby atmosphere of The Physiological Society (see the observation by Katz in Chapter 4). In the outside world, they were interpreted as, and had the effect of, doing unnecessary harm.

During the 1950s his laboratory in Canberra was a magnet for a new generation of cellular neurophysiologists from around the world. Over 100 of his approximately 200 students and collaborators came from that time. The several experimental rigs were in use around the clock, experiments often lasting through the night and sometimes through the next day (as in other electrophysiological laboratories of that era). For social variety there were the famous parties at Eccles' home, where he and his wife would entertain the group with square dancing, party games, and sports.

In the 1960s Eccles broadened his interests from the spinal cord to other brain regions and spent the last 30 years of his career on the cerebellum, hippocampus, and eventually the neocortex. These provided the experience to extend his philosophical attempt to reconcile the facts of brain function with his religious beliefs as a Catholic. Eccles published many articles and several books on resolving the mind–body problem (106 of his 588 publications, according to Andersen and Lundberg, 1997), his most extensive attempt in a dialogue between himself, a dualist, and his old friend Popper, an agnostic, laid out in the book *The Self and Its Brain: An Argument for Interactionism* in 1977 (see Popper and Eccles, 1977). It continued his attempt to probe the neural basis of consciousness, which has lately become a fashionable topic in cognitive neuroscience. So he can be called a pioneer in this field as well. He died on May 2, 1997.

Perspective on Eccles. In summing up Eccles' career, several themes are of interest to modern-day scientists. One is his odyssey, as he described it himself, across the oceans, from Australia to Britain, back to Australia, to New Zealand, back to Australia, to the United States, and finally to Switzerland; a scientist goes where the opportunities are greatest to realize his or her career goals. Another is his life as an educator: He was willing in Dunedin to assume overwhelming teaching responsibilities that not only served his institution but grounded him in the fundamentals of his field. He was also an educator through his research: His 200 students and collaborators populated academia and industry with the new science. Scientists are supposed to write original research articles, not books; yet his books were instrumental in shaping modern neuroscience.

In addition to these accomplishments, there was the sheer dynamism of the man. To those who knew him, his was a personality truly larger than life. He had a vigorous physique, with prodigious stamina at the experimental rig, at his desk writing up the results or a new book, and traveling the world with his message. The voice was penetrating, with a broad Aussie accent, overwhelming in debate and naturally dominating in conversation. He had a wide mouth, ready instantly to break into a broad grin or hearty laugh to express a life-embracing sense of humor. There was total engagement in whatever issue was being discussed, with an encyclopedic grasp of the literature. He was courteous, loyal, and generous to his friends and colleagues. Finally, he was a scientist who reserved a place in his life for his spiritual side. To those who knew him, he was the embodiment of a great era in the creation of modern neuroscience.

In summary, in the space of a few years in the 1940s and 1950s, the main pathways involved in reflexes in the spinal cord became known, thus closing a chapter that had begun with the classical descriptions by Sherrington of the nature of spinal reflexes 50 years earlier. With this, the focus for understanding brain mechanisms moved on from the spinal cord to the rest of the nervous system.

Retinal Processing: Lateral Inhibition and Contrast Enhancement

An attractive model for working out response properties and neural pathways at the cellular level was the visual system. A key characteristic of our visual experience is that it gives a selective representation of our environment. This is exemplified by the enhancement of contrast we see at a sharp border between a light and a dark area in our visual field.

The phenomenon of *contrast enhancement* was first described and explained by Ernst Mach in the late nineteenth century (Mach, 1897). At the light–dark border there occurs an enhancement of contrast, such that the dark edge appears darker and the light edge appears lighter. This implies that each site in the receptive field has inhibitory interactions with its neighbors. At the border, this means that on the light side there is less inhibition from the dark side, making it lighter, and on the dark side there is more inhibition from the light side, making it darker. This phenomenon was well-known among psychophysicists, who called it "Mach bands."

When physiologists began to carry out experiments on the visual system with the new electronic equipment of the 1920s, the cellular basis of contrast enhancement, starting in the retina, was one of the first phenomena to attract their attention. There were several pioneers in this work.

Ragnar Granit. Granit was a Finn of Swedish extraction. In the late 1920s he trained briefly with Sherrington in Oxford and then carried out psychophysical experiments on visual processing at the University of Pennsylvania before returning to Finland. He was then stimulated by the pioneering studies of Edgar Adrian and his students who were recording impulse responses from sensory end organs. These started with the single-fiber recordings of impulse responses of muscle spindles by Adrian and Yngve Zotterman (1926a, 1926b) (see Chapter 7). For the retina, the key experiment was the recording of impulse responses from fibers of the optic nerve from the retina of the eel by Adrian and his student Rachel Matthews (1927a, 1927b, 1928).

Granit hypothesized that in processing visual stimuli excitation of the retina is always accompanied by inhibition. He proposed to demonstrate this by examining the frequency at which a flickering light undergoes perceptual fusion (flicker fusion frequency) in two half–visual fields (this apparently drew on his acquaintance with the work of Sherrington; the last chapter of *The Integrative Action of the Nervous System* [Sherrington, 1906] was on flicker fusion in the visual system). The results supported the hypothesis

> "With adjacent fields at different levels of brightness the fusion frequency rose in the brighter and fell in the darker field..., a fact interpreted as demonstrating a mechanism of contrast" (Granit, 1967, 256). The theoretical significance of the observation seems to be that the inhibitory system is excited relatively more and more as the intensity of the excitatory process in a group of neurones increases. Consequently the inhibitory effect passing from the more stimulated area to the adjacent less stimulated area will be greater than the inhibitory effect passing in the opposite direction [Graham and Granit, 1931,p. 671]. "Today this sounds like a description of Hartline's ... lateral inhibition in the *Limulus* eye or of recurrent inhibition in the motoneurons..." (Granit, 1967, 256).

These were the first clues to the role of inhibition in neural processing. Back in Finland, Granit pursued how to prove inhibition in the retina by hypothesizing that under some conditions it could be shown that light caused a reduction in retinal activity. To test this hypothesis he used the electroretinogram (ERG), the massed field potential that can be recorded by electrodes on the eyelids, similar to the massed recordings of cellular activity underlying the electrocardiogram (EKG) and electroencephalogram (EEG) (see Chapter 7). He was able to confirm the hypothesis by showing a suppressive effect of light stimulation on the off response of the ERG (Granit and Therman, 1935). He also used microelectrode recordings from the retinas of different species (Granit and Svaetichin, 1939).

> With my background in the physiology of the central nervous system, acquired in Sherrington's laboratory, I now knew for certain that the details of the visual image were elaborated by the interplay of excitation and inhibition in the nervous centre of the retina itself.
>
> (Granit, 1967, 257)

Keffer Hartline. These results, while intriguing, required clearer testing at the cellular level, which was being pursued at about the same time by Haldan Keffer Hartline. Hartline's philosophy is contained in his later comment (Hartline, 1967, 274):

> Can we understand how these diverse and complex response patterns, highly specialized for specific tasks, are generated in the retina? Broad Sherringtonian principles can guide us—the interplay of excitatory and inhibitory influences in convergent and divergent pathways, with various spatial distributions, thresholds, time courses. But the application of broad principles to specific cases of such complexity is not easy. It is here that comparative physiology can help. The animal world is rich in its variety of visual systems, built in different ways and with different degrees of complexity, although all governed, we are confident, by the same universal, basic principles.

In this statement are two principles that became the underpinning of the use of simple systems for modern electrophysiology: invertebrate preparations for their apparent simplicity and for their accessibility to single-cell techniques. Also, we again see the influence of Sherrington on work in other parts of the nervous system.

Hartline graduated in 1927 from Johns Hopkins University Medical School, where he began his studies of retinal electrophysiology in a variety of species, including insects, frogs, cats, rabbits, and humans. After studying abroad, including with physics giants Werner Heisenberg and Andrew Sommerfeld in Germany, Hartline joined the Eldridge Reeves Johnson Foundation for Medical Physics at the University of Pennsylvania, under Detlev Bronk, one of the pioneers of the early electrophysiology of the nervous system in his studies with Adrian (Chapter 7). There, inspired by the work of Rachel Matthews and Adrian in the eel optic nerve (the same study that had inspired Granit) and by a single-fiber study of Adrian and Bronk, he began his "application of unitary analysis to the receptors and neurons of the visual system" (Hartline, 1967).

For this he chose the visual system of the horseshoe crab, *Limulus poly-phemus* (Hartline and Graham, 1932). In this animal, the light-sensitive receptor cells are arranged around a central dendritic process of a neuron called the "eccentric cell." Stimulation of the receptor cells activates the central dendrite, which sets up impulses in the axon to send the message to the central nervous system. *Limulus*, as a "living fossil," with visual responses limited mainly to signaling differences between light and dark, might not seem a promising preparation for study of the fine points of visual responses. However, it had the great advantage that its optic nerve could be dissected down to single fibers, allowing impulses to be recorded from single eccentric cells in response to light. Simple electrodes attached to a string galvanometer sufficed for this purpose.

This preparation and recording apparatus permitted Hartline to identify many basic properties of the visual response. These included the fact that a wide range of luminosity was compressed into a smaller range of frequencies of impulse discharges. Responses to changes in light intensity were more vigorous than those to steady illumination, a property that emphasizes sensitivity to change, as Adrian had first shown for various sensory receptors. This means that processing of sensory signals begins in the receptors themselves. Hartline went on to demonstrate these principles in recordings from the frog optic nerve as well, including evidence for inhibitory as well as excitatory effects, as Granit's results had indicated.

To analyze the inhibitory effects further, he returned to *Limulus* (Hartline et al., 1952). When a single spot of light was used to stimulate a single receptor, the nerve response was graded in frequency with the light intensity. However, when a test pattern consisting of a dark and a light region was used and moved over the site of the recorded cell, the light side of the border gave a higher response than expected and the dark side gave a lower response. In other words, there was an enhancement of "contrast" between the light and dark sides. This implied that there were inhibitory connections between eccentric cells such that at a border more strongly stimulated cells had less inhibition from weaker neighbors and more weakly stimulated cells had more inhibition from their stronger neighbors (Appendix 9.2).

This result implied that there existed below the *Limulus* retina a set of interconnections between the eccentric cell axons that mediate inhibition between them. Such connections were finally demonstrated with the electron microscope by Fahrenbach in 1985.

Stephen Kuffler. Contrast enhancement was extended to the mammal in an elegant and persuasive demonstration at the cellular level in the study of Stephen Kuffler in 1953.

Kuffler was born in 1913 and grew up in his native Hungary, went to medical school in Vienna in the 1930s, and escaped the Nazis after the *Anschluss*, making his way to England and then to Australia. There, he chanced to meet Eccles, who invited him to join his group and work on the neuromuscular junction. He was also much stimulated by the arrival of Bernard Katz from England. We have already enjoyed the photograph of the three of them on a stroll in Sydney (Chapter 7). In Eccles' laboratory he devised an isolated nerve–muscle preparation, which produced one of the three classical studies that established the chemical nature of transmission at this junction (Chapter 4).

After the war Kuffler was recruited to the Wilmer Institute of Ophthalmology at Johns Hopkins University. There, he continued to develop his reputation for devising elegant preparations to demonstrate physiological principles.

One such set of experiments was on the physiology of the muscle spindle with Cuy Hunt. He then initiated a study of the mammalian retina.

The results were first published briefly in the Cold Spring Harbor symposium on the neuron in 1952 and in full in "Discharge Patterns and Functional Organization of the Mammalian Retina" in the *Journal of Neurophysiology* in 1953 (Appendix 9.3). In this paper he began by acknowledging the work he was building on: the first single-spike recordings from the eel optic nerve by Adrian and Matthews in 1927 and 1928, the cell responses of *Limulus* by Hartline and his colleagues in the 1930s (summarized in Hartline, 1940), the more recent demonstration in the frog retina of inhibitory interactions (Hartline et al., 1952) at the same symposium, and the studies by Granit and colleagues in the 1930s and 1940s of excitation and inhibition using field potentials and microelectrode recordings in several vertebrate species (summarized in Granit, 1950).

Kuffler proposed to extend these studies in two new ways. With S. A. Talbot he invented a new ophthalmoscope through which the retina could be stimulated with two small light or dark spots so that he could analyze interactions between two stimulated areas of differing extents. He also devised a preparation of the in vivo cat retina in which the optics were largely undisturbed while a metal microelectrode was inserted at the edge of the eyeball. Through his previous training with Eccles, he of course was closely familiar with the unfolding story in the spinal cord (Kuffler, 1953, 39):

> The present set-up also furnishes a relatively simple preparation in which the neural organization resembles the spinal cord and probably many higher centers of the nervous system. Many analogies have been found with discharge patterns in the spinal cord which are currently under study.

His long-time colleague John Nicholls (1998) related the following:

> Once again in one series of experiments in which he was sole author, Steve revealed a fundamental mechanism. A key feature was to use natural stimuli to define the receptive field properties of individual ganglion cells and their optic nerve fibers. The major conclusion was that these cells responded primarily to contrast and to moving stimuli rather than to diffuse light. These properties in turn depended on the

convergence of excitatory and inhibitory inputs arising from cells in preceding layers of the retina.

Kuffler's paper heralded the start of a new era in the study of mammalian vision and of excitatory and inhibitory interactions in general throughout the nervous system. More than any other, the image in the paper (reproduced in Fig. 9.2) of a micropipette on a retinal ganglion cell surrounded by two concentric circles representing an excitatory ("on") center and an inhibitory ("off") surround stood as a beacon to neurophysiologists, showing with consummate elegance what it was possible to reveal of the functional organization underlying information processing in a nervous structure of a mammal.

Students were drawn to Kuffler's laboratory, attracted by the elegance of his experiments and by his wonderful personal qualities of absolute integrity combined with modesty and self-deprecating humor.

> In addition to doing his own research he recruited a group of brilliant, independent young scientists, including David Hubel, Torsten Wiesel, Edwin Furshpan, and David Potter, together with an outstanding electronics engineer, Robert Bosler, with whom he was to work closely for the rest of his life. Steve also began to spend summers at the Marine Biological Laboratory at Woods Hole with his family and co-workers and started the first experimental lab courses devoted to the nervous system (the "Nerve–Muscle Program," later to become the neurobiology course). These intense lab and discussion courses had immense influence on generations of young graduate students and postdoctoral fellows coming from a variety of disciplines.
>
> (Nicholls, 1998)

The way his work on the retina inspired his students Hubel and Wiesel is described in Chapter 10.

This group of young investigators around Kuffler is mentioned also because in 1959 a far-seeing head of pharmacology, Otto Krayer, attracted Kuffler to move this entire unit of neurophysiologists to Harvard Medical School. A remaining gap in the group was filled by hiring a biochemist, Ed Kravitz, who we have already met in his pioneering work on the neurotransmitter γ-aminobutyric acid (GABA) (Chapter 4). This is widely regarded as the world's first department of neurobiology.

Horace Barlow. An important member of the new generation of retinal physiologists was Horace Barlow. Born in 1921, a great grandson of Charles Darwin, he was educated at Cambridge, England, another member of the extraordinary genealogical web cast by the descendants of Darwin (see Huxley and Keynes, Chapter 6). While a student he became interested in visual physiology and psychophysics. In 1953 he published an instant classic paper, "Stimulation and Inhibition in the Frog's Retina," in the *Journal of Physiology*, which built on Sherringtonian principles:

> It is certain that there is convergence, and probable that there is overlap, in the nervous pathway leading from receptor cells to optic nerve fibres. This is reminiscent of the convergence onto ventral horn cells that occurs in the spinal cord, and Sherrington's concepts suggest that the convergence may bring about some kind of "sensory integration.(70)"

His experiments showed properties similar to those reported earlier by Granit and Hartline and to the new ones reported contemporaneously by Kuffler:

> The inhibitory action of light falling outside the receptive field of "on–off" fibres has not been described before. It is not surprising that it has not been observed in threshold experiments on man, for any units which were uninhibited would have lower thresholds, and would therefore be responsible for the threshold. Simultaneous contrast effects are presumably caused by an inhibitory mechanism similar to the one described; a white spot surrounded by black looks brighter (more impulses) than a white spot of the same intensity surrounded by grey, because the grey falls on the inhibitory fringe of the ganglion cells, and so inhibits their discharge (causes fewer impulses).
>
> Hartline did not observe inhibition because his stimulus spots did not extend outside the receptive field. . . . It is probably also related to the various forms of temporal inhibition postulated by Granit (1947); his experiments were done with large stimuli which would cover both excitatory and inhibitory regions of the retina, and the results he observed would represent the excess of the excitatory over the inhibitory process.
>
> (Barlow, 1953, 85)

Kuffler had made similar observations. From this time, the definition of "receptive field" of a neuron included all of the parts of a field that could affect the excitability of a cell, including inhibition as well as excitation. Barlow also observed responses to moving stimuli, the first evidence for "movement sensitivity" as a property of visual cells.

Further experiments by Kuffler and Barlow, independently and in collaboration, as well as other laboratories, made the 1950s a dramatic time for retinal studies. They provided the basis for the identification of the wiring of the retina in the 1960s (Chapter 7) and the first explorations of central visual processing later in the decade (Chapter 10).

Expanding the Reflex Concept

As we have seen, the work of Eccles and others in the 1950s detailed the sensory and motor pathways for specific reflexes first revealed by Sherrington. The concept of the reflex, however, implied the existence of mechanisms to generate and coordinate it. We consider here the first steps toward enlarging the concept of the reflex to embrace the coordinated actions underlying integrative activity.

One of the first ideas came from work on alternating flexion and extension of the limbs involved in walking, by Thomas Graham Brown in England. He obtained evidence (Graham Brown, 1911) for intrinsic mechanisms of excitation and suppression within spinal cord neurons that could generate these patterns. As summarized by Adrian (1966, 26) in his memoir of Graham Brown:

> The conception is that of a single reflex movement regarded as the product of a potentially rhythmic nervous apparatus like that involved in walking or running. In his earlier work he was at some pains to analyse what he called "Narcosis progression"—the rhythmic kicking of the hind legs of a rabbit under ether—and he had found it occurring in deafferented limbs. This led to the conception of "rhythmic half centres" in the spinal cord linked together and capable of beating rhythmically under balanced excitatory and inhibitory stimulation, though the rhythm could be altered by afferent impulses or by cerebral control and the same half-centre could produce isolated movement as well as the repeated discharge.

Such central mechanisms for automatic behavior are obviously "hard-wired" into the interactions between motoneurons and the local interneurons and propriospinal neurons at the segmental level in the spinal cord. The cerebral control mentioned by Adrian was evidenced by Graham-Brown's experiments with Sherrington, which showed by stimulating the motor cortex how these "automatic" spinal cord centers could be controlled and modulated by higher centers (Graham Brown 1914).

The concept of the reflex was further enlarged and extended by placing it in a developmental context. George Coghill was an early leader in this work. He saw reflexes emerging not as individual responses to specific stimuli, as in the adult, but rather out of integrated responses of the emerging embryo to its environment (Coghill, 1930):

> ... reflexes begin as total action patterns in response to a comparatively general field of stimulation and acquire their restricted function or specificity on both sensory and motor sides secondarily (641).
>   ... This law has been demonstrated in the origin of unconditioned reflexes, and it appears also to apply to the formation of conditioned reflexes, instincts and the so-called process of trial and error (638).

... [As an example] The particular acts of feeding, which may appear to be severally discrete, are actually only phases of a reaction which is fundamentally unitary. Chain reflexes are fundamentally total reactions under the dominance of the mechanism of the total pattern of action (640).

The "half-center" concept was revived and elaborated by Soviet workers— Bernstein, Severin, Orlovsky, Shik—in the 1960s and 1970s and by Lundberg, Grillner, and their colleagues in Sweden. The larger developmental and behavioral context for viewing reflexes was carried forward by biological psychologists and ethologists, as we shall see (Chapter 11).

Command Neurons and Central Pattern Generators

We have seen how invertebrate nervous systems provided models such as the squid axon for understanding the action potential, the stretch receptor cell for sensory reception and neuronal integration, and the retina for studies of early visual processing. They also provided some of the first insights into how neurons interact to generate specific kinds of behavior.

A good idea can have many parents, and such is the case with central pattern generators.

This idea in invertebrates arose from experiments on the crayfish initiated by C. A. G. ("Kees") Wiersma in the 1930s. He was interested in using the crayfish as a simple system for studying reflex behavior. He found that the crayfish has several giant axons that extend through the body to innervate ganglion cells to the muscles of the body (the body is the "tail" of the crayfish if you're thinking of it during dinner). In 1947 he reported that a single shock to a giant axon elicits a "tail flip" that simulates the coordinated escape response of the crayfish from danger. Clearly, the crayfish nervous system is wired for coordinated reflexes, similar to the centers for reflex behavior and locomotion in the vertebrate spinal cord.

Wiersma and colleagues continued to explore these mechanisms through the 1950s, which led (Wiersma and Ikeda, 1964) to the concept of the "command neuron" (Appendix 9.4).

Edwards et al. (1999, 153) noted on the fiftieth anniversary of Wiersma's original report:

Fifty years ago C. A. G. Wiersma established that the giant axons of the crayfish nerve cord drive tail-flip escape responses. The circuitry that includes these giant neurons has now become one of the best-understood neural circuits in the animal kingdom. Although it controls a specialized behavior of a relatively simple animal, this circuitry has provided insights that are of general neurobiological interest concerning matters as diverse as the identity of the neural substrates involved in making behavioral decisions, the cellular bases of learning, subcellular neuronal computation, voltage-gated electrical synaptic transmission and modification of neuromodulator actions that result from social experience. This work illustrates the value of studying a circuit of moderate, but tractable, complexity and known behavioral function.

These studies implied a stereotyped central circuit activated by the command neuron, and thus arose the allied concept of the "central pattern generator," or CPG (Appendix 9.5). There is obviously a close similarity with the "half-center" concept developed for spinal cord control of the limbs in the vertebrate.

It did not take long, however, to discover that what seemed like a simple division between command neuron and CPG was actually much more complicated: The CPG contains elements that are both generators and drivers, and the driving elements can be generators as well as modulators. In addition, the giant fiber systems parallel other fiber systems which contribute to, and play essential roles in, eliciting the reflex behavior. These issues are still with us today (see Kuperfermann and Weiss, 1978; Edwards et al., 1999); for similar issues in vertebrates, see Korn and Faber (2005); Jordan et al. (2008).

The advantages of the simple invertebrate system suggested to the first explorers in the 1950s that it should be possible to know each cell of such a system and therefore to predict entirely its behavior. This idea was tested in the lobster cardiac ganglion, which contains only nine cells with the specific function of controlling the heartbeat. It turned out that this simple system was also too complicated because of the overlapping functions including pacemaking, pattern generation, oscillatory behavior, facilitation, and other properties (Maynard, 1955; see Bullock, 1977, 419). This gave rise to skepticism that the simple system approach could ever succeed at the neural system level. Out of this period emerged a multidisciplinary approach, eventually including genetic techniques, in which each cell could be isolated and analyzed for its multiple contributions to the entire system (see Selverston, 1985).

When ethologists came to study instinctive behavior, they developed similar concepts, as we shall see in Chapter 11.

Chapter 10

Neural Circuits: Cortical Columns and Cortical Processing

The 1950s was a golden age of discovery in the cerebral cortex, witnessing the first steps by the pioneers pushing their recording microelectrodes into the unknown territories of the major cortical systems. From knowing next to nothing about cortical functional organization, neurophysiologists by the end of the decade had the cortical column as an organizing principle. The homunculus for the somatosensory and motor cortex was revealed, the visual cortex was opened up for a parallel approach to identifying visual stimuli and feature detectors, there were tantalizing hints that the auditory cortex contained a frequency map, and the motor cortex was found to contain circuits for lateral excitation and inhibition within the motor homunculus. An outgrowth of the cortex, the olfactory bulb, was found to represent odors by spatial activity patterns analogous to the spatial organization of the sensory cortical systems. These findings set the agendas for the next half-century of cortical studies.

In the neuroanatomy course in my first year at Harvard Medical School in 1956, I looked forward eagerly to the lectures on the cerebral cortex, anticipating my first glimpse into how cortical cells might give rise to mental activity (today, we would say the "neural basis of cognition," but it's the same thing). Alfred Pope, an outstanding early neurochemist, was the lecturer. He meticulously took us through the anatomy of the cortex, cell by cell, as described by Ramón y Cajal using the Golgi stain a half-century before, starting at the surface—the small pyramidal cell in layer 2, the slightly larger pyramidal cell in layer 3, the stellate (star-shaped) cell in layer 4, the large pyramidal neuron in layer 5, and the large polymorphic cell in layer 6. Then, he went through the interneurons: the Martinotti cell in layer 1, the bipolar cell in layers 2 and 3, and other types in the deeper layers. It was all organized beautifully. When he had laid this all out in detailed diagrams of the cells, he stepped back from the blackboard, admired his handiwork, turned to us, and said, "And of course we don't have a clue what they do."

The Cortical Column

Rafael Lorente de No. In contrast to this layer-by-layer account, a different conceptual framework had been put forward by one of Ramón y Cajal's former students, Rafael Lorente de No. In 1938 he had been invited by John Fulton to contribute a chapter on the cerebral cortex to the *Physiology of the Nervous System* (Appendix 10.1). de No provided not only a masterly account of the neuronal elements of the cortex (Fig. 10.1) but also took the opportunity to formulate a new hypothesis for their functional organization (Appendix 10.1). He wrote,

> Save for layers I and II, all cortical layers contain cells having synaptic contacts with the specific afferents, so that it would be improper to call any one layer "receptor." On the other hand, every layer except I has axons reaching the white matter, and therefore no layer may be called "effector (312)."

With regard to the all-important intrinsic connections—those between cells within and between the cortical layers—Lorente de No proposed that they took place within vertical cylinders of cells, each cylinder having a specific afferent fiber as its axis:

> All the elements of cortex are represented in it, and therefore it may be called an *elementary unit*, in which, theoretically, the whole process of transmission of impulses from the afferent fiber to the efferent axon may be accomplished (311).

One can see that this was essentially identifying the radial cylinder as an input–output unit, equivalent to the elementary reflex unit of the spinal cord, the difference being that the cortical unit was embedded in a far more complex information-processing environment.

The key to Lorente de No's concept was that the connections within the radial unit were organized in loops which could set up reverberating circuits, that is, circuits within which impulses would activate cells that would feed back excitation, maintaining the excitation indefinitely. A mechanism of this type seemed to be required for the maintained activity that would be needed as the basis for both short-term and long-term memory. Note that this maintained activity within a cortical unit resembles the maintained activity within a central pattern generator (CPG), as discussed in Chapter 9.

To have this remarkable hypothesis within a textbook was unusual, but as we shall see, it did not lie dormant. In this respect it presaged the textbook by Donald Hebb a decade later, which contained a suggestion for a wiring scheme that laid the basis for circuits for learning and memory (Chapter 12).

Vernon Mountcastle. At the time of my class in neuroanatomy, investigators in both North America and Europe were beginning to use the new microelectrode methods to explore the cortex. Herbert Jasper, Penfield's colleague at the Neurological Institute in Montreal, was one of the first, inserting a microelectrode into the cortex of the anesthetized cat to record different types of cell activity in different layers. Another was Denise Albe-Fessard in Paris. But the key breakthrough came with the discovery of the cortical column by a neurophysiologist at Johns Hopkins University Medical School, Vernon Mountcastle.

Mountcastle (Fig. 10.2A) was born in 1918 in Kentucky and trained at Johns Hopkins University Medical School. After service in World War II he returned to Hopkins to work in the Bard Laboratory for Neurophysiology, which had been set up by Phillip Bard, an early leader in the physiology of motor and emotional behavior. In the early 1950s Mountcastle carried out a series of studies of microelectrode recordings of the central representation of tactile responses. This started with the thalamus and, the thalamus being the gateway to the cortex, led on to the cortex.

In a recent interview (Grauer, 2007), Mountcastle recalled the dramatic day in 1955 when he

was studying the results of tests on the brains of cats, recording the character of each cell from successive penetration layers. "I was writing them down vertically on a yellow piece of paper," he recalls. Suddenly the vertical note taking helped him see the stunning pattern in the brain: Skin cells lay atop skin cells, joint cells atop joint cells and so on, extending in columns from the brain's surface all the way down through six layers of cortex. "That was my 'aha' experience."

His experimental strategy was to make penetrations that were entirely in a radial direction into the cortex. In these cases, as described in his recollection above, he found that all of the "units" (i.e., cells) he encountered tended to fire impulse responses to the same type of skin stimulus (i.e., light touch, deep touch, joint movement, etc.). By contrast, when his electrode was inserted obliquely so that it passed across the cortex, he encountered a series of cells responding to different types of stimuli. In his paper of 1957, the last section (pp 430–431) of the discussion put forth his conclusion regarding these findings:

IV. AN HYPOTHESIS OF FUNCTIONAL ORGANIZATION OF CORTEX

The data reported in these papers support the view that there is an elementary unit of organization in the somatic cortex made up of a vertical group of cells extending through all the cellular layers. The neurons of such a group are related to the same, or nearly the same, peripheral receptive field upon the body surface. They are activated by the same type of peripheral stimulus, i.e., they belong to the same modality subgroup. It follows from this last observation that they should show the same discharge properties, which they do, especially as regards adaptation to steady stimuli. Finally, all the cells of such a vertical column discharge at more or less the same latency to a brief peripheral stimulus. They are thus grouped into an initial firing pattern. It is emphasized that this analysis is based strictly upon the first response of cortical cells to a peripheral stimulus, the early repetitive response, which our experiments as well as those of others (3) have shown to be extraordinarily sensitive to the parameters of the stimulus. It seems likely that even the light state of anesthesia in our preparations has severely suppressed the later and more complex discharge patterns, which we have seen only very rarely (19, Fig. 9-f). It suggests, however, that the cortical cells will be arranged sequentially in time into a variety of firing patterns, and a principal experimental objective at present is a detailed analysis of this later activity.

Our data should not be interpreted to indicate that all the cells of this vertical column are necessarily activated monosynaptically by the specific thalamocortical afferents, although the anatomical studies of Lorente de No (15), including among other regions the somatic cortex of the mouse, and of Sholl (22) on the visual cortex of the cat, have indicated that this is possible for neurons of all the cellular layers, except perhaps the second. But the powerful synaptic connections of the cells with short and ascending axons, which make up such a large percentage of the cells of the cortices of higher mammals, indicate that elements of all the cellular layers will receive spatially multiplied synaptic impingements after one or more additional synaptic transfers. Our data are compatible with these anatomical observations.

The hypothesis that such a vertically linked group of cells is the elementary unit for cortical function is not new. Such a conclusion was reached by Lorente de No from his extensive studies on synaptic linkages of cortical neurons. He emphasized from the pattern of those linkages that the vertical chains of neurons were capable of input–output activity without necessarily wide horizontal spread. That such a horizontal spread is not required for even rather high order functioning of the cortex is indicated by recent experiments reported by Sperry (26). He showed that cats after widespread vertical subpial dicing of the visual cortex, the incisions extending through the grey and into the white matter, were then still capable of very fine visual pattern discriminations. This capacity survived the subsequent removal of the superior colliculi. Sperry had previously found (25) that monkeys after similar vertical dicing of the sensory and motor cortices were capable of what appeared to be normal motor activity. It follows from his experiments that rather small vertical columns of cortex are capable of integrated activity of a complex order. This conclusion fits the results of the present experiments, and the hypothesis of functional organization proposed.

It is fair to say that every investigation of the cortex since then has built on those paragraphs. A key claim was that the physiology of the cortical cells was intimately tied to the anatomical entity of the column. Since such narrow columns were not evident in the anatomy of the cortex, it was important to demonstrate this correlation. This was the subject of four papers published by Mountcastle and his collaborators in 1959. In these he was joined by Tom Powell from Oxford University, who devised a method for recovering the electrode tract and correlating the route of the electrode and the precise location of each recorded cell, in both radial and oblique penetrations. This classic demonstration (Powell and Mountcastle, 1959) (see Fig. 10.3, Appendix 10.2) cemented the hypothesis; from then on there could be no doubt that the cerebral cortex contains a columnar organization. (Powell adapted this technique for identifying the electrode tract and recording sites of responses in our subsequent work in the olfactory bulb.)

The *cortical column* thus became the central organizing principle of the neocortex and one of the key tools for subsequent analysis of all cortical areas. Initially believed to be restricted to primary sensory areas, columnar structures were later shown to be present in callosal projections to cortical association areas (Jones et al., 1975; Goldman-Rakic, 1981). After over a half-century of serving as an organizing principle for cortical studies, the columnar hypothesis is being reassessed from new perspectives (Horton and Adams, 2005).

Central Visual Processing and Feature Detectors

While Mountcastle was developing his approach to the somatosensory cortex, David Hubel and Torsten Wiesel were developing their approach to the visual cortex, building on the studies in both the cortex and the retina.

David Hubel. David Hubel (Fig. 10.4) was born in the United States in 1926, the son of a chemical engineer whose job took the family to Montreal. As he recalled later (Hubel and Wiesel, 2005, 9), his boyhood in the 1930s was filled with pursuing different hobbies such as chemistry, electronics, reading in science, piano, Latin, and working on a farm in the summer. "With parents who didn't organize our lives [chauffeuring to one organized activity after another] it was much easier to reach the level of boredom necessary to think up things to do for ourselves [a sentiment that applied as well to my generation growing up in the 1940s, before the car culture and television changed life in the United States]."

The way he got into neurophysiology was typical of the tortuous paths people took before the institutionalization of graduate training in neuroscience and is well described in his memoir (Hubel and Wiesel, 2005). He received undergraduate and medical training at McGill University in Montreal, where around 1950 he first met Penfield and Jasper. During residency training he began to do research in neurophysiology, beginning in the electroencephalography (EEG) laboratory under Jasper at the Montreal Neurological Institute. A friend then urged him to transfer to Hopkins because of the research being done there by Mountcastle and Kuffler, which he did in 1954. With dual citizenship, he was subject to the draft in the United States, so after the residency ended the next year he took a position at Walter Reed Army Institute of Research in Washington, D.C. Although this meant leaving the stimulating atmosphere of Hopkins, it was compensated for by the stimulating environment at Walter Reed, with Michael Fuortes (before he joined Kay Frank at the National Institutes of Health—see Chapter 7), Robert Galambos, and Walle Nauta (Chapter 11), among others, under David Rioch.

Free to do research full time, Hubel, on a suggestion by Fuortes, designed some wire electrodes to do single-unit recordings in the cat cortex. Though without previous experience in either single-unit recordings or the cat cortex, he developed a tungsten electrode that was better than the previous steel ones. Soon the world—at least a subset of the neurophysiology world—took notice. Next came a chamber to seal the opening over the cortex and reduce arterial and respiratory pulsations, and finally, he developed a method to pass current through the electrode to leave metallic deposits to show a recording site.

With this combination, he was able to begin recording from the cortex. He chose the visual cortex, drawing on conversations he had had with Kuffler. He applied his new recording instrumentation to recording from cells in the primary visual cortex (V1) in response to flashes of light. This got a little boring, and he began to explore whether cortical cells were more interested in more complicated stimuli. In desperation one day he started waving his hand in front of the cat's eye and was astonished to see that one cell responded to movement in one direction and another in the opposite direction.

To pursue this work, he was encouraged to contact Kuffler at Hopkins. Mountcastle then invited him to join the physiology department there. So after a final year at Walter Reed, he moved to Hopkins in the summer of 1958 to begin work in the Kuffler laboratory with a new colleague, Torsten Wiesel. They were given a 225–square foot laboratory plus office space for both of them and a small budget for their experiments. (At the present writing, laboratory plus office space in the United States starts at around 1000 square feet for one assistant professor, with a startup package of up to $1 million or so for research.)

Torsten Wiesel. Torsten Wiesel (Fig 10.4) was born in 1924 in Uppsala, Sweden, and grew up on the grounds of a mental hospital headed by his father, a psychiatrist. Observing bizarre behavior among the patients was a frequent and normal occurrence. He grew up excelling in athletics and immersing himself in reading, especially philosophy, which stimulated his first thoughts on the mind and how it worked (Hubel and Wiesel, 2005, 27).

In 1946 he began medical training at the Karolinska Institute in Stockholm, where he came under the tutelage of Ulf von Euler, a leading biochemist and physiologist, and Carl Gustav Bernhard, a leader in neurophysiology. Wiesel especially prized the informality of Bernhard and his laboratory, which contrasted with the traditional rigid formality in Sweden. (I too admired Bernhard for this when I spent 2 years in his department in the mid-1960s; everyone within the laboratory was on an informal "du" basis, from the professor down to the glass washers, at a time when the formal "de" and "ni" were still standard almost everywhere.)

As his training was ending, he tried a year of child psychiatry; but the analytical emphasis turned him off. He knew he wanted to focus on the physiology of the brain. Fortunately, Bernhard appointed him as an instructor in the Department of Neurophysiology at the Karolinska Institute. His first research project was to work with Bernhard on testing the effects of local anesthetics on severe epilepsy. This did not seem to be leading in a very exciting direction. Good fortune smiled again when Bernhard told him that he had been contacted by Professor Kuffler in America, who was looking for a postdoctoral fellow to pursue work he had started on the visual system. Wiesel read the 1952 version of Kuffler's receptive field study in the Cold Spring Harbor volume (libraries subscribed to these series, so they were immediately available around the world, though instead of pushing a key on the computer keyboard, one had to walk a few hundred feet to the library) and decided that was what he wanted to do.

He arrived at the Wilmer Institute at Johns Hopkins in August 1955. By then Kuffler had assembled a group that included Ed Furshpan, David Potter, Josef Dudel (from Germany), and Taro Furokawa (from Japan). The Wilmer was an institute for eye research, so Wiesel and Kenneth Brown were designated to continue the eye research. Over the next 3 years Brown worked on the cellular basis of the electroretinogram, while Wiesel wrote several papers extending Kuffler's work on the receptive field properties of retinal ganglion cells.

Hubel and Wiesel. At this point the two stories merge. Kuffler brought the two together for lunch and suggested that they collaborate. From Walter Reed Hubel would bring his recording methods applied to the cortex, while Wiesel would bring his extension of Kuffler's approach to receptive field properties applied to the retina. Together they would attack the mystery of the functional organization of the visual cortex.

The experiments began in the spring of 1958, in anesthetized cats, stimulating the recorded cells in the visual area of the cortex with spots of light shone on the retina. The initial results were disappointing; the cortical cells showed little responsiveness to these stimuli.

> The break came one long day in which we held onto one cell for hour after hour. . . . Suddenly, just as we inserted one of our glass slides into the ophthalmoscope, the cell seemed to come to life and began to fire

impulses like a machine gun. It took a while to discover that the firing had nothing to do with the small opaque spot—the cell was responding to the fine moving shadow cast by the edge of the glass slide as we inserted it into the slot. It took still more time and groping around to discover that the cell gave responses only when this faint line was swept slowly forward in a certain range of orientations. Even changing the stimulus orientation by a few degrees made the responses much weaker, and an orientation at right angles to the optimum produced no responses at all. The cell completely ignored our black and white spots. When finally we could think of nothing more to do with this cell, we discovered we had worked with it for nine hours. The 1959 paper of course gives no hint of our struggle. As usual in scientific reports we presented the bare results, with little of the sense of excitement or fun.

(Hubel and Wiesel, 2005, 60)

The 1959 paper was entitled "Receptive Fields of Single Neurones in the Cat's Striate Cortex," submitted in April 1959 and published in the *Journal of Physiology*. Its elegance of presentation carried forward the tradition of the Kuffler approach (Fig. 10.5, Appendix 10.3).

The opening of a new era in studies of vision and of the cortex was conveyed by the clarity of the figures. Each told its own story.

Cells were driven from only one eye or the other, the first demonstration of ocular dominance cells. These were subsequently found to be organized in ocular dominance columns.

The cells were driven by spots, arranged not concentrically, as in the retinal cells, but along a line acting as a border separating excitatory and inhibitory responses. These were later called "simple cells."

Cells were "tuned" to a specific orientation. This was the harbinger of orientation columns; different cells were tuned to different orientations.

Cells were particularly sensitive to movement of a border in one direction, expressing movement sensitivity.

No cell showed a center-surround organization as in the cat retina. Only half the cells responded to diffuse light.

In summary, even using the simple stimuli of spots and slits of light, it was obvious that cortical cells were selective for one eye or the other, arrangements of stimuli into borders between light and dark, orientations of the borders, and movement of the borders. The impact of these findings was not only the novelty of the results but also the simple and systematic methods for demonstrating them. Hubel and Wiesel subsequently emphasized how a key to their success lay in how simple the methods were, using only the spots and slits, rather than sophisticated instrumentation for grids of different wavelengths. The advantage they stressed was that they had the flexibility to explore different unpredicted response properties such as the full range of 360° of orientation or movement. The quantitation could come later in others' hands.

Another point they emphasized was that they paid no attention to latency measurements of the responses, such as had been essential for Eccles' approach to using recordings in the spinal cord to identify pathways and synaptic connections. They focused on response properties rather than on the possible circuits that could mediate them. As we have discussed in Chapter 9, these two approaches are complementary in revealing the neural basis of behavior.

Even with this initial paper they had accumulated much additional data, which led to their paper in 1962 in which they were able to distinguish between "simple cells," such as those in the 1959 paper, and "complex cells," those with additional properties of selectivity. These results belong to the rapidly expanding field of visual processing in subsequent decades, all within the framework of the initial study (see Hubel and Wiesel, 2005).

The fact that Kuffler brought them together, shaped the strategy of their collaboration, provided them with the space and facilities, and was the initial guiding force of the work is worth a comment. In most laboratories, he would have been the senior author on at least their first papers together and in most cases all of them, sharing credit for the giant step forward that he had organized and funded. But that wasn't the way Steve ran his laboratory. Despite his close involvement in the life of the laboratory, each person or group, including his own, had his or their own project and received all the credit.

Their early papers were published in The Journal of Physiology, much desired by neurophysiologists. That journal had a policy of authors listed strictly alphabetically, which dictated the order of Hubel and Wiesel (just as it did Hodgkin and Huxley). That policy later changed. In other journals of the time the order could be varied to reflect better the contributions of each to the particular study. Women were identified only by their initials, which contributed even further to their anonymity in a male world.

Jerry Lettvin. Some of these response properties had been seen by Horace Barlow in the frog optic nerve in 1953, including the possibility of complicated forms such as "bug detectors." Even more elaborate forms were seen by Jerry Lettvin and his collaborators at MIT and were reported in their paper on recordings from the frog optic tectum that also came out in 1959. The group at MIT was one of the most interesting in the early days of neuroscience.

Jerry Lettvin was born in 1920 in Chicago. He trained in neurology and psychiatry and saw action in World War II. After the war, he continued his training at the Boston City Hospital on the neurology service of Derek Denny-Brown (see Chapter 13) and then joined the faculty at MIT to work full-time on research in neurophysiology. He was a close companion there of Warren McCulloch, an early pioneer in experimental and theoretical neurophysiology; McCulloch was a collaborator with Walter Pitts on one of the most famous articles in neuroscience and computer science (see Chapter 16).

Jerry is a larger-than-life character of great warmth, humor, empathy, joy, and intellect. He is a great polymath, always juggling a variety of subjects.

In the middle 1950s he and his colleagues McCulloch, Pitts, and Humberto Maturana (Fig. 10.6) undertook a study of the responses of the retina to complex objects, recording the responses from optic nerve endings in the optic tectum, a cortical structure in the midbrain. In their classic paper "What the Frog's Eye Tells the Frog's Brain" (Lettvin et al., 1959), they showed that the retinal ganglion cells respond selectively to different complex types of visual stimuli, ranging from simple edges to curves to even complex shapes they likened to "bug detectors" (Appendix 10.4).

The study was published in the proceedings of a meeting and so did not have the immediate wide readership of the Hubel and Wiesel study. However, it was well known to most visual system investigators. It provided a model for central circuits acting as "feature detectors," which became important in popularizing that term and concept in sensory neuroscience. This approach to analyzing central visual mechanisms with more elaborate stimuli anticipated studies much later for selectivity for complex shapes in higher visual association areas such as those by Tanaka and colleagues.

Intracellular Recordings from the Brain

Eccles' intracellular recordings were from the motoneurons of the spinal cord. Intracellular recordings from the brain were more difficult because of the problems of vascular and respiratory pulsations and the smaller sizes of the neurons. The first attempts were made by several investigators at about the same time. It is instructive to consider these attempts because they give insight into the problems faced by investigators in Germany, France, and England in the years after World War II, which nonetheless enabled them to participate in the great strides forward of the 1950s.

Richard Jung. One of these was Richard Jung (1911–1986) in Germany. After medical training, he was drawn to research on the brain, inspired by Adrian's single-nerve recordings, Hans Berger's discovery of EEG waves in 1929, and the electrical stimulation experiments of deep structures of the brain by W. R. Hess and of the cortex by Ottfried Foerster. He was one of the first in Germany to carry out research on the EEG and in 1937 discovered the theta-rhythm in the hippocampus in response to sensory stimulation (Kornmuller and Jung, 1938).

His training in England gave him contacts, which helped reestablish German neurological science after the war. In 1951 he set up the Department of Neurology and Neurophysiology at Freiburg, reflecting his desire to bring basic brain research to bear on neurological disorders, very much in line with similar efforts in the United States and United Kingdom (see Chapter 13). In 1952 he reported the first single-unit recordings from the visual cortex of the cat in response to light (Jung et al., 1952). He particularly pursued the relations between neurophysiology and behavior, such as the neural basis for epilepsy, the sleep–waking cycle, and attention and perception (Creutzfeldt, 1986); this included the proposal of a search light model as the neural basis for attention, a concept that was later taken up by Francis Crick and others.

Denise Albe-Fessard. Meanwhile, in France, Denise Albe-Fessard was also interested in the cortex. She had been born Denise Albe in 1916 in Paris. Although an outstanding student, she was advised against medicine as a career because of the limited prospects for women at that time and chose instead to study physics and chemistry in order to become an engineer (Albe-Fesssard, 1996). However, when she graduated in 1937 there were few jobs for female physicists in industry, so she reoriented her career to biology by becoming a technical assistant in a laboratory in the Centre National de la Recherche Scientifique (CNRS), working under Daniel Auger on recordings of action potentials in the seaweed *Nitella* (see Chapter 6). During this work she learned of the EEG and brain research through visits to the laboratory by Alfred Fessard, one of the first in France to study the EEG. An indication of the early state of electronics at that time can be gained from her recollection that Fessard, for recording the action potentials from nerve and muscle,

> ...had obtained a CRO [cathode ray oscilloscope], a French model in which the vacuum had to be re-established in the tube before each measurement. German tubes without this inconvenience had just appeared on the market, but it was still necessary to build the time base and amplifier.
>
> (Albe-Fessard, 1996, 8)

During the war (1939–45) Fessard set up a small electrophysiology laboratory at the Institut Marey, which was to play a central role in the revival of French neurophysiology. Albe joined him there as a technical assistant and became Madame Albe-Fessard in 1942. Research was carried forward on a limited scale during the war and didn't much improve afterward; as she observed (1996, 12), "The first years after liberation were difficult, with laboratory supplies almost impossible to obtain."

The International Physiological Congress in 1947 was held in Oxford and was a signal step toward repairing the connections broken during the 1930s and the war and building new ones. Albe-Fessard met E. G. T. Liddell, Charles Phillips, and David Whitteridge, establishing connection with the Sherrington school at Oxford as well as with physiologists at Cambridge.

A constant thorn in the side was having to communicate in English, a problem that dogged French scientists of the prewar generation for years, limiting them at first to delivering their talks at international symposia and writing their papers in French. It held back acknowledgment of their achievements and led to misunderstandings, as Madame Albe-Fesssard ruefully notes.

...even after improving my English [in the 1960s] thanks to American collaborators, I have always had some difficulty of expression in that language, above all in replying quickly to questions. It is always difficult to be subtle in a foreign language, and the necessary simplicity of my oral expression has often led me to be accused of aggressiveness. I think that those who have so misjudged me ought to have had to present their own work in a language not their own—they would have understood me better.

(Albe-Fessard, 1996, 24)

It was not until 1950 that the Institut Marey began to receive American visitors. For foreign connections, she made annual visits to Brazil to work with colleagues there.

Albe-Fessard's early studies had been on the electrical activity of electric fish (Gymnotes). In the 1950s she began a second line of work on microelectrode recordings from the cerebral cortex of the cat. This resulted in one of the first intracellular recordings from the cortex (Buser and Albe-Fessard, 1955), from pyramidal neurons in the sigmoid gyrus responding to somatosensory stimulation in the cat. The paper was entitled "Activites intracellulaires receuilles dans la cortex sigmoide du chat: participation des neurones pyramidaux au potentiel evoque somesthesique" ("Intracellular Activity Recorded in the Sigmoid Cortex of the Cat: Participation of Pyramidal Neurons in the Somatosensory Evoked Potential").

This was a singular achievement, among the first intracellular recordings in the mammalian brain, after Eccles and others in the spinal cord. However, it had limited impact as a brief communication in French in a French journal not widely read outside France. As a first communication of a new method, there were concerns raised that the recordings contained artifacts, though she was defended by Jung, who was one of the other pioneers in cortical recordings, as we have noted. Finally, this work was not followed up by a longer paper or series of papers to test and extend the initial findings, always critically important in opening a new field.

Charles Phillips. The person who was most recognized for the first intracellular recordings from the cortex, indeed, from the brain above the spinal cord, was Charles Phillips (Fig. 10.7). He was born in 1916 and came to Oxford in 1935, the year when Sherrington retired. He studied under Eccles, Sherrington's last student, before Eccles left for Australia. Phillips went into neurology, serving on the home front in World War II. After the war, he returned to Oxford to begin research in neurophysiology. In the early 1950s he carried out studies with Liddell, examining movements of the extremities in response to focal shocks to motor cortex; this gave rise to the interpretation that the stimulation activated small populations of pyramidal cells—"congeries of neurons," in their terminology—to the muscles.

He then tackled the challenge of recording intracellularly from these pyramidal neurons. He reported recordings in 1956 in the cat and in 1959 from the baboon. (I heard Phillips describe these results at a meeting on cortical physiology in Philadelphia in 1958 and, impressed with the results and the energy with which he described them, joined him for graduate study in 1959 to study the intracortical circuits that control the pyramidal cells, what we now would call "microcircuits.")

In these studies he tested the motoneuron model and found that the largest motoneurons, the Betz cells, showed similar properties of action potential generation, synaptic potentials, and integration of excitation and inhibition. In addition, he showed recurrent excitation as well as lateral inhibition, presumably mediated by cortical interneurons in analogy with the spinal cord circuits demonstrated by Eccles (Appendix 10.5). *Recurrent inhibition* confirmed the general prevalence of this type of feedback as high as the cerebral cortex. *Recurrent excitation* was a new finding, which came to be recognized as special to the cortex. These studies laid the basis for future studies of the local excitatory and inhibitory circuits that control the output from the cortex.

Two Motor Systems

During this period, the distinction was emphasized between the *pyramidal motor system*, in which cortical pyramidal cells send their axons through the pyramidal tract to make direct synapses on motoneurons in the spinal cord for control of fine movements of the digits in primates, and the *extrapyramidal system*, in which cortical connections are made to brainstem centers which connect to interneurons in the spinal cord controlling the motoneurons. This distinction was particularly important clinically in distinguishing between motor defects due to lesions at the level of the spinal cord, midbrain, white matter, or cerebral cortex.

Human Cortex and the Homunculus

The human cortex was not a subject for physiological study until the 1950s. Wilder Penfield, a neurosurgeon who trained under both Sherrington and Ramón y Cajal, founded the Montreal Neurological Institute in 1934 and became one of the most prominent people in midcentury neurological sciences (see Chapters 10, 12–14).

Penfield became particularly known for developing operative procedures for removal of cortical tissue for *relief of epilepsy*. In the course of these operations he carried out a systematic mapping of the human cortex, verifying the presence of the motor strip in the frontal lobe along the rolandic sulcus with successive representation of the head, shoulders, arms, trunk, and legs. These findings became widely known through the diagram of the *homunculus* ("little man"), a caricature who had large lips, hands, and feet, representing the larger amounts of cortex devoted to controlling the fine movements of those muscles (Penfield and Rasmussen, 1950) (Fig. 10.8, Appendix 10.6). The motor homunculus in turn was parallel to a similar somatosensory homunculus across the Rolandic sulcus, representing the higher sensory innervation of those regions.

Penfield found that shocks to the cortex could evoke not only movements but also memories, laying the foundation for the study of *cortical mechanisms in memory*. These studies also pointed to the importance of the hippocampus in memory. Through these studies Penfield and the Montreal Neurological Institute became a magnet for students interested in studying the human brain and human cognitive functions, which included Herbert Jasper and Brenda Milner. Jasper led a group of neurophysiologists that made some of the first single-unit recordings of cells in the cortex (Li et al., 1956). Brenda Milner carried out the study of the patient H. M. that played a central role in the rise of cognitive neuroscience (see Chapter 12). Penfield's role in supporting this research is discussed further in Chapter 12 and his role in the development of neurosurgery, in Chapter 14.

Auditory Cortex: An Auditory Map?

Thus, during the 1950s the idea of mapping of sensory space in the cortex was established for the visual and somatosensory systems. What about the auditory system? The possibility that the frequency selectivity along the cochlear basilar membrane, laid down by the traveling wave demonstrated by von Békésy (Chapter 7), is represented by a corresponding mapping of frequency in the auditory cortex was reported by Archie Tunturi in 1952. These results remained unconfirmed, however, until the 1970s, when it was shown that the mapping is highly sensitive to the actions of the anesthetics used in the experiments.

The Pattern Theory of Olfaction

The mechanisms for processing olfactory stimuli were the most elusive of all. Nothing was known about brain mechanisms in vertebrate olfaction until Edgar Adrian, a pioneer in single-unit analysis of sensory receptors (as we saw in Chapter 7) and in the early studies of the physiological basis of the EEG, turned his attention to them in the 1940s. In the early 1950s he reported multiunit recordings from the olfactory bulb of the rabbit, which showed that different odors elicit different patterns of activity across the olfactory bulb. We can do no better than quote his own words:

> So far then it looks as though Acetone molecules will produce an excitation coming mainly from the front of the organ and from the particular groups of receptors in that area which have this specificity to it. A strong concentration may bring in other groups but, owing to the structure of the organ, there will always be critical regions where the concentration is only just strong enough to excite and here the specific effect will show

itself. And there will be critical times. At each inspiration the amount of material which enters the nose will increase progressively to a maximum and at the beginning and end of each inspiration the concentration is near the threshold value. The physical and chemical properties of the substances will therefore determine the time course of excitation. For instance, a large spike unit may have a specific sensitivity to Xylol. As the concentration of Xylol in the air is increased, other units will begin to come in during the later part of the discharge. With pyridine and eucalyptus the smaller spikes appear first and the large ones come later on. The result is that the photographic reproduction of the discharge has a characteristic shape for each substance, and this shape is reproduced with remarkable constancy each time the substance is presented in the nose.

The result is that the electrophysiologist, looking at a series of these records, could identify the particular smell that caused each one. We must not conclude that the brain identified the smell by the same criteria but we can at least see how a great variety of smells might be distinguished without the need for very great variations in the receptors.

(Adrian, 1953, 12–13)

On this basis he suggested a *pattern theory of odor representation,* in which different odors are encoded by different spatial and temporal activity (Fig. 10.9, Appendix 10.7).

Adrian's experiments suggested that there is a systematic relation between the olfactory epithelium and the olfactory bulb that gives rise to the activity patterns, which received support from anatomical tracing studies by Wilfred le Gros Clark at Oxford (summarized in Clark, 1957). Mozell (1958) suggested that the patterns could arise in part from different gradients of absorption of odor molecules across the olfactory epithelium, which became known as the *chromatographic theory* of spatial patterning of odor responses.

Testing for the cellular basis of activity patterns in olfaction was much more difficult than in vision, where the stimulus can be controlled in a precise way in space to give insight into the spatial response. In olfaction, stimulus control is not as precise and there are no a priori guides to what the patterns will look like. Application of the 2-deoxyglucose method to the olfactory system by Frank Sharp and his collaborators finally showed that the basis of the activity patterns is *selective glomerular activation* (Sharp et al., 1975; Stewart et al., 1979). These patterns are key to understanding the neural representation of the information carried in the odor molecules. They are currently being pursued by a variety of molecular (Mombaerts, 1996) and imaging (Xu et al., 2000) techniques.

Chapter 11

Neural Systems: The Neural Basis
of Behavior

*Until well into the twentieth century brain activity was believed to be domi-
nated by electrical activity in specific neural pathways. Research at midcentury revealed for the first time widely distributed systems involved in global
functions underlying behavior. The first evidence was also found that the
brain is a gland as well as a computer. The reticular activating system in the
brainstem was shown to provide for arousal of the cortex as an accompani-
ment to sensory perception. Rapid eye movements were demonstrated in
sleep, leading to an entirely new understanding of sleep as a complex active
brain state. Operant conditioning was demonstrated, introducing a new paradigm for studying brain mechanisms in motivation and learning. The two-
state theory for the brain mechanisms involved in the control of feeding was
introduced, which has guided subsequent research on feeding behavior. The
relation of the brain to the pituitary body as the master gland for control of
hormones in the body was solved, both the neural control of the posterior
pituitary and the portal system controlling the anterior pituitary. The long
domination of behavioral studies by laboratory manipulations was finally
challenged by studies of the brain mechanisms underlying behavior and the
rise of ethology through studies of natural behavior.*

In contrast to the pathways and circuits mediating specific types of perception
and behavior are the systems that have more global effects, involved in releasing
and responding to circulating hormones or in setting the behavioral state of the
organism. The midcentury was a time of extraordinary advances in revealing
these systems, too.

Arousal and the Reticular Activating System

Sherrington had shown that low transections of the brainstem in the cat render the muscles paralyzed and flaccid, whereas high transections, above the red nucleus, produce a state of tonic hyperactivity, called "decerebrate rigidity." These differing states aided the analysis of spinal cord pathways and functions, as we have seen in his classic monograph *The Integrative Action of the Nervous System* (1906).

In the 1930s Frederick Bremer (1937) of Belgium turned his attention to the state of the brain above these transections. He showed that low transections ("encephale isole," or isolated encephalon) had no effect on normal waking and sleeping patterns, whereas high transections ("cerveau isole," or isolated brain) produced permanent deep sleep. These experiments pointed to the midbrain-pontine region as a site of mechanisms of *arousal.*

In the 1940s, Robert Morrison and colleagues at Harvard carried out experiments in which different regions of the thalamus were stimulated electrically and the effects on electrical activity of the cerebral cortex observed. Stimulation of sensory relay nuclei produced responses limited to the cortical projection areas, whereas stimulation of interposed nuclei produced widespread activation of the cortex, which increased with increasing repetitive stimulation. These were identified as *nonspecific thalamic nuclei,* and their responses were termed *recruiting responses.*

The link between the brainstem system and the thalamic system was discovered by Giuseppe Moruzzi of the University of Pisa and Horace Magoun of UCLA in 1949 (Appendix 11.1). They found that high-frequency stimulation in the core of the brainstem produces arousal in the cerebral cortex. The sites in the brainstem were found to correlate with a diffuse system of cells extending from the medulla to the diencephalon. It appeared that this *reticular formation* functions as a *reticular activating system.* Lesions of the reticular formation produce a state of deep sleep and block the arousal that is usually produced by stimulation of specific somatosensory pathways, which send collaterals to the brainstem reticular formation and to the thalamic nonspecific nuclei.

Putting all of this together, sensory stimulation activates the specific sensory pathway leading to perception and the nonspecific pathway through the reticular activating system to the arousal that alerts the cortex so that conscious perception can take place, as summarized in the diagram from the classic paper of Starzl et al. (1951) (Fig. 11.1).

This characterized the phenomena of arousal, attention, and consciousness studied in global terms, which is relevant to the understanding and clinical management of patients in coma and the assessment of brain death. In the 1990s the neural basis of consciousness began to be taken as a serious subject for research at the level of the cortex itself, due to the work of Francis Crick, Christof Koch, and others. Current work is focused on more specific aspects of consciousness related to conscious movement and perception.

Sleep and Rapid Eye Movements

The traditional view of sleep, expressed by Shakespeare in the words of Macbeth, was that it is a passive restorative state of the brain.

> Sleep, that knits up the ravelled Sleeve of Care,
> The death of each day's Life, sore Labor's Bath,
> Balm of hurt Minds, great nature's second course,
> Chief nourisher in Life's Feast.
>
> *(II, ii)*

As such, it attracted relatively little interest among physiologists. One of the few was Nathaniel Kleitman at Chicago, whose research in the 1930s and 1940s gave physiological support to the traditional view. However, experiments by one of his graduate students, Eugene Aserinsky, overturned this view, showing for the first time the alternating states of activity that occur in the brain, starting the modern study of sleep. The way this came about gives revealing insights into how graduate research was carried out in the 1950s, in contrast to today, and is a case study in the sometimes strained relations between a student and his mentor.

Eugene Aserinsky. Eugene Aserinsky (Fig. 11.2) was about as unlikely a prospect to play the role of revolutionary, or in fact any role at all, in science as one could imagine, as he himself records in a memoir (Aserinsky, 1995). Born in Brooklyn in 1921, he grew up in a borderline poor family. He graduated from high school at 16 and started college but lost interest. Over the next 12 years he tried several jobs, was in the army briefly, married, and had a child. Finally, in 1949, with the help of the G.I. bill, he decided on a career in science. Though without a college degree, he persuaded the University of Chicago to let him take the graduate entrance exam, performed brilliantly, and was admitted. (Our modern rigidly structured admissions procedures would have made this impossible.)

Most of the faculty at that time were cell physiologists, participating in launching the new era of research at the cellular level; but Aserinsky wanted to do organ physiology (not the first nor the last time he went against the grain). The only faculty member available for this was Kleitman. Aserinsky was immediately uncomfortable in the presence of this senior professor with an authoritative manner and never developed a normal working relation with him. Kleitman had read a casual observation that falling asleep by an infant was associated with blinking movements of the eyelids and suggested that Aserinsky follow this up. For equipment Aserinsky was given an empty laboratory room, a reclining chair, and an ancient smoked drum apparatus (kymograph) for mechanical recording of blinking. From then on he was on his own: no collaboration, no other students to work with, no graduate courses, no journal clubs, etc.—a common experience in graduate training in those days, as we have noted.

For several months he attempted to observe and quantitate blinking movements in infants, but no pattern emerged. He then decided in desperation to observe all movements of the eyes throughout the night. It became an exhausting project, requiring not only staying up all night but also analyzing the recording data during the day. Meanwhile, at home, life was difficult: a second child was born, his wife was suffering depression, there was frequently not enough food. At times he was about to give up.

However, at the laboratory, he began to get indications of 20-minute "no eye movement" periods. These results in infants emboldened him to begin experiments on adults, for which he was able to find an aging electronic polygraph, with channels for multiple recording electrodes to record the movements of the eyes (the electro-oculogram) and the brain waves from the scalp (the electro-encephalogram, EEG). The polygraph was so unreliable that for a long time it was not clear whether deflections of the pens during the all-night sessions were due to specific signals from the eyes and scalp, to electrical artifacts from the machine or the electrodes, or to movement artifacts of the body muscles. When those problems were sorted out, the evidence began to emerge that the eyes were undergoing periods of saccadic-like movements, *saccades* being the way our eyes jump when we are watching a moving object go by.

Aserinsky was aware of the long history of people linking movements of the body and the eyes in sleep to having dreams (as if the sleeper is watching an internal movie or acting it out) and began waking up his subjects when they were having eye movement episodes and querying them on whether they were dreaming. He began to be able to identify specific "rapid eye movement periods" of around 20 minutes, associated with the dreaming state. He reported his progress to Kleitman, who encouraged him to be sure to eliminate any possibility of artifacts in the recordings. Kleitman also assigned a medical student, William Dement, to help him with the all-night experiments and provided them with a movie camera to record the sleep sessions. The pattern began to come together of an initial period of falling asleep, followed by "rapid eye movement" periods alternating with "no eye movement" periods.

In the spring of 1953 Aserinsky and Kleitman briefly reported their finding at the annual meeting of biologists in Atlantic City. A short report was published in *Science* on September 4 of that year: "Regularly Occurring Periods of Eye Motility, and Concomitant Phenomena, During Sleep" (Aserinsky and Kleitman, 1953; Appendix 11.2). They note for the first time eye movements during sleep as "rapid, jerky, and binocularly symmetrical (273)." They correlate these statistically with dreams: "the ability to recall dreams is significantly associated with the presence of the eye movements (274)." They further correlate these periods with increased rate of respiration and heart rate as well as bodily movements. They conclude (274):

> The fact that these eye movements, EEG pattern, and autonomic nervous system activity are significantly related and do not occur randomly suggests that these physiological phenomena, and probably dreaming, are very

likely all manifestations of a particular level of cortical activity which is encountered normally during sleep. An eye movement period first appears about 3 hr after going to sleep, recurs 2 hrs later, and then emerges at somewhat closer intervals a third or fourth time shortly prior to awakening. This method furnishes the means of determining the incidence and duration of periods of dreaming.

A full paper in the *Journal of Applied Physiology* in 1955 by Aserinsky and Kleitman, entitled "Two Types of Ocular Motility Occurring in Sleep," provided fuller documentation of these patterns (Fig. 11.3, Appendix 11.3). In the opening paragraph the authors formulate an anatomical and physiological rationale for the presence of eye movements during sleep:

> One is led to suspect that the activity of the extra-ocular musculature and the lids might be peculiarly sensitive indicators of CNS changes associated with the sleep–wakefulness cycle. The disproportionately large cortical areas involved in eye movements, the well-defined secondary vestibular pathways to the extra-ocular nuclei, and the low innervation ratio of the eye muscles point to at least a quantitative basis for their reflection of general CNS activity. A more specific relationship of ocular motility to fluctuations in the sleep–wakefulness cycle is suggested by the anatomical proximity of the oculomotor nuclei to a pathway involved in maintaining the waking state [the reference here is to an anatomy textbook] and by the oddity that the orbicularis oculi contracts during sleep while other skeletal muscles relax (p 1) . . .

The authors conclude that they have described "A new type of ocular activity termed 'rapid eye movements' during sleep," associated with a 10% increase in heart rate, a 20% increase in respiratory rate, a low-voltage EEG pattern over the frontal and occipital areas of the brain (a pattern resembling that during waking), increased activity of the body musculature including the face, and occasional vocalizations. "Through interrogation of the subjects and from other indications, it is believed that the rapid eye movements were involved in visual imagery accompanying dreaming."

In this paper the term "rapid eye movements" is used routinely for the first time to describe the jerky saccade-like eye movements. The acronym "REM" sleep soon followed in the literature, as well as other terms such as "dream sleep" and "paradoxical sleep" (the paradox being the heightened arousal occurring during the sleeping state). Dement and Kleitman (1957a, 1957b) soon correlated more precisely the successive periods of deep and REM sleep with characteristic changes in the EEG, which became a valuable tool in sleep research, with Dement becoming a leading authority.

By then Aserinsky had left sleep research. In need of a job, he left immediately after receiving his degree in 1953 and found one on the faculty of Jefferson Medical College. Later in the 1960s he returned to the field he had created,

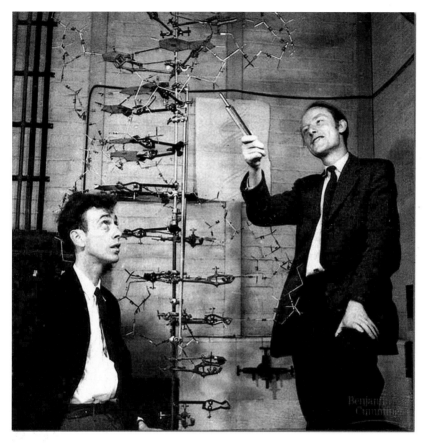

Figure 2.1 James Watson, Francis Crick, and DNA model, 1953. With permission from A. Barrington Brown / Photo Researchers, Inc.

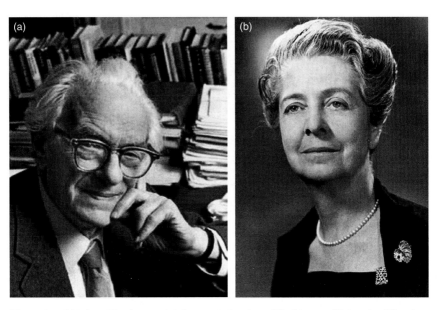

Figure 3.1 *(a)* Viktor Hamburger. With permission from Washington University Libraries, Department of Special Collections, University Archives. *(b)* Rita Levi-Montalcini. With permission from the Becker Medical Library, Washington University School of Medicine.

An *in vitro* Assay: the Halo effect

Chick embryonic tissue + ganglia

Sarcoma + ganglia at 24 hours

Sarcoma + ganglia at 48 hours

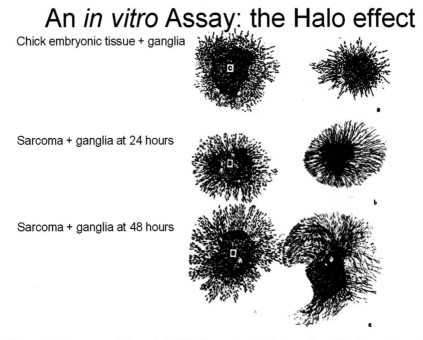

Figure 3.2 Nerve growth factor's (NGF) effect on isolated tissue. From Hamburger V., and Levi-Montalcini R., 1949, with permission from John Wiley & Sons Ltd.

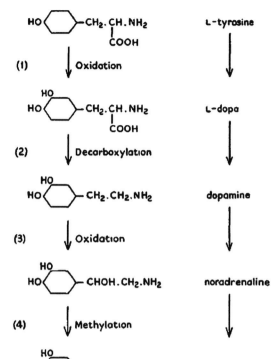

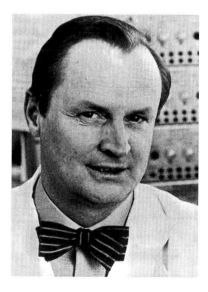

Figure 4.1 Catecholamine synthesis pathway. Blaschko (1957), with permission.

Figure 4.2 Arvid Carlsson. © AP Images.

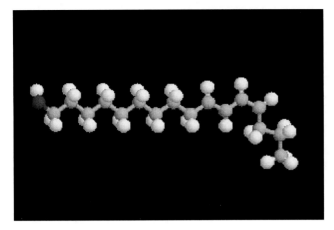

Figure 4.3 Bombykol molecule: the first identified pheromone. With permission from Gerard DuPuis: http://www.faidherbe.org/site/cours/dupuis/accueil.htm.

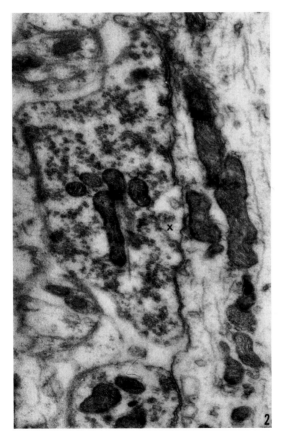

Figure 5.1 Electron micrograph of a synapse. © Palay (1956), with permission.

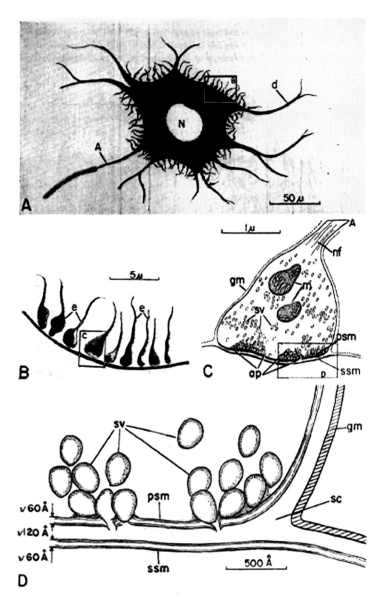

Figure 5.2 Diagrams summarizing the structure of the synapse. A. Representative motor neuron covered with synaptic terminals. B. Higher magnification of synaptic terminals. C. Fine structure of a synaptic terminal. D. High magnification of a presumed site of vesicle release. De Robertis (1959), with permission from Elsevier.

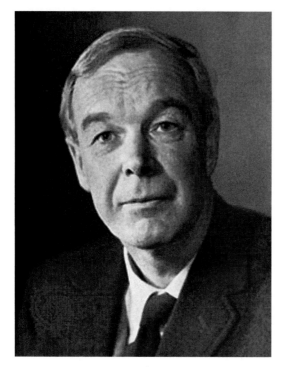

Figure 6.1A Alan Hodgkin.
© The Royal Society with
permission.

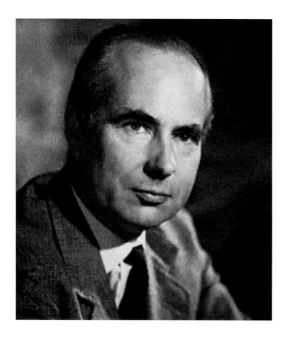

Figure 6.1B Andrew Huxley.
© The Royal Society with
permission.

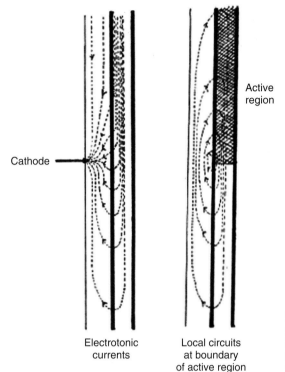

Cathode ──

Active
region

Electrotonic
currents

Local circuits
at boundary
of active region

Figure 6.2 Diagram of local circuits in a nerve fiber. Hodgkin (1937b), with permission from John Wiley & Sons Ltd.

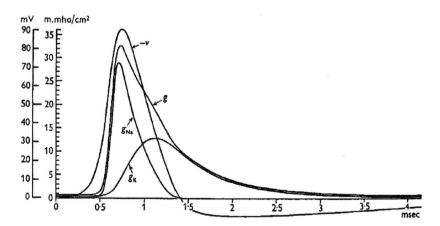

Figure 6.3 The Hodgkin-Huxley model of the action potential. Key to abbreviations: v, action potential; g, overall change in membrane conductance underlying the action potential; g_{Na}, sodium ion conductance; g_K, potassium ion conductance. Hodgkin and Huxley (1952d), with permission from John Wiley & Sons Ltd.

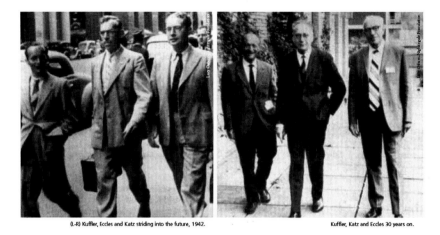

(L-R) Kuffler, Eccles and Katz striding into the future, 1942.   Kuffler, Katz and Eccles 30 years on.

Figure 7.1 *Left* (*left* to *right*), Steven Kuffler, John Eccles, and Bernard Katz in Sydney, Australia, during World War II. *Right*, Kuffler, Eccles, and Katz 30 years later. Used with permission.

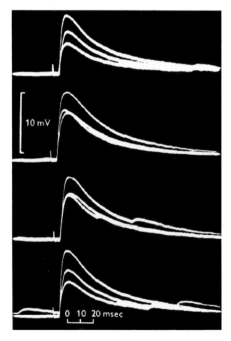

Figure 7.2 End-plate potentials and miniature end-plate potentials. del Castillo and Katz (1954b), with permission from John Wiley & Sons Ltd.

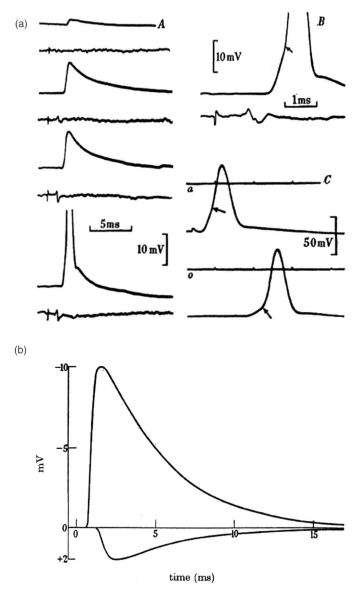

Figure 7.3 (a) Excitatory postsynaptic potentials (EPSPs) giving rise to an action potential (next to bottom trace). B, C. Rise of an action potential from an EPSP. (b) Comparison of an excitatory postsynaptic potential (above) and inhibitory postsynaptic potential (below). Time in milliseconds (thousandths of a second). Brock et al. (1952), with permission from the Royal Society.

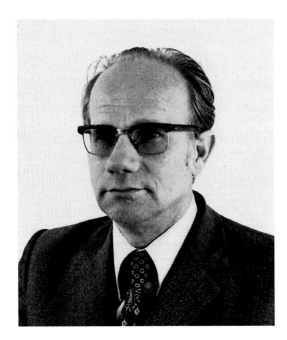

Figure 7.4 Ladislav Tauc. From Israel, M., 2000, with permission from Elsevier.

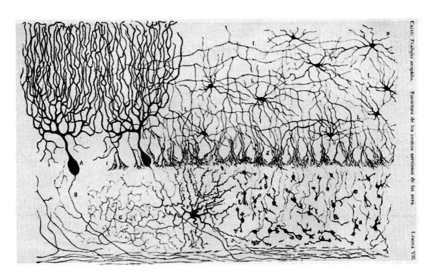

Figure 8.1 Classical Golgi stain of the cerebellum by Ramón y Cajal (1911). Copyright by Herederos de Santiago Ramón y Cajal. Used with permission.

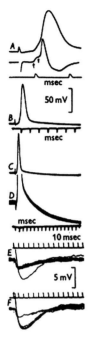

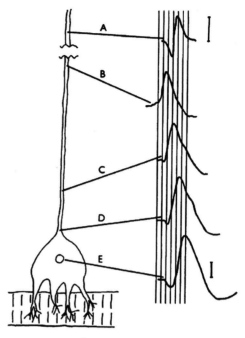

Figure 8.2 Summary of synaptic integration in the neuron, leading to action potential initiation in the initial segment of the axon of the spinal motor neuron. Eccles (1957), with permission from Springer Science + Business Media.

Figure 8.3 Impulse initiation in the axon (site B) in the crayfish stretch receptor. Edwards and Ottoson (1958), with permission from John Wiley & Sons Ltd.

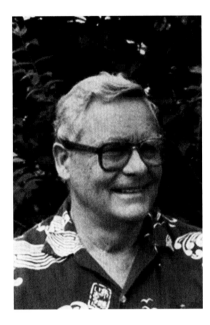

Figure 8.4 Wilfrid Rall. Photo Courtesy of Madelyn Rall Badger.

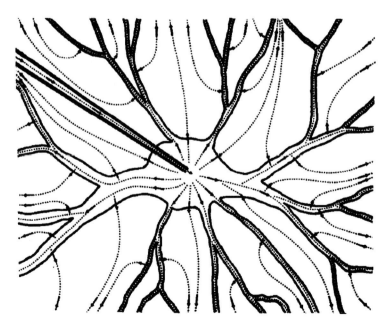

Figure 8.5 Local current spread from an intracellular electrode in neuronal dendrites. Rall (1959), with permission from Elsevier.

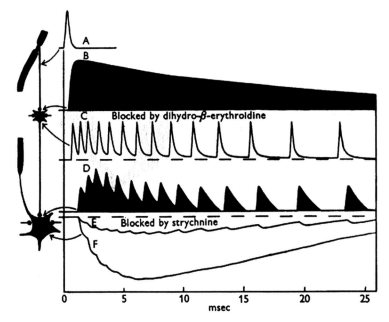

Figure 9.1 Demonstration of the pathway for Renshaw inhibition in the spinal cord. *A.* Incoming impulse in the dorsal root fiber. *B.* EPSP in an interneuron. *C.* Prolonged impulse discharge of an interneuron. *D.* Prolonged EPSP in a motoneuron. *E.* Weak inhibitory postsynaptic response to a weak incoming input. *F.* Strong inhibitory postsynaptic response to strong input. Eccles et al. (1954), with permission from John Wiley & Sons Ltd.

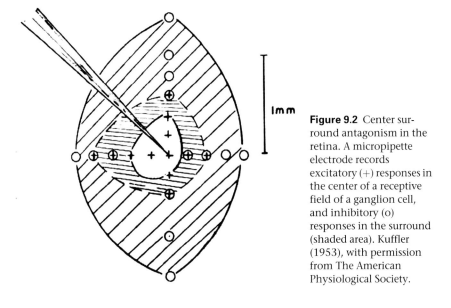

Figure 9.2 Center surround antagonism in the retina. A micropipette electrode records excitatory (+) responses in the center of a receptive field of a ganglion cell, and inhibitory (o) responses in the surround (shaded area). Kuffler (1953), with permission from The American Physiological Society.

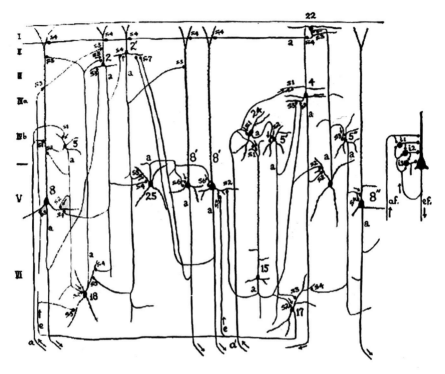

Figure 10.1 Summary of neuronal connections in the cerebral cortex. Lorente de No (1938), with permission.

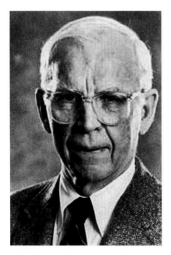

Figure 10.2 Vernon Mountcastle. Photo used with permission from Vernon Mountcastle.

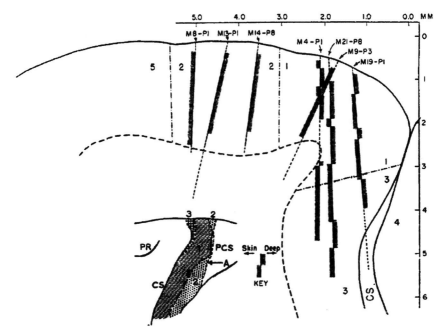

Figure 10.3 Demonstration of the cortical column in the somatosensory cortex. Powell, Thomas, and Mountcastle, 1959, reprinted with permission of The Johns Hopkins University Press.

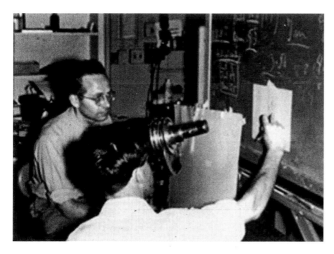

Figure 10.4 David Hubel and Torsten Wiesel, experimenting at the rig. With permission from David Hubel.

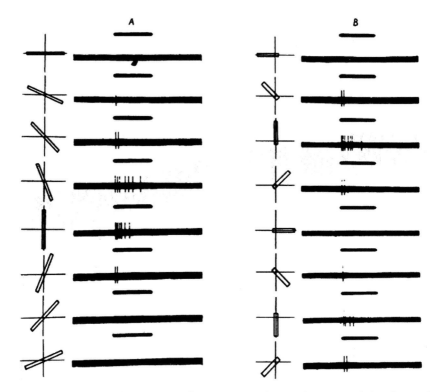

Figure 10.5 Directionally selective cell responses in the visual cortex. Hubel and Wiesel (1959) with permission from John Wiley & Sons Ltd.

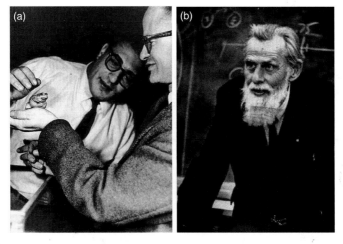

Figure 10.6 *(a)* Jerome Lettvin and Walter Pitts. Copyright © 2000, 2001, 2002 Free Software Foundation, Inc. *(b)* Warren McCulloch. From Moreno-Diaz, R and Moreno-Diaz, A., 2007, with permission from Elsevier.

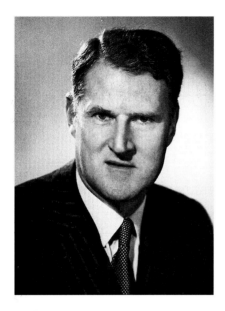

Figure 10.7 Charles Phillips. © The Godfrey Argent Studio.

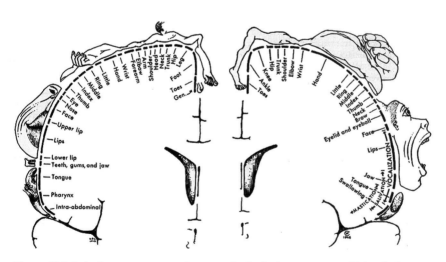

Figure 10.8 Left, the somatosensory homunculus in the human cortex. Right, the human motor homunculus. Penfield and Rasmussen © 1950 Gale, a part of Cengage Learning, Inc. Reproduced by permission. www.cengage.com/permissions.

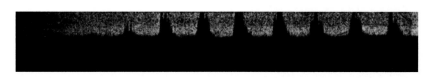

Figure 10.9 Cell responses in the rabbit olfactory bulb to odor stimulation. Adrian (1953), with permission from John Wiley & Sons Ltd.

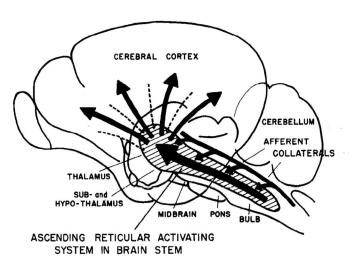

Figure 11.1 Diagram of reticular activation system. Starzl et al. (1951), with permission from The American Physiological Society.

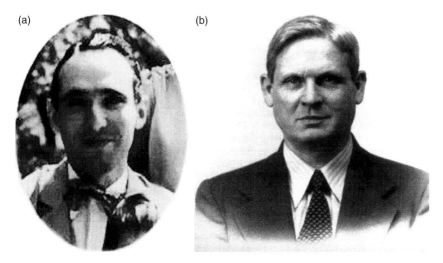

Figure 11.2 *(a)* Eugene Aserinsky. With permission from Le Sommeil, les Reves et l'Eveil. *(b)* Nathaniel Kleitman. Photo Courtesy of William Dement. http://ead.lib.uchicago.edu/view.xqy?id=ICU.SPCL.NKLEITMAN&q=Samuel+-King&page=7

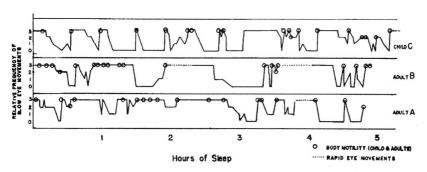

Figure 11.3 Recordings of periods of rapid-eye movement (REM) sleep. Aserinsky and Kleitman (1955), with permission from The American Physiological Society.

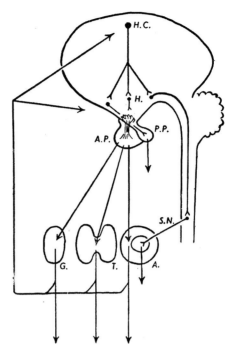

Figure 11.4 Diagram of the hypothalamic–pituitary portal system. Abbreviations: H.C.- human cortex; H.- hypothalamus; A.P.- anterior pituitary; P.P.- posterior pituitary; S.N.- spinal nerve; G.- growth hormone target; T.- thyroid gland; A.- adrenal gland. Harris (1955), with permission.

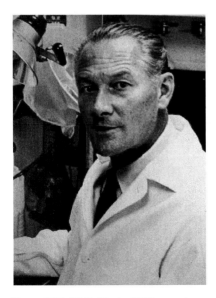

Figure 11.5 Walle Nauta. With permission from The National Academies Press.

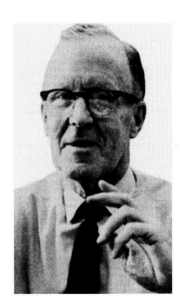

Figure 12.1 Donald Hebb. Reprinted from *The Cerebral Code* by William H. Calvin, published by the MIT Press.

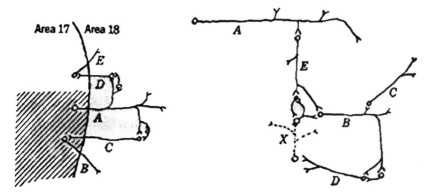

Figure 12.2 The cell assembly and the Hebbian synapse. Hebb (1949), with permission.

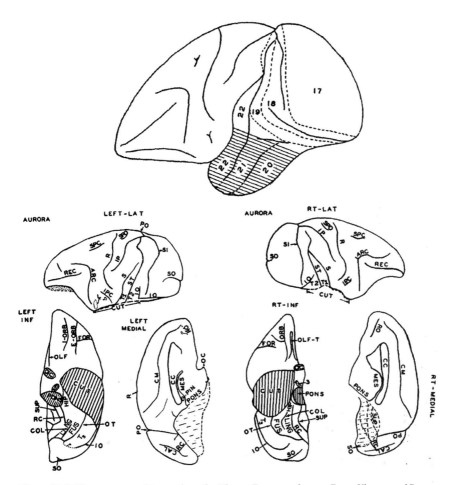

Figure 12.3 Tissue removed to produce the Kluver-Bucy syndrome. From Kluver and Bucy, 1955, with permission from John Wiley & Sons Ltd.

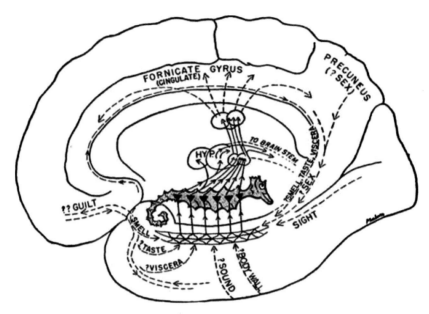

Figure 12.4 Diagram of the limbic system. MacLean and Delgado (1953), with permission from Elsevier.

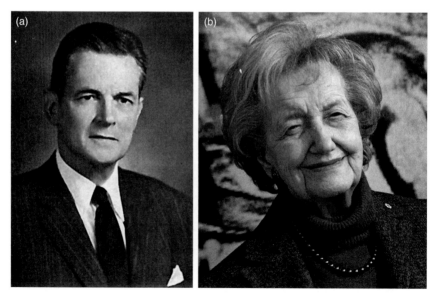

Figure 12.5 *(a)* William Scoville. With permission from Massachusetts General Hospital. *(b)* Brenda Milner. Photo with permission from Brenda Milner.

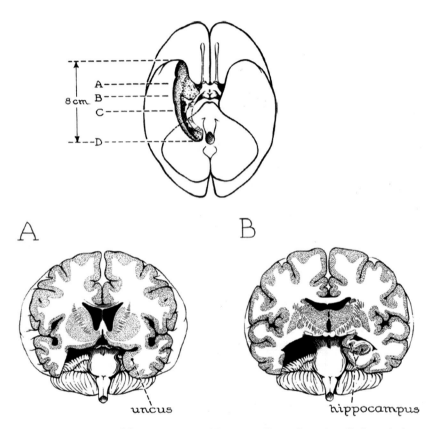

Figure 12.6 Diagrams of the tissue presumably removed by William Scoville from the brain of H. M. Scoville and Milner (1957), with permission from BMJ Publishing Group Ltd.

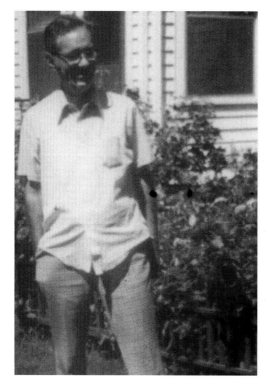

Figure 12.7 Photo of H. M. Photo courtesy of Suzanne Corkin.

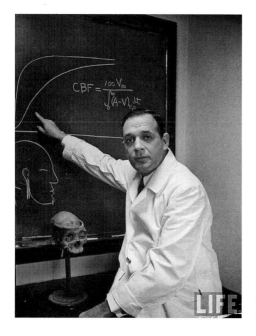

Figure 13.1 Seymour Kety. Alfred Eisenstaedt / Getty Images used with permission.

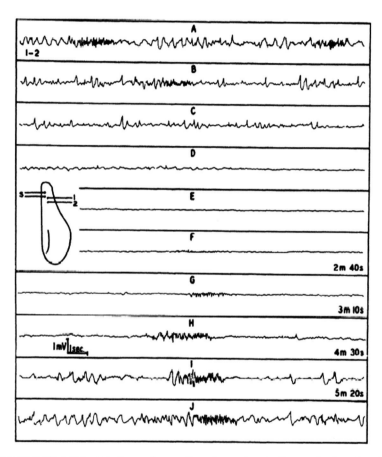

Figure 13.2 Electrical recordings of spreading depression in the cerebral cortex. Leão (1944a), used with permission from The American Physiological Society.

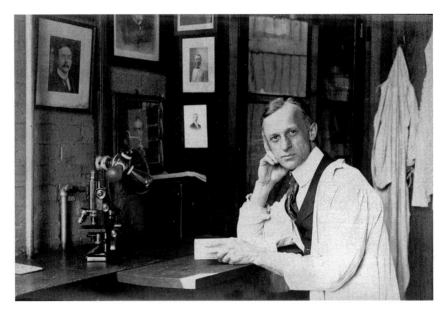

Figure 14.1 Harvey Cushing. Courtesy of The Alan Mason Chesney Medical Archives of the Johns Hopkins Medical Institutions.

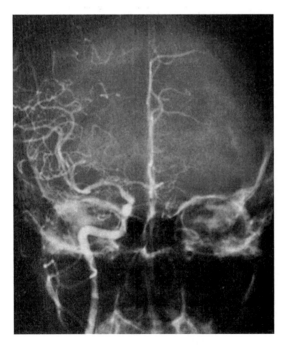

Figure 14.2 X-ray of cerebral angiography. Petty et al., 1996, used with permission from Dowden Health Media.

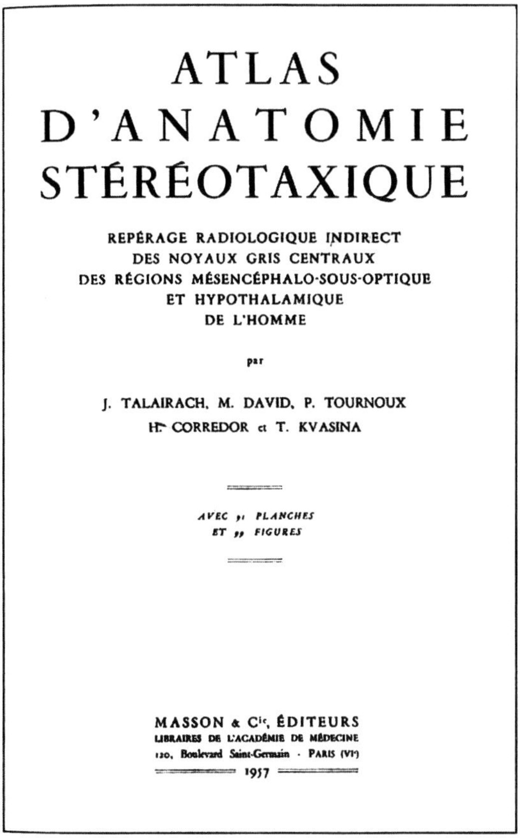

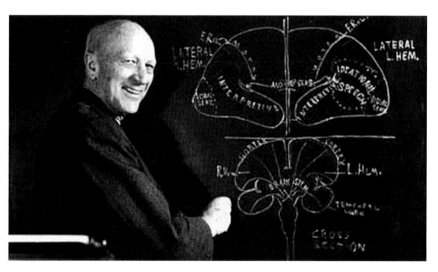

ATLAS D'ANATOMIE STÉRÉOTAXIQUE

REPÉRAGE RADIOLOGIQUE INDIRECT
DES NOYAUX GRIS CENTRAUX
DES RÉGIONS MÉSENCÉPHALO-SOUS-OPTIQUE
ET HYPOTHALAMIQUE
DE L'HOMME

par

J. TALAIRACH, M. DAVID, P. TOURNOUX
H. CORREDOR et T. KVASINA

AVEC 91 PLANCHES
ET 99 FIGURES

MASSON & Cie, ÉDITEURS
LIBRAIRES DE L'ACADÉMIE DE MÉDECINE
120, Boulevard Saint-Germain · PARIS (VIe)
1957

Figure 14.3 Title page of Talairach's brain atlas. With permission from Elsevier.

Figure 14.4 Wilder Penfield. With permission of the curator of the Wilder Penfield Archive, Montreal Neurological Institute.

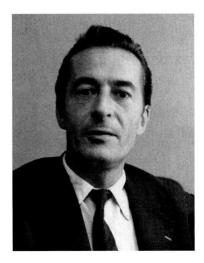

Figure 15.1A Henri Laborit. With permission from the Laborit family.

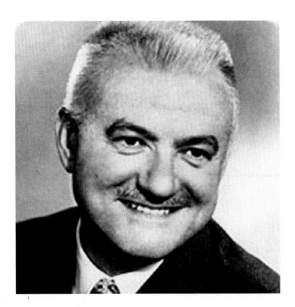

Figure 15.1B Pierre Deniker. Courtesy of the Albert and Mary Lasker Foundation.

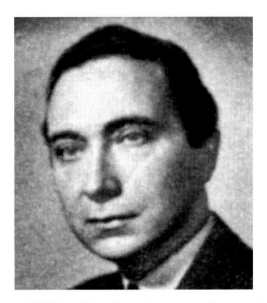

Figure 15.1C Jean Delay. From histrecmed with permission.

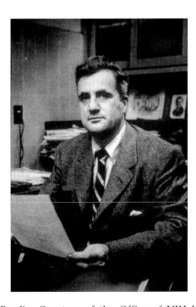

Figure 15.1D Bernard Brodie. Courtesy of the Office of NIH History at The National Institutes of Health, Bethesda, MD.

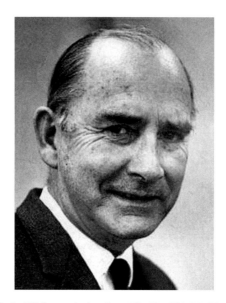

Figure 15.2A John Cade. With permission from *The Herald & Weekly Times Limited* and the State Library of Victoria.

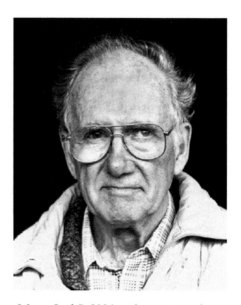

Figure 15.2B Mogens Schou. Grof, P. 2006, with permission from Nature Publishing Group.

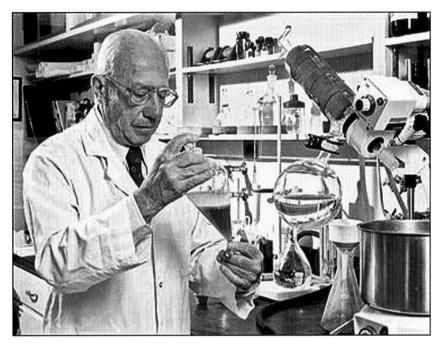

Figure 15.3 Leo Sternbach. With permission from the Associated Press.

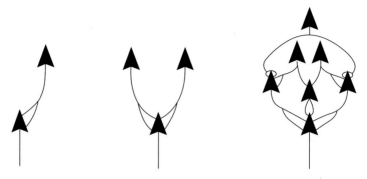

Figure 16.1 Diagrams of oversimplified neurons and neuronal connections performing logic operations. From McCulloch and Pitts (1943), with permission from Springer.

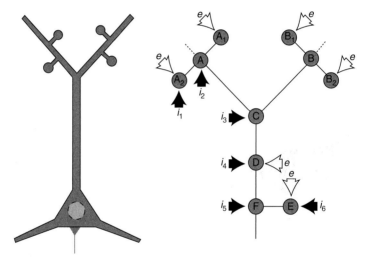

Figure 16.2 *Left* Schematic diagram of a cortical pyramidal neuron with branching dendritic tree and representative synaptic spines. *Right* Pyramidal neuron as a branching system of nodes for logic operations. e, excitatory synapse; i, inhibitory synapse; A–F, sites for integration of dendritic logic gates. Adapted from Shepherd, 1989 with permission from Elsevier.

working on physiological differences between REM and non-REM sleep; but the field had forgotten him. He had turned his back on the field and on keeping up contacts with people doing sleep research. As a consequence, "out of sight, out of mind." Kleitman, Dement, and others became recognized as the pioneers of sleep research, a fact that Aserinsky deeply resented. It was only in the 1990s that reconciliation and recognition came, shortly before his death from a traffic accident.

In summary, Aserinsky's graduate studies, carried out largely single-hand-edly, radically changed our understanding of sleep, from a passive resting and restoration of the brain to an alternation of actively interacting brain regions and circuits. Ironically, Kleitman, for his part, never gave up the Shakespearean view, continuing to think of REM sleep as simply a modified period of restoration during normal sleep. "Kleitman died still believing there was only one state of sleep," Dement told an interviewer (Brown, 2003, 97). But for most brain scientists and neurologists, it was the opening of a new world. In the 1960s and 1970s Michel Jouvet in France characterized the different brain regions and their neurotransmitters involved in sleep. This was followed by identification of alternating brain circuits supporting the different stages of sleep by Alan Hobson, John McCarley, and others.

At the 1995 meeting of the Associated Professional Sleep Societies, 2000 sleep investigators were in the audience when Aserinsky, Kleitman, and Dement came together to be honored. And at the meeting of those same societies in 2003, on the fiftieth anniversary of the discovery, the audience had grown to nearly 5000 and Dement invoked Lincoln's Gettysburg Address to mark the occasion in semiseriousness (Brown, 2003, 97): "Two score and ten years ago Aserinsky and Kleitman brought forth on this continent a new discipline conceived at night and dedicated to the proposition that sleep is equal to waking." The audience enthusiastically agreed.

Operant Conditioning by Brain Self-Stimulation

During the early twentieth century, operant conditioning emerged as the dominant form of behavioral analysis, exemplified by the Skinner box, in which a thirsty animal pressed a lever to learn a behavior and receive a liquid reward. A new approach to learning was introduced by another graduate student, working at the same time as Aserinsky but in another country, Canada, and under more collegial circumstances.

This was James Olds, working on his graduate thesis with Peter Milner in the laboratory of Donald Hebb at McGill University in Montreal. In their classical paper (Olds and Milner, 1954; Appendix 11.4), they let the animal press a lever to deliver electrical stimulation to different parts of the core of the brain. With the stimuli in certain areas, the rats would press the bar repetitively many times, presumably indicating that the shocks were functioning as rewards, in other words were "reinforcing," in a way equivalent to that in classical conditioning experiments. The acquisition and extinction curves compared favorably with those produced by conventional operant conditioning. By mapping out the central brain structures, Olds and Milner found that reinforcement was highest in central basal regions of the forebrain roughly corresponding to the medial forebrain bundle, most sensitive in the septal area but extending up to the cingulate gyrus of the cerebral cortex. The method was called *operant conditioning by brain self-stimulation*.

The finding of Olds and Milner has been characterized as "one of those rare scientific discoveries that starts a new field" (Rosenzweig et al., 1996, 540). We are seeing that the 1950s were full of these rare events. The rewarding effects of brain self-stimulation were shown in many different species, including humans, who reported feelings of pleasure, warmth, and even sexual excitement (Breedlove et al., 1996, 540). There has been speculation that brain self-stimulation identifies specific "reward circuits" that use dopamine as their transmitter, but the evidence has been controversial (Rosenzweig et al., 1996, 541).

Hypothalamus and Feeding Behavior

Classical concepts about neural mechanisms involved in feeding originated in studies in which lesions were created in different hypothalamic regions.

"Dual-Center" Hypothesis of Feeding. It was first found that lesions of the ventromedial hypothalamus (VMH) produced an animal that overeats and becomes obese (Hetherington and Ranson, 1940). This was demonstrated initially in the rat and subsequently in many species. It was therefore concluded that the VMH is a "satiety center" that is normally activated by eating to satiety, which shuts down eating. Further studies by John Brobeck at the University of Pennsylvania found that lesions of the lateral hypothalamus (LH) produce animals that stop eating (Anand and Brobeck, 1951a, 1951b). This suggested that the LH is a "feeding center." The two findings were put together by Eliot Stellar at Penn in the *dual-center hypothesis of feeding*, in which feeding is due to LH activity, which becomes increasingly suppressed by VMH activity as eating reaches satiety (Stellar, 1957) (Appendix 11.5).

It was soon realized that the centers are not easily defined and consist instead of cells concentrated in the hypothalamic region but spreading out widely in the brain. The fibers of the medial forebrain bundle run through these regions, confounding attempts to localize specific functions. Other mechanisms have also risen to prominence, such as the individual controls of carbohydrate, fat, and amino acids. Nonetheless, hunger and satiety define the axis of feeding behavior, and the dual-center hypothesis has to a great degree defined the problem of feeding control and stimulated most of the research in this area for the past 50 years.

Feeding Control: Jacques Le Magnen. This pioneer of the behavioral analysis of feeding behavior was born in France in 1916. In 1929, at the age of 12, he contracted encephalitis in a world epidemic and lost the sight in both eyes. For many years he was home-taught and developed a prodigious memory. Finally receiving his baccalaureate degree in 1944 in wartime Paris, he was taken on by Henri Pieron, director of the Laboratory of Sensory Physiology at the Collège de France, where he began studies of human olfaction. At that time "it was a field almost devoid of experimental data and procedures, mostly just a few theories" (Le Magnen, 2001, 376). Le Magnen developed olfactometers for measuring volatility, concentration, and rate of inhalation of an olfactory stimulus and applied them to studying differences in smell sensitivity between the sexes. Around 1950 he moved to new quarters in the Collège de France and began studies on the influence of olfaction on feeding behavior in rats, the experiments being carried out by technical assistants. According to Bellisle, Laffort and Köster (2003, 85):

> Beginning in 1950, Jacques Le Magnen put forward a series of revolutionary concepts. His ideas have inspired and still inspire generations of scientists. He was the first to develop instruments that made it possible to register food and water intake in the rat across the whole 24 h day, and to show how the behavior and its determinants change under the influence of circadian cycles. During the phase of activity (the night in the rat), intake permits the build up of bodily reserves which will be used in the resting phase, during which consumption is reduced to a minimum. This day/night alternation is one of the cornerstones of energetic and hydro-mineral regulation. During the daily active period, meals alternate with fasting in response to metabolic signals that are generated by the acquisition of the ingesta and by the composition of bodily reserves. In all this, the role of the sensory characteristics of food, olfactory of course, but also gustatory and visual, was not forgotten. In what he called "learning of palatability," Jacques Le Magnen showed how the sensory characteristics of food transform themselves into a complex conditioned stimulus that guides behavior, permits the formation of food preferences and aversions, and determines the size of a meal depending on the anticipated metabolic consequences of ingestion. Furthermore, his laboratory confirmed that the same sensory and metabolic factors also function in humans.

Food as a "complex conditioned stimulus" meant that intake is the outcome of a balance between hunger and satiating factors in the sensory qualities of the food: He found that removal of an odor in a food to which the animal has been conditioned elicits an immediate increase in intake (the odor becomes a satiating factor), as does changing the odor of a food (which acts to stimulate the appetite). Food intake is thus dynamically controlled by food flavor, a fact not lost on the food and flavor industries in their efforts to maximize food consumption. Le Magnen's pioneering concepts became better known worldwide after he began to attract graduate students in the 1960s (including Paul Laffort, Stylianos Nikolaidis, and Patrick MacLeod) and from the 1970s published in English.

I experienced Le Magnen's prodigious memory at the International Society for Olfaction and Taste meeting in Paris in 1977. Although I came for a visit unannounced, he instantly recognized me and discussed some of my work, aided no doubt by the 30,000 Braille cards he is reported to have assembled from the literature. In addition to his memory, his other great asset was his wife Regine, who was always by his side.

Neurosecretory Cells: The Brain as a Gland

In 1928, Ernst Scharrer reported (see Scharrer, 1987) that in the hypothalamus of a teleost fish there were nerve cells which resembled gland cells in containing large amounts of material similar to that of known secretory cells such as the insulin-producing beta cells of the pancreas. Scharrer called these *neurosecretory cells* and suggested that they function as endocrine cells inside the nervous system and that their secretions might be related to the nearby pituitary gland.

At the time ideas about nervous activity were exclusively in terms of electrical activity. As recalled by Berta Scharrer (1987, 2) (Appendix 11.6),

> ... initially the idea that neurons may be capable of dispatching neurohormonal, i.e. blood-borne, signals, an activity heretofore attributed only to endocrine cells proper, met with powerful resistance. It did not conform with the tenets of the neuron doctrine, and the fact that it was proposed on the basis of cytological evidence was considered preposterous.

Comparative studies showed that groups of neurosecretory cells are present in the nervous systems of both invertebrates and vertebrates, including humans. The analogy between the hypothalamic–hypophyseal system of vertebrates and the brain–corpus cardiacum–corpus allatum system of insects was recognized (Scharrer and Scharrer, 1944), indicating the presence in both invertebrates and vertebrates of master glands coordinating brain control over multiple hormones. With the advent of the electron microscope it was possible to visualize clearly the large electron-dense secretory granules in the secretory cells and their similarity with granules in gland cells of the body and to understand how in both cases the granules (dense-core vesicles) arise from the Golgi body (Scharrer and Brown, 1961).

From that time on, there has been an evolution of the concept of the nervous system, from being dominated almost entirely by electrical activity to a view of the brain as containing cells with all the properties of secretory cells as well as their electrical activity. Today, we realize increasingly that the brain is a gland as well as a computer.

The Hypothalamic–Neurohypophyseal System

Although in this new concept all nerve cells are secretory as well as electrical, the pituitary gland is recognized as the master gland and as being controlled by the activity in a deep region of the brain overlying it called the "hypothalamus." It was long recognized that the pituitary body has two parts, an anterior part that appeared to be glandular and a posterior part that appeared to be an extension from cells in the hypothalamus. The solution to how control over these parts of the pituitary body is exerted was one of the great sleuthing stories of the 1950s.

The relation between the hypothalamus and the underlying pituitary gland has a long and complicated history. The nerve fiber tract arising in cells of the hypothalamus and connecting through the pituitary stalk to the posterior pituitary was described by Ramón y Cajal (1894), who suggested that the fibers carry sensory signals from the posterior pituitary to the hypothalamus. However, the hormonal nature of the posterior pituitary gland quickly gained attention because at about the same time it was shown that extracts of the posterior pituitary increased vascular tone and blood pressure (Oliver and Schafer, 1895). The active substance in such an extract came to be called a "hormone," from the Greek for "arouse into activity, to urge on." The term was suggested by W. B. Hardy "and although the property of a messenger is not suggested by this term, it was finally adopted" (Harris, 1955, 1),

Identifying the posterior pituitary hormones became part of the new field of *endocrinology*, concerned with identifying the hormones secreted by different glands and actions on their target tissues and organs. During the early part of the twentieth century, these studies were carried out in parallel with the studies of neurotransmitters in the autonomic system (see Chapter 4). In both cases, methods were limited to the organ level, either making extracts of the gland to test its positive effects or, particularly in endocrinology, removing the gland to test for effects of its absence.

A series of studies showed multiple effects of the posterior pituitary extracts, which required the first half of the twentieth century to sort out. Kamm (1928) purified the crude extract and identified two main fractions, each with multiple actions, clarifying the terminology for them. One was an antidiuretic action in both sexes, coupled with the increase in vascular tone as first noted. The active principle of this extract was termed *antidiuretic hormone* (ADH).

The other type of action was in females and related to reproductive behavior. This involved increased uterine motility during coitus (related to transportation of sperm to the ovaries), promoting uterine contractions during parturition and causing contraction of the myoepithelial cells of the mammary glands to cause milk-letdown in response to sensory stimulation of the nipples. This hormone was named *oxytocin* ("quick birth"). Crude extracts were first prepared by Dale (1909) and Ott and Scott (1910). For many years it was difficult to separate the actions of ADH from oxytocin. Were they due to one hormone or several?

It was not until the availability of new biochemical methods around 1950 that Lawler and Du Vigneaud (1953) were able to demonstrate enzymatic cleavage of glycinamide from vasopressin to produce ADH and show that its structure consists of an eight–amino acid peptide. Oxytocin was also synthesized, by Popenoe and Du Vigneaud (1953), and shown to have the expected action on rat and human uterus and human mammary gland. Its structure differed by two amino acids from that of ADH. The identification of these two hypothalamopituitary peptide hormones was a tour de force, following closely the more widely known synthesis of the longer polypeptide insulin by Sanger and Tuppy (1951) see Chapter 4), both preceding the synthesis of nerve growth factor by Stanley Cohen in 1960 (Chapter 3).

How these hormones get to the posterior pituitary gland was also a controversial matter. Bargmann (1951), using the Gomori stain that marks neurosecretory products, was able to trace the fibers arising in the neurosecretory cells of the preoptic and paraventricular nuclei in the posterior hypothalamus through the fiber tract to the posterior pituitary. From that time it has been understood that the hypothalamic cells synthesize hormones in their cell bodies and transport them through their axons in the pituitary stalk to secrete them from their axon terminals in the posterior pituitary into the bloodstream. Even then it needed to be established that the hormones themselves were distinct from the substance visualized by the Gomori stain. Parallel experiments showed that similar principles apply to neurosecretion in the insect (Scharrer, 1952).

Neurophysiological evidence for the functional properties of posterior pituitary cells began with the study of Eric Kandel. After his pioneering study of the hippocampal pyramidal cell with Alden Spencer (Spencer and Kandel, 1961), he undertook while a house officer in psychiatry at Harvard a study of the posterior pituitary cells in the fish. These were the first recordings to show that these cells generate action potentials, which propagate through the axon to bring about release of their peptide hormones in a manner similar to that of neurotransmitter release (Kandel, 1964). He describes in his memoir (Kandel, 2006) how, despite the novelty of this finding, it wasn't going to lead to insights into cellular mechanisms of memory, so he was off to Tauc's laboratory in France to record from *Aplysia* neurons (Chapter 7).

The Hypothalamic–Adenohypophyseal Portal System

The anterior part of the pituitary gland presented an even greater puzzle because it had no direct connection with the overlying hypothalamus. Many experiments involving extirpation (removal) and grafting of the gland into various locations were carried out in the first part of the twentieth century to determine its function. Out of this came the designation of the pituitary as the master gland controlling multiple body functions. These include growth of body cells, salt balance through regulating the adrenal cortex, energy and growth through regulating thyroid function, spermatogenesis and testosterone levels through regulating the testes, and the menstrual cycle and pregnancy through regulating the ovaries. This work belongs more properly to the field of endocrinology. Here, we focus on studies related to identifying the mechanism by which the brain controls this gland.

It was not until 1940 that David Rioch and his collaborators introduced the standard nomenclature for the separate parts of the pituitary gland. In simplified terms, the pituitary stalk protrudes from the hypothalamus, giving rise to hormone-secreting cells of the adenohypophysis situated in the *pars distalis* and hormone-secreting endings of the neurohypophysis in the *infundibular process*.

Blood vessels were found on the pituitary stalk by Fr. I. Rainer (Harris, 1955, 20) in Bucharest. His student G. T. Popa described these vessels and the key point that they terminate in capillaries in both the hypothalamus and the adenohypophysis (Popa, 1930;). Which way does the blood flow in these vessels? They suggested that it flows from the pituitary to the hypothalamus. George Wislocki of Harvard suggested instead that blood flows from the hypothalamus to the pituitary gland, ending in the adenohypophysis (Wislocki and King, 1936). Geoffrey Harris in Oxford then carried out a series of studies which provided definitive evidence for this direction of flow. This included direct microscopic observation of the blood flow in the vessels in anesthetized animals (Green and Harris, 1949). This established the concept of the *hypothalamic–hypophyseal portal system* through which the hypothalamus can regulate anterior pituitary function. These studies are summarized in Harris' classic monograph *Neural Control of the Pituitary Gland* (1955) (Fig. 11.4, Appendix 11.7).

Harris suggested that neurons in the hypothalamus liberate factors into this local vascular system to "regulate the rate of secretion of the anterior pituitary hormone" and asked, "are there as many humoral mechanisms involved as there are hormones?" (Harris 1955, 177) Thus were united, in a stroke, the great systems: nervous system, neuroendocrine system, and endocrine system.

For this work, Harris has been regarded as the "father" of neuroendocrinology; we have seen that the Scharrers have a claim to be co-parents. As noted by Charles Sawyer (1975, 97):

"Harris was not the first to suggest that the adenohypophysis might be controlled by a humoral mechanism involving the hypophysial portal system, but it was the force of his intellect, personality and multifaceted research approach to the problem in the late 1940's and early '50's which really established the neurovascular concept."

Also in suggesting that the hormone is the secreted factor, Harris recognized that it was produced by a precursor and that there was a need for a term to represent the precursor in order to characterize the formation of the hormone and the secreted hormone itself. By 1973 the peptides luteinizing hormone–releasing hormone, thyrotropin-releasing hormone, and somatostatin had been identified as the humoral mechanisms postulated by Harris. Subsequent work has identified all of the anterior pituitary controlling factors and characterized the central humoral and neural pathways that control their release.

Founding Modern Neuroanatomy

While these investigations of the deep structures and functions of the brain were taking place, another quiet revolution was beginning in the form of attempts by a young investigator working almost in isolation to develop a better method to trace the fiber pathways in these regions.

Walle J. H. Nauta. Walle J. H. Nauta (Fig. 11.5) was born in 1916 to Dutch missionaries and community activists on the Malacca Strait in Sumatra, Indonesia (Jones, 2006). He was educated at the University of Leiden, completing his preclinical training in 1937. As a student assistant in the anatomy department, he became interested in brain anatomy and found the hypothalamus particularly fascinating. His description (Nauta, 1993, 1337) of how this interest led to his life's work is interwoven with several other stories in our account of those times:

> The first publications of the Scharrers had just come out, reporting their astonishing observation that cells of the magnocellular nuclei of the hypothalamus combine neural with secretory characteristics [see earlier section, "Neurosecretory Cells: The Brain as a Gland," for the studies of the Scharrers]. The laboratories of S. W. Ranson in Chicago and W. R. Hess in Zurich were reporting a steady stream of intriguing novel findings about the involvement of the hypothalamus in autonomic and endocrine functions, as well as in the sleep–wakefulness cycle. I had also read with admiration Philip Bard's classical paper on "sham rage," a phenomenon clearly implicating the hypothalamus in at least the outward manifestations of anger. And from G. B. Wislocki's laboratories at Harvard had come evidence that the long-sought last link in the efferent pathway connecting the hypothalamus with the anterior pituitary was vascular rather than neural [see earlier section, "The Hypothalamic–Adenohypophyseal Portal System," for the studies of Wislocki]. I thought that these recent findings provided a good reason for an expanded search for the intrinsic and extrinsic fiber connections of the hypothalamus. It seemed to me, moreover, that several of the recent physiological findings were raising anatomical questions that could not be answered in terms of existing anatomical knowledge. And that realization, in turn, led me to think that the anatomy of the brain was a neglected rather than an exhausted subject.

Nauta decided on a project to trace the fiber connections of the hypothalamus by the method of degenerating myelinated fibers introduced many years previously by Vittorio Marchi. This project was delayed by the need to finish his medical studies; then, in May 1940, Holland was overrun by the Nazis as they occupied Europe during World War II, so he was not able to pick up the work until 1942. Unfortunately, the Marchi method gave no results when applied to the hypothalamus because most of the fibers are unmyelinated and the Marchi method stains only the degenerating myelin. What was needed was a method to stain degenerating axons themselves, not the degenerating myelin sheaths. He reasoned that the best chance would lie with a method using deposition of silver in the degenerating axons. Such methods, especially that of Bielschowsky, had been used to demonstrate nerve fibers and terminal structures; but they gave variable results, and Ramón y Cajal's difficulties with them had led him to doubt even the existence of "bouton terminaux" in the cerebral cortex (Nauta, 1993).

In the years after the war, Nauta made a series of attempts to adapt silver methods to degenerating axons but with little luck. While working in Zurich, he came across a paper by Paul Glees, a neuroanatomist at Oxford, who reported a modification of the Bielschowsky method that gave better staining of degenerating axons and terminals. However, Nauta's attempt to reproduce these results failed, possibly because of differences in the tap water of Zurich and Oxford used to make the solutions.

The resolution of the problem came when a chemist graduate student, Paul Gygax, worked with him to adjust the solutions so that there was better staining, but the sections remained murky. How to clear them? It is worth recording Nauta's (1993, 1341) account of how it happened as it illustrates perfectly Pasteur's dictum (Chapter 1), "In the fields of observation, chance favors only the prepared mind":

> After months of frustrating attempts to improve the clarity of the sections, the resolution of the problem finally materialized, suddenly and quite by accident. On a Saturday afternoon in the spring of 1949, I discovered that I had used up all of my fresh formalin and had to make up the reducing solution from a half-empty, cork-stoppered bottle of 10% formalin that I found in an out-of-the-way place, where it had been stored for at least six years. In the reducer made up from this stale formalin the sections to my astonishment slowly turned light brown, and when I examined them in the microscope I saw, for the first time in all those years, a picture of axon degeneration that resembled the one I had been hoping for. I excitedly called Paul Gygax, who arrived a short time later, carrying a fresh supply of formalin and a small bottle of formic acid; it had not taken him more than a minute to figure out that the stale formalin I had mentioned must have had a high concentration of formic acid. A few quick trials with fresh formalin acidified with formic acid bore him out.
>
> With this denouement, the project changed from a series of frustrations to a joyride

The new method was published by Nauta and Gygax in 1951. Several years ensued during which improvements were made (Nauta and Ryan, 1952). By 1952 Nauta had moved to the Walter Reed Army Institute of Research in Washington, D.C., with its renowned laboratory for histology and pathology and a group of outstanding electrophysiologists, (Chapter 10). There, Nauta and Gygax (1954) reported modifications which gave a higher selectivity of staining for degenerating over normal axons. In this form the Nauta method stimulated a new generation of investigators tracing fiber connections in the brain. Nauta's own early studies provided new understanding of the connections of the fornix, amygdala, basal ganglia, and spinothalamic tract (Jones, 2006). Further modifications of the solutions produced enhancements of the selectivity for degenerating fibers and, combined with electron microscopy, enabled identification of the actual degenerating terminals onto postsynaptic targets. Ultimately, a wide range of nondegeneration methods emerged that are used today to identify axons of selected neuron types and their synaptic connections.

Nauta's role in the rise of modern neuroscience has been summarized by Jones (2006):

> his influence was broad, not only on account of his modernizing, almost single handedly, the whole field of experimental neuroanatomy but also because of the influence that he had over so many students and fellow scientists as a collaborator or teacher or as an author of some of the most fundamental papers in neuroscience.

When the Neurosciences Research Program awarded him the F. O. Schmitt Medal and Prize in Neuroscience for 1983, it said (Nauta, 1994) that he

> devised new experimental methods that ... established systems neuroanatomy as a leading discipline in neuroscience.... He more than any other has created the modern science of neuroanatomy.

And to those who were fortunate to know him, he was one of the finest gentlemen to grace any field of science.

Psychology

I end this chapter with brief observations on the contributions of experimental psychology to the conceptual basis of modern neuroscience. Much of the early background is covered by the definitive monograph of Edgar Boring, *A History of Experimental Psychology* (1950).

In brief, learning theory in the early part of the last century was dominated by behavioral psychologists who studied learning by observing laboratory animals carrying out tasks devised by the experimenter. Pavlov's dogs, Watson's conditioning experiments, and Skinner's boxes are leading examples. For these investigators, the brain was a black box, and explanations were sought at the level of abstract principles defined exclusively in psychological terms.

Peter Milner at McGill, a pioneer of biological psychology (see Operant Conditioning by Brain Self-Stimulation), calls this a "bad period" of psychology (Milner, 1999), which persisted in many psychology departments until recently. The "good period" in this view may be said to have begun at midcentury, with the publication of the book of Donald Hebb (1949; see Chapter 12) and the experimental approach to brain mechanisms exemplified by Olds and Milner and others, as noted earlier in this chapter. A big impetus came from studies of brain-damaged patients, which are covered in the next chapter.

Ethology

With the rise of behavioral psychology in the early part of the century the study of natural behavior in the field faded from view. However, this trend was reversed by ethologists whose work became well known at midcentury. First came **Karl von Frisch**, an Austrian zoologist who studied the senses and behavior of bees. He discovered their ability to sense polarized light and deciphered the waggle dance through which a forager bee communicates with its colony. **Konrad Lorenz** was a professor of psychology in Germany who devoted his early career to studying geese, comparing wild, domestic, and hybrid varieties. He was a prisoner of war of the Soviets during 1942–48. After repatriation, he became known to the general public through his summary of his studies of animal behavior in *King Solomon's Ring* (1949; see English translation, 1952), the ring symbolizing Solomon's (and Lorenz's) ability to speak to animals. There is a famous photograph of geese imprinted on Lorenz, waddling in a line after him on his daily walk. A close contemporary was **Niko Tinbergen**, a Dutch biologist who also studied natural behavior. In 1951 he published *The Study of Instinct*, which laid out the case for the importance of instinctual behavior in the wild.

The combined effect of these three pioneers and their books turned attention once again to inbuilt behavior. The culmination of this work in the 1950s was thus a critical step toward the synthesis provided by Edward Wilson in 1975 that gave rise to the new field of *sociobiology*. This in turn merged naturally with, on one hand, the evidence for inbuilt neural systems for central pattern generation, and on the other, the increasing understanding of genes, particularly those that determine or control specific types of behavior. Current concepts of brain function thus combine nature and nurture in order to understand the neural basis of behavior.

Chapter 12

Learning and Memory: Donald Hebb, Brenda Milner, and H. M.

Learning and memory are fundamental to all animal species and the basis for much of human cognitive abilities. The leading hypothesis for the neural basis of learning and memory is due to Donald Hebb, as presented in a textbook in 1949; the activity-dependent Hebb synapse is still the focus of much current research. Research in the 1950s extended cortical studies to the limbic lobe, reporting the first evidence for neural mechanisms in the amygdala and other subcortical structures related to emotional behavior. A new chapter in studies of the brain opened with surgical operations for the relief of epilepsy, which showed the critical role of the hippocampus in memory. Bilateral removal of the hippocampus for relief of chronic debilitating epilepsy rendered a patient, H. M., unable to form new memories. A series of studies of H. M. beginning in 1957 and lasting for half a century by Brenda Milner delineated the role of the hippocampus in the formation of memories and launched the new field of cognitive neuroscience.

As we have seen, much of the research on the nervous system has been motivated by an interest in the neural basis of perception. Other major interests have been in the neural mechanisms of emotion and of learning and memory. Midcentury was a time for revolutionary advances in those mechanisms as well, showing that the parts of the brain mediating these types of behavior are closely linked.

Learning and Hebb's Postulate

Few names resonate more widely in modern neuroscience than that of Donald Hebb. His theory of the neural basis of learning goes back, not surprisingly for readers of this history, to the mid-twentieth century. Since so much of neuroscience as well as psychology is focused on mechanisms of learning and few investigators take the trouble to understand what Hebb was really about, we outline this history in more detail.

As mentioned in the previous chapter, learning theory in the early part of the last century was dominated by the behaviorists, who treated the brain as a black box and argued that studies of the brain had no relevance to studies of the mind. In contrast, a few learning theorists carried out experiments with the motivation to understand the underlying neural mechanisms.

Karl Lashley was one of the leaders. Lashley was at Harvard in the 1920s and 1930s and the Yerkes Laboratory of Primate Biology in the 1940s. Milner observes that Lashley "retained a sensible approach to psychology as it passed through a bad period, and raised important questions that are still valid" (Milner, 1999, point 1).

Lashley carried out a series of studies of rats doing various types of visual learning tasks and of the effects of lesions of the cerebral cortex on the learning. A key finding for him was that learning deficits were proportional to the amount of cerebral cortex that was removed, independent of the location. This result was reported in a paper entitled "In Search of the Engram" (Lashley, 1950), as celebrated at the time for its dramatic title as for its negative (and soon to be disproved) finding. To explain his results, Lashley hypothesized that much of the function of the neocortex is expressed through subcortical integrative mechanisms.

The main problem Lashley wrestled with was the neural representation of what is learned. Here, another approach enters the arena. One of Ramón y Cajal's students, Lorente de No, carried on the Golgi method in a series of studies of the neocortex. (In one of these he identified clusters of cells in the somatosensory face area of the rat, calling them *cortical glomeruli*. These later were rediscovered by Tom Woolsey and Henrik van der Loos [1970] at Johns Hopkins University and renamed *cortical barrels,* which have become one of the main models for cortical organization and learning.)

Lashley was impressed by a diagram of cortical organization based on Golgi-stained cells in one of Lorente de No's papers (1934). This diagram represented cells forming reverberatory circuits through their axon collaterals within the cortex, the schema Lorente de No was to repeat in his classic chapter on the cerebral cortex in *The Physiology of the Nervous System* by John Fulton at Yale in 1938 (discussed in Chapter 10). Lashley picked up on this concept and postulated that "From such a structural organisation functional properties may be inferred with some confidence" (Milner, 1999, point 7). This without any idea of the properties of either the neurons or their synapses! Lashley's view was that the neurons act as resonators, tuned to different frequencies; the sensory impulses enter the cortex in waves, which spread and interfere with each other, producing standing wave patterns that represent the stimuli. These wave patterns represented the stimulus; a subsequent learning process related the percept embodied in the standing wave pattern to a sensory response (Milner, 1999, point 9).

Donald Hebb (Fig. 12.1) was a student of Lashley. He had studied at McGill, tried being a school principal for several years, and was drawn back to graduate studies in psychology by reading William James, James Watson, and Sigmund Freud. He worked under Lashley to obtain his PhD in 1936 on how early visual deprivation affects visual perception in the rat. Wilder Penfield then invited him to join the Montreal Neurological Institute (see Chapter 10), where he studied the effects of frontal lobe injury on human behavior, concluding that the minimal effects indicated widely distributed neural systems. Next, on the faculty at Queen's University, he developed intelligence tests for rats and humans. By 1942 he was convinced that learning was a more important factor in intelligence than commonly recognized.

In that year Hebb joined Lashley at Yerkes and began studies of the behavior of chimpanzees. There, he began to pull together his experiences in a book, as he was to write in the introduction, that would develop "a general theory of behavior that attempts to bridge the gap between neurophysiology and psychology." A draft was prepared by around 1945. The intellectual atmosphere at Yerkes was a great stimulus in writing the book. The contributions of Lashley and others to the ideas in the book have been the subject of lively debate (see Orbach1999; Milner, 1999; Haider, 2008). Hebb returned to McGill, where he was named chair of psychology in 1948. His book, entitled *The Organization of Behavior: A Neuropsychological Theory*, came out in 1949.

Just what was contained in this book, the concepts of which are at the center of modern neuroscience more than half a century later? Remember, in the late 1940s there still was no information about the properties of central neurons and synapses, no membrane physiology, no cell fine structure, no neurotransmitter systems, not a single recording from a cortical cell, no bioactive substances, and none of the other advances of the 1950s that we have covered in the preceding chapters.

A key point of departure for Hebb was a book by Hilgard and Marquis (1940), pointing out that Lorente de No's diagrams of recurrent cortical circuits could be related to a mechanism for learning. This "may well have been the moment of Hebb's epiphany" (Milner, 1999, point 11). In contrast to Lashley, Hebb ignored the analogy of interference patterns and focused directly on the synapses connecting a population of neurons.

There were several essential ideas contained in Hebb's chapter 4 (Fig. 12.2, Appendix 12.1):

1. *The Hebbian synapse.* "When an axon of cell A is near enough to excite B and repeatedly or persistently takes part in firing it, some growth process or metabolic change takes place in one or both cells such that A's efficiency, as one of the cells firing B, is increased" (62). In other words, learning occurs when correlated increases occur in both pre- and postsynaptic activity.

(Although activity-dependent potentiation was known at the neuromuscular junction and was later found at other synapses, it was too brief to qualify as a candidate to serve as a basis for long-term learning. However, the discovery subsequently of long-term potentiation by Bliss and Lomo [1973] immediately identified a synaptic mechanism for long-term memory and a model synapse [the connection between Schafer collaterals and CA1 dendrites in the hippocampus]. The Hebbian synapse was born. It also provided the basis for learning by connectionist artificial neural networks.)

2. *The cell assembly.* Cells that are active together form what is called a "cell assembly." This is also reflected in the popular litany that "cells that fire together wire together." According to Milner (1999,), the cell assembly may be Hebb's most important conceptual contribution:

3. *Reverberatory activity.* In Hebb's schema, the reverberatory activity implicit in Lorente de No's diagrams persists after the initial input, thereby enabling the cell assembly to continue to represent the triggering event.

(It may be noted that, conceptually, the reverberatory activity in Lorente de No's hypothetical cortical circuits builds directly on the representations of circular circuits underlying circus movements of cardiac muscle believed to underlie auricular and ventricular fibrillation in the heart. These schemas were already recognized in the early part of the century. Currently, sustained reverberatory activity in cortical neuronal circuits is still unproven. Long-term changes in cell firing patterns, reflecting long-term Hebbian synaptic changes, have become the main model for the neural substrate underlying learning and memory.)

4. *Mental activity.* Different cell assemblies activated in different sequences form the neural substrate of thinking.

The Organization of Behavior appeared at a propitious moment. The ideas of Skinner were in ascendance, persuading psychologists that physiological facts had no relevance to psychological concepts. An *idea*, by a psychologist's definition, was a psychological concept divorced from a neural substrate.

"Ideas had been considered to be purely mental by most psychologists up to that time (even by behaviourists, which is why they refused to talk about them). Hebb gave ideas a neural basis and opened the door to a cognitive neuroscience" (Milner, 1997, point 10).

Hebb's ideas thus had their first effects within psychology, helping to counterbalance pure behaviorism and stimulate the rise of physiological psychology and psychobiology in the 1960s and 1970s.

(As an experimental and computational neuroscientist, I paid little attention to Hebb's ideas themselves as synapses with long-term changes, ill-defined cell assemblies, and speculative reverberating circuits had little experimental support. Long-term potentiation changed all that in the 1970s, and by the 1980s connectionist networks with Hebbian properties were entering the field of neuroscience. All of these developments led to the rise of cognitive neuroscience, as exemplified by the first Summer Workshop in Cognitive Neuroscience in 1985, organized by Stephen Kosslyn, Michael Posner and myself.)

Summary. Donald Hebb brought about a revolution in cognitive neuroscience. The legacy of his theory of learning, formulated at the very outset of the rise of modern neuroscience, is still unfolding (see Brown and Milner, 2003). A strong claim for the importance of this revolution has been made by Raymond Klein:

> When philosophy and physiology converged in the 19th century, Psychology emerged with the promise of a science of mental life (Boring, 1950). By providing a neural implementation of the Associationists' mental chemistry, Hebb fulfilled this promise and laid the foundation for neoconnectionism which seeks to explain cognitive processes in terms of connections between assemblies of real or artificial neurons. Let me risk the charge of "hero worship" by predicting that as our relatively young science matures, the stature of Hebb's ideas within psychology and behavioural neuroscience will grow to match the stature of Darwin's ideas within biology.
>
> (Klein, http://www.cpa.ca/cpasite/userfiles/documents/
> publications/cjep/special_eng.html)

This assessment was echoed by others:

"...the greatest tribute to Hebb was probably paid by Adams (1998),who stated that 'Two of the most influential books in the history of biology are Darwin's *On the Origin of Species* (1859/1964) and Hebb's *The Organization of Behavior* (1949)' (Milner, 1999, see online)."

The Limbic System

Although most interest was focused on the cortex, other parts of the nervous system were discovered to play critical roles in the higher cortical functions underlying cognition and behavior. Among the great advances in the 1950s was the recognition of the importance of the limbic system and the first evidence for the functional roles of the hippocampus and amygdala within it.

Limbic Lobe. The "great limbic lobe" was first suggested by Paul Broca in France in 1878 as a ring formed by the cingulate gyrus, a ring of cerebral cortex, and the hippocampus encircling the central core of the forebrain. He proposed that this border, "placed at the entrance and exit of the cerebral hemisphere," was like the threshold of a door; hence, the term "limbic," the Latin for threshold being *limen*. He considered that this limbic lobe was the seat of lower faculties compared with the higher faculties of the rest of the cerebral cortex.

Papez Circuit. This idea lay mostly dormant until given new life in 1937 by James Papez, a neurologist in Chicago. Emotional outbursts by patients with damage to the hippocampus and cingulate gyrus stimulated him to reassess the anatomical relations of these regions within the brain. This led him to a novel hypothesis for the neural circuit underlying emotions, described in his paper "A Proposed Mechanism of Emotion" (Papez, 1995) (Appendix 12.2).

In this scheme, *emotional expression* arose from the hypothalamus, deep within the core of the brain, through projections to the brainstem which controlled the motor output (muscles and glands) of emotional expression. But how did the rest of the brain know about this output? This was conveyed by the mammillary bodies of the hypothalamus to the thalamus and on to the cingulate gyrus, the center for *subjective interpretation* of the emotional state. The cingulate gyrus in turn connected to the hippocampus, which combined this information with different inputs coming from other parts of the brain and sent this *emotional output* back to the mammillary bodies. In this scheme, the pathway from cingulate to hippocampus to mammillary bodies provided a means whereby the subjective experience of emotion at the highest cortical level could be combined with the emotional content of the hypothalamic output for emotional expression.

No one had previously conceived of how these structures of the brain might be meaningfully related, and the *Papez circuit* was taken up with great enthusiasm and became a powerful stimulus to further research. An attractive feature was that it gave an interesting function to the hippocampus, which up to then had been considered to be part of the rhinencephalon ("nose brain"), related in some unknown way to smell.

Kluver-Bucy Syndrome. In the same year that Papez published his circuit, Heinrich Kluver and Paul Bucy at Chicago reported the preliminary results of experiments in which they bilaterally removed the temporal lobe in monkeys. Although preliminary, the report was widely known and cited in subsequent years. Publication of the full report was delayed by World War II and finally occurred in 1955 (see Bucy and Kluver, 1955) (Fig. 12.3, Appendix 9.3). They noted five main effects:

1. *Overattentiveness*: The animals are restless; they have an urge to orient toward or respond to all stimuli.

2. *Hyperorality*: The animals compulsively examine all objects by putting them in their mouths.

3. *Psychic blindness*: The animals see but do not understand; they indiscriminately approach and examine objects even though harmful (such as a lighted match).

4. *Sexual hyperactivity*: The animals increase their sexual activity, also indiscriminately, even toward inanimate objects.

5. *Emotional changes*: Monkeys previously wild and aggressive are rendered tame and placid and can be handled easily.

This complex of features came to be known as the *Kluver-Bucy syndrome*. The psychic blindness has subsequently been shown to be due to loss of temporal lobe neocortex. The hyperactivity may be due in part to discharging neurons on the borders of the lesion. The sexual hyperactivity (which originally was one of the most sensational aspects of the syndrome) seems to be so undirected as to be part simply of the general hyperactivity of these animals. Finally, the emotional changes in the Kluver-Bucy syndrome have been especially linked to the *amygdala*.

Amygdala. This complex of cells is located in the cerebral cortex at the base of the forebrain in lower mammals and on the medial wall of the base of the temporal lobe in higher mammals. Although the Kluver-Bucy ablations gave the first clues as to the relation of the amygdala to emotions, the changes varied, depending on the species; cats, for example, are rendered savage instead of placid after amygdala destruction. Some research connected the hypersexuality with the increased aggression in these cases. However, ablation is such a crude tool and there are so many uncertainties about the extent of damage in different studies that no firm conclusion could be reached.

A more precise way to study the amygdala was to use focal electrical stimulation. Paul MacLean was one of the pioneers in these studies. His studies of the amygdala and related parts of the Papez circuit helped lead to the modern concept of the limbic system.

Paul MacLean was born in 1913; educated at Yale, with an interest in philosophy; and then received his MD there in 1940. After World War II, he began a private practice in psychiatry but was soon stimulated to uncover the brain mechanisms underlying psychiatric disease and took a fellowship with Stanley Cobb at Massachusetts General Hospital (MGH) in Boston (we will see how the MGH served as a training ground for neuropsychiatrists in Chapter 13). In studying patients with epilepsy, he became interested in their emotional experiences and their possible relation to the temporal lobe and the hippocampus. This led him to James Papez and the "Papez circuit." Greatly stimulated by a visit with Papez, MacLean drew together his studies of patients in a paper in 1949 entitled "Psychosomatic Disease and the Visceral Brain: Recent Developments Bearing on the Papez Theory of Emotion" (Appendix 12.4). According to Kelly Lambert (2003, 344):

> MacLean avoided referring to the circuit as the rhinencephalon because he wanted to downplay the olfactory function and emphasize the emotional function. He subsequently decided to use the term *visceral* because of its original 16th century definition referring to strong inward feelings. The significant aspect of this paper was MacLean's suggestion that mammalian brains may have a common feature of a rather primitive system responsible for integrating sensory information, suggesting a dichotomy between our intellectual behavior and emotional, nonverbal, behavior.

This paper brought MacLean to the attention of John Fulton, whose work with Carlyle Jacobsen at Yale on the frontal lobe and its relation to emotion had led to the development of psychosurgery (see Chapter 14). At Yale, MacLean became interested in Broca and his idea of the "limbic lobe." According to Lambert, 344:

> Because Broca emphasized the limbic lobe's role in olfaction, a function thought to be of little importance to humans, this anatomical circuit had become the unwanted child of brain anatomy books and lectures. MacLean wrote that one author conveyed that this area of the brain likely contributed very little to the evolution of the human brain and, consequently, should not be considered further in the text. After reviewing Broca's use of the term limbic, he felt that this term was more appropriate than the term visceral and he began referring to the emotional circuit as the *limbic system* because this new term had only descriptive connotations as opposed to the functional connotations associated with the term visceral.

These and further studies in the 1950s played an important role in bringing a wider appreciation of the limbic system, both for the public and for research and clinical practice. MacLean eventually developed his ideas into the concept of a "triune brain", composed of a reptile, lower mammal and human, united but with the verbal human cortex unable to communicate effectively with the non-verbal primitive reptile and lower mammal brains (see MacLean, 1990).

MacLean's research brought a new focus on studies of the structures and functions of the individual components of the limbic system, particularly the hippocampus and amygdala. For example, with Jose Delgado, MacLean carried out a study in 1953 showing that focal electrical stimulation of the brain in the region of the cells of the amygdala complex evoked different types of visceral and emotional expressions (Fig. 12.4). This helped to start the investigation of the functional characteristics of this part of the brain, which has become of intense current interest for its key role in the emotional life of mammals.

Delgado also achieved more public notice when, to demonstrate the ability of deep brain stimulation to control behavior, he implanted electrodes in the brain of a bull and confronted the bull in a bull ring. A movie shows the bull moving menacingly toward him but turning away when Delgado pushed the buttons that turned on the current through the electrodes. The movie achieved instant fame as an example of how humans stood on the threshold of brain control. However, follow-up investigations showed that the electrodes were not placed where they were supposed to be, an infection occurred around them, and the turning of the bull was a very general aversive response to the bull's brain being subjected to a lot of electrical current.

Rhinencephalon vs. Limbic System. As can be seen from the quotation, MacLean's work also began the demotion of the rhinencephalon from its traditionally dominant role in concepts of comparative neuroanatomists about the evolution of the forebrain in favor of new functions related to emotion and ultimately memory. While this facilitated the new research, it also consigned smell to an even less significant role in mammalian, and human, behavior than its apparently already small role in comparison with vision and hearing. For example, anatomical studies showed that removal of the olfactory bulb caused degenerating fibers that reached only into the area of the piriform cortex, stopping short of the hippocampus.

The conclusion was that the hippocampus was removed from playing a significant role in smell and that its key functions were related to central connections from other brain areas comprising the limbic system. MacLean himself never lost his initial interest in the olfactory system and later (see Yokota et al., 1970) carried out a pioneering study using intracellular recordings from hippocampal pyramidal neurons to distinguish between unconditioned responses to septal inputs near the cell body and conditioned responses to olfactory inputs in the distal dendrites. But for most neuroscientists the sense of smell faded into insignificance in the mammalian brain, until the revival of interest toward the end of the century by the discovery of the olfactory genes (Buck and Axel, 1991).

Memory and the Hippocampus

If the relevance of work that took place in the golden age of the 1950s needed more justification, it would be sufficient to recount the case of H. M., the initials of the most famous patient in the history of modern brain science. The report of this patient, whose neurosurgical operation resulted in loss of the ability to form new memories, was made by Scoville and Milner in 1957. Against the oft-repeated mantra that the half-life of a scientific paper is a few months before it sinks into oblivion, consider the following statistics. As noted by Suzanne Corkin (2002), since 1957 this paper has been cited 1744 times. Even more notable, since 1998 it has been cited 258 times, nearly as often as the 284 times for one of the highest-profile papers in modern neuroscience, on stem cells (Gage, 1998).

We have here another example of a discovery in the 1950s which is still an unsolved problem, still a signal point of reference, influencing the agenda of research on memory today. It makes it all the more important to be sure what the case of H. M. was really about and why it is still so important.

There were three actors in this drama: H. M., his neurosurgeon, and his psychologist.

H. M. The first actor was H. M. These are the initials of a person born in 1926 in Connecticut who had a normal childhood until the age of 9, when he had an accident with a bicycle that knocked him briefly unconscious. He began to have occasional minor seizures, which his doctors considered to be possibly due to his accident. At the age of 15 he developed major (grand mal) seizures, with convulsions of his whole body and falling to the ground with loss of consciousness. He completed his education and got a job, but the seizures became more frequent (approximately twice a day). At that time (early 1950s), the only medications were narcotic drugs, which were addictive and made one drowsy; so it was impossible to continue to work, and he had to quit his job and stay at home. He and his family discussed with his doctors what could be done.

William Scoville. Enter the neurosurgeon, William Scoville (Fig. 12.5A). The line to Scoville started in the 1930s with a chimpanzee named Becky. Becky was the subject of a study of the effects of removal of the frontal lobe of the brain on behavior. It was carried out by Carlyle Jacobsen in the laboratory of John Fulton, as we have seen, a leading brain scientists at Yale University. The frontal lobes were already recognized as being the part of the brain that is responsible for the evolution of higher intelligence in monkeys, culminating in humans. Jacobsen removed the frontal lobes in the hope of understanding better the contribution that this key part of the brain makes to both intelligence and emotion. He observed that Becky, who had been easily frustrated to turn quite vicious, became after the surgery docile and pleasant, though still seemed to behave normally.

Jacobsen presented these dramatic results at a neurological meeting in 1935, where, so legend has it, a Portuguese neurologist, Egaz Moniz, rose in the audience and asked whether a similar removal of frontal lobe tissue in human psychotic patients would have a similar beneficial behavioral effect. Returning home, he proposed to his neurosurgical colleague Pedro Almeida Lima a similar surgical approach to treating schizophrenics by alleviating them of their disturbed, violent, and suicidal impulses. In 1936 Lima performed the first operation in a schizophrenic patient by undercutting the nerve fibers that connected the frontal lobe to other parts of the brain. This undercutting operation became known as a "frontal leucotomy" (*leuc*, "white matter," i.e., fibers). The approach quickly spread to other centers around the world. Many proceeded from a limited frontal leucotomy to a full frontal lobotomy, removing entirely both frontal lobes. Because of the aim to change the disordered mental state of the patient, the approaches were dubbed "psychosurgery."

Psychosurgery immediately held out hope as the only available method for treating severe schizophrenia and other types of severe mental disorders. It was particularly taken up in the United States, where by the early 1950s some 10,000 operations had been performed (including on the sister of future President John Kennedy). Similar statistics applied to the United Kingdom. Although many patients were cured of the worst symptoms of their disease, many were recognized as having undergone marked personality changes by the more extensive operations (see the discussion of psychosurgery in Chapter 14).

Scoville was an undergraduate at Yale, took his medical degree at Penn, and trained in neurosurgery at Harvard and Baltimore. After World War II, he started the neurosurgery department at Hartford Hospital and was affiliated with the head of neurosurgery at Yale, William German. He published many papers and became known for innovations in neurosurgical practice. Behind this sober academic record, however, was a colorful personality, characterized by "wild activity," "insatiable ego," and sometimes "unchecked emotions," together with "espousing new ideas," someone who "commends the . . . good works of others," and was disciplined to "long hours of hard work with few vacations" (Whitcomb, 1979).

Scoville's practice included psychosurgery. H. M. was brought to him for evaluation. An examination of brain waves was carried out with an electroencephalogram, in which multiple electrodes were placed over the skull to record the resting electrical activity of the different parts of the brain. The expectation was that this would show localized abnormal activity somewhere, suggesting that this was where the intense bursts of nerve cell activity arose that led to the unchecked firing in the motor pathways and the loss of consciousness; but no abnormalities were seen. Although Scoville's experience with psychosurgery had been mainly with patients with schizophrenia or severe depression, he believed that he could use a similar approach of surgical removal of suspected disordered brain tissue for relief of these epileptic symptoms.

The operation was carried out on September 1, 1953. The operative report was that small parts of the hippocampal formation were observed to be atrophic (degenerated), supporting the idea that these were involved in the disease process. A bilateral medial temporal lobe resection was performed, removing most of the hippocampal formation, the neighboring parahippocampal gyrus (equivalent to the entorhinal cortex), and the nearby amygdala.

The postoperative recovery was normal, and it seemed that the operation was a success. However, it was soon apparent in the days after the operation that H. M. had suffered severe memory loss. This took the form of an inability to remember to whom he had just talked. A person would come into the room and introduce him- or herself by name, he would greet the person by name, the person would go out and a few minutes later return, and H. M. would have no memory of having met him or her. This type of memory loss was called "anterograde amnesia" (*antero*, "in front") because it was loss of memory for new events. It was known to occur in certain types of neurological disorders. One was Korsakoff syndrome, found often in severe alcoholics but due not to the alcohol per se but to the malnutrition, particularly lack of vitamin A, causing degeneration of central brain regions.

H. M. also had retrograde amnesia for events up to about 3 years before the operation. But the anterograde amnesia was the devastating type because it meant he could form no new memories.

Scoville and his associates were stunned and distressed by this turn of events. After reporting these results of "a very grave, recent memory loss" at a meeting in 1954, he determined to seek the aid of a professional psychologist who could thoroughly evaluate H. M. in order to relate as closely as possible the symptoms to the areas removed.

Brenda Milner. Enter Brenda Milner (Fig. 12.5B). She had been born and educated in England, studying psychology under the psychologist Oliver Zangwill, who trained her to analyze the effects of brain lesions for the insights they could give into brain mechanisms underlying normal behavior. During World War II she came to Canada with her husband, Peter Milner (see Chapter 11). In 1949 she persuaded Donald Hebb, then at McGill, to take her as a graduate student; and he in turn persuaded Wilder Penfield (see Chapters 10 and 14) to take her, to carry out psychological testing of patients to correlate brain regions removed at surgery with their behavioral effects. She completed her thesis under Hebb in 1952. (It may be recalled that Peter Milner was making his own mark in physiological psychology during this time with his collaboration with Olds on brain stimulation learning [Olds and Milner, 1954; see Chapter 11].)

Brenda Milner was pursuing her work with Penfield when William Scoville asked her for advice on psychological testing of H. M. She agreed, and so began one of the longest associations between scientist and subject in the history of science and medicine.

In the 1957 paper Scoville and Milner published the first results of their collaboration. Since this paper has been cited so many times, it will be worthwhile to examine exactly what was reported in "Loss of Recent Memory After Bilateral Hippocampal Lesions."

Given the dire effect on the patient, the authors were understandably concerned to begin by explaining the reasons for the operation. Some 300 psychosurgical operations had been carried out by Scoville on patients with severe schizophrenia who had not responded to other forms of treatment. His strategy was to use "fractional lobotomies," that is, undercutting only limited parts of the orbital surfaces (just over the eyes) of both frontal lobes, in the hope of avoiding "undesirable side effects." It was found that this had "an appreciable therapeutic effect in psychosis" without producing any significant personality deficit.

Scoville wanted to explore further what other parts of the brain could be partially resected (removed) to achieve even better results. This took him into the territory of the limbic lobe. At this time, interest in the limbic lobe was reviving, thanks to Paul MacLean (1952) and others. In reviewing the anatomy of the limbic lobe, he found that some areas appeared to be transitional, between the simplest three layers of the olfactory cortex and hippocampus and the six layers of the neocortex (see Pribram and Kruger, 1954). In this scheme orbital frontal cortex and mesial (toward the midline) temporal cortex were considered to be closely related. On this basis, "it was hoped that still greater psychiatric benefit might be obtained by extending the orbital undercutting so as to destroy parts of the mesial temporal cortex bilaterally" (Scoville and Milner, 1957, 11).

Supported by this reasoning, such surgeries were carried out on a total of 30 patients, with partial removal of mesial parts of the temporal lobe bilaterally, with or without undercutting of the orbital frontal lobe, and duly reported (Scoville et al., 1953). Various amounts of hippocampal tissue were removed in the different patients. The 1957 paper with Milner reports on a subset of 10 patients in which psychological testing was carried out (Fig. 12.6, Appendix 12.5). Within this subset, H. M. was in a group with the most "radical bilateral medial temporal lobe resection." This was despite the fact that his electroencephalogram showed only "diffuse abnormality." In a key statement for subsequent concern about the ethics of the procedure, the authors note that although there were no signs localizing the disturbance to the hippocampus,

> This frankly experimental procedure was considered justifiable because the patient was totally incapacitated by his seizures and these had proven refractory to medical approach. It was suggested because of the known epileptogenic qualities of the uncus and hippocampal complex and because of the relative absence of post-operative seizures in our temporal-lobe resections as compared with fractional lobotomies in other areas. The operation was carried out with the understanding and approval of the patient and his family, in the hope of lessening his seizures to some extent. At operation the medial surfaces of both temporal lobes were exposed and recordings were taken from both surface and depth electrodes before any tissue was removed; but again no discrete epileptogenic focus was found. Bilateral resection was then carried out, extending posteriorly for a distance of 8 cm. (about 3 inches) from the temporal tips.

In these 10 patients there were no significant neurological deficits and no gross changes in personality; H. M. was described as retaining his characteristic "cheerful placidity." In the psychotic patients, the resections limited to the medial portions of the lateral lobe had no significant therapeutic effect. In the case of H. M., the seizures were sharply reduced for about a year, after which they returned (both major and minor), though they left him "less stuporous" so that his medications could be reduced. Hardly a dramatic achievement.

The general intelligence of the patients could be assessed accurately only in the case of H. M. because the psychotic patients were too disturbed preoperatively for "finer testing of higher mental function to be carried out." Here, we begin to see why, of all patients subjected to psychosurgery and who suffered memory loss, H. M. has been of special interest. Postoperatively his intelligence appeared to be raised slightly, perhaps due to the lower amount of medication required. But, as the authors point out,

> There has been one striking and totally unexpected behavioral result: a grave loss of memory in those cases in which the medial temporal-lobe

resection was so extensive as to involve the major portion of the hippo-campal complex bilaterally.

This was not recognized at the time in the most severely affected psychotic patient "because of her disturbed emotional state." This again is why H. M. became of special importance; his mental state could be assessed without complications of a "disturbed emotional state."

Of the 10 patients, H. M. was in the group with the severest memory loss. It was described as follows:

> ...the loss was immediately apparent. After operation this young man could no longer recognize the hospital staff nor find his way to the bathroom, and he seemed to recall nothing of the day-to-day events of his hospital life. There was also a partial retrograde amnesia, inasmuch as he did not remember the death of a favourite uncle three years previously, nor anything of the period in hospital, yet could recall some trivial events that had occurred just before his admission to the hospital. His early memories were apparently vivid and intact.
>
> ...Ten months ago the family moved from their old house to a new one a few blocks away on the same street; he still has not learned the new address, though remembering the old one perfectly, nor can he be trusted to find his way home alone. Moreover, he does not know where objects in continual use are kept, for example, his mother still has to tell him where to find the lawn mower, even though he may have been using it only the day before. She also states that he will do the same jigsaw puzzles day after day without showing any practice effect and that he will read the same magazines over and over again without finding their contents familiar. This patient has even eaten luncheon in front of one of us (B. M.), without being able to name, a mere half-hour later, a single item of food he had eaten; in fact, he could not remember having eaten luncheon at all. Yet to a casual observer this man seems like a relatively normal individual, since his understanding and reasoning are undiminished.

Other findings were that H. M., like other patients with severe memory deficits, was able

> to remember a three-figure number or a pair of unrelated words for several minutes, if care was taken not to distract them in the interval. However, they forgot the instant attention was diverted to a new topic. Since in normal life the focus of attention is constantly changing, such individuals show an apparently complete anterograde amnesia.

Further,

> On the Wechsler Memory Scale ... his immediate recall of stories and drawings fell far below the average level and on the "associate learning" subtest of this scale he obtained zero scores for the hard word associations, low scores for the easy associations, and failed to improve with repeated practice. These findings are reflected in the low memory quotient of 67. Moreover, on all tests we found that once he had turned to a new task the nature of the preceding one could no longer be recalled, nor the test recognized if repeated.

Before the operation there had been scant indication of a relation between the hippocampus and memory. A clinical study (Glees and Griffith, 1952) had suggested that bilateral destruction of the hippocampus in humans causes recent memory loss as well as, in some cases, anterograde and retrograde amnesia. So there were few warning signs against bilateral hippocampal removal. After the operation, Milner and Penfield (1955) described two cases of memory loss in patients who had had removal of the hippocampus on only one side but in whom it was later shown that the remaining hippocampus was damaged, thereby supporting the results in H. M.

Summary. H. M. represents a historical turning point in understanding human memory. Before him, there was little evidence for the brain mechanisms in memory. The leading idea, coming from a leading authority, Karl Lashley, was that memory was a unitary phenomenon that was a function of the entire cerebral cortex. After H. M., it was recognized that there were different types of memory, beginning with the distinction between short-term and long-term memory. The different types reflected contributions from different regions of the brain: Short-term memories depend on the hippocampus, and long-term memories depend on other regions. The different types also depend on different sequences of mechanisms, starting with acquisition, proceeding through storage and maintenance to recall. H. M. disproved Lashley in showing that a particular brain region could be associated with a particular type of memory; that is, a particular type of memory is associated with a particular region of the brain. However, the studies of H. M. and other similar patients agreed with Lashley at a local level that the extent of memory deficit was correlated with the amount of cortex removed.

Thus, beginning in the 1950s, the careful studies of H. M. by Brenda Milner began the systematic study of the biological basis of memory and thus provided the foundation for the growth of these studies as a major focus of modern neuroscience (see Kandel, 2006). We have seen that Donald Hebb has been claimed to have been the founder of modern cognitive neuroscience; it appears that he has two additional co-founders: Brenda Milner and H. M.

H. M. died on December 2, 2008, at the age of 82. The obituary in the *New York Times* on December 5 revealed to the world that H. M. was Henry Gustav Molaison (Fig. 12.7), recognized

as the most important patient in the history of brain science. As a participant in hundreds of studies, he helped scientists understand the biology of learning, memory and physical dexterity, as well as the fragile nature of human identity.

Chapter 13

Neurology: Foundations of Brain Imaging

Clinical neurology was early combined with psychiatry in the nineteenth century and only began to emerge as a separate specialty around 1900. In North America, the Neurological Unit of the Boston City Hospital was one of the early seeding places for the new discipline. At midcentury, a succession of neurologists in Boston, including Stanley Cobb, Tracy Putnam, Derek Denny-Brown, Raymond Adams, and C. Miller Fisher, laid the basis for modern clinical neurology as an independent discipline. The first effective drug for treatment of epilepsy was introduced. Spreading cortical depression was discovered by Leão and linked to migraine. The role of dopamine and the substantia nigra in Parkinson disease was recognized. Carl Schmidt and Seymour Kety at Penn developed methods for measuring the vascular circulation of the brain, the first key step toward the development of positron emission tomography and the new era of brain scans. The development of a polio vaccine, which caused the virtual elimination of that dread paralytic disease, was one of the great medical and neurological achievements of the century. In these modern advances, clinical neurology became increasingly built on a rigorous basis of animal research.

Clinical neurology had its beginnings in the United States, United Kingdom, and France, in the late nineteenth century. The history is rich and deep and available in various accounts. While recognizing this history, with our focus on the origins of modern neuroscience, we will begin in North America.

The origins of neurology (see Scott and Toole, 1998 for summary) began in England in 1861 with the opening of the National Hospital for the Relief and

Cure of the Paralyzed and Epileptic at Queen's Square in London. In the U.S., Weir Mitchell in Philadelphia published "Gunshot Wounds and Other Injuries of Nerve in 1864" (based on his experience during the American Civil War), and William Hammond, also in Philadelphia, published "A Treatise on the Diseases of the Nervous System", generally regarded as the first textbook of neurology. The first professor of neurology anywhere was the renowned Jean-Martin Charcot in Paris, appointed in 1882. This was followed in England by the appointment of John Hughlings Jackson, generally regarded as the "father of British neurology" (Scott and Toole, 1998), to Queen's Square in 1884.

American medicine began to emerge as a profession in the late nineteenth century, led by the medical faculty of the new Johns Hopkins University. There, William Osler in medicine and William Halsted in surgery established new standards for training and practice in what was a largely unregulated system of medical schools and hospitals. Disorder persisted into the twentieth century to such an extent that the Carnegie Institution finally commissioned a nonmedical person, Louis Flexner, an English professor, to review the state of American medicine and make recommendations. Out of that review came the "Flexner report" (1910), a school-by-school review of medical education and medical practice. One of the main recommendations was for medical schools to maintain a full-time faculty to teach medicine. This provided the foundation for the rise of the research-based academic medical school faculty and, with it, the rise of the clinical specialties and biomedical research.

Diseases of the nervous system were traditionally taught among other diseases in medical schools and treated by internists. After Mitchell and Hammond, the first professors of neurology appeared, as did the founding of the American Neurological Association (Talley, 2005). Many diseases of the nervous system were difficult to diagnose; for example, it was not until 1868 that Charcot identified multiple sclerosis as a specific nervous disease. By 1900 most large medical schools had departments of nervous and mental disease, but there was not yet any hospital specialized in treating nervous disorders.

Well into the early twentieth century, neurology in the United States tended to be merged with psychiatry, both in clinical practice and in combined neuropsychiatry departments in medical schools and hospitals. There was not a clear differentiation along the continuum of nervous and mental diseases. There were few who made a living from a neurological practice alone. In the absence of effective treatments for neurological disorders, the practice was limited to descriptions of symptoms and logical pinpointing of the brain site and nature of the pathology underlying the symptoms.

After the Flexner report, neurology, along with other specialties, began to form. By the 1930s there were still fewer than 100 board-certified neurologists in the United States; by 1950 there were more than 1400 (Talley, 2005). This upsurge was accompanied by an increase in the credibility of diagnoses of neurological diseases. As an example, Talley (2005, 390) notes that

> Throughout the 19th century, doctors considered hysteria the most common neurological condition that affected women between menarche and menopause. . . . As hysteria gradually declined as a neurological diagnosis in the first half of the 20th century, physicians interpreted increasing numbers of these patients, especially women, as having multiple sclerosis.

(During my medical training a woman with hysteria was presented on rounds on Denny-Brown's neurology service at the Boston City Hospital in the late 1950s.)

Psychiatry began its independent rise in the early twentieth century, given a large impetus by Sigmund Freud and his psychoanalytic methods. The view from neurology (see Aird, 1994) was that these methods gave psychoanalysis a professional identity that was attractive to the patient as well as being remunerative to the analyst. This growth of psychiatry had the effect of slowing the independent emergence of neurology.

Neurologists began to achieve their own identity when they started to acquire tools of their own. The electroencephalogram (EEG) led the way (see Chapter 8). After its discovery in 1929 by Hans Berger in Vienna, a number of laboratories during the 1930s began to study the electrical waves recorded from the scalp, carrying out basic research on the nature of the waves as well as using them to differentiate between types of epileptic seizures. Although the waves represent only the summed activity of many neurons, the EEG was the first tool to provide neurologists with objective data regarding the functional state of the brain in health and disease.

The Neurological Unit of the Boston City Hospital

Many developments fueling the rise of neurology began in the Harvard Neurological Unit of the Boston City Hospital, the first neurological teaching unit in the United States (Aird, 1994, 233), set up under Stanley Cobb in 1925 and supported by grants from the Rockefeller Foundation.

Stanley Cobb. Stanley Cobb was early interested in the basis of epileptic seizures and first tested the hypothesis that they were due to cerebral anoxia following cerebrovascular spasm. (Cerebral anoxia was being actively investigated in the late 1950s; I recall work by John Barlow in the unit when I was a medical student there.)

Brain waves had been confirmed and investigated in animal experiments in the 1930s by a number of investigators, including Edgar Adrian at Cambridge, England. William Lennox, a fellow in neuropathology in the Neurological Unit, joined with Cobb and Frederic and Erna Gibbs to test a hypothesis that seizures were due to changes in cerebral neurochemistry. For this work, new equipment for multiple recordings from the scalp was developed by the technician Albert Grass. This led to the formation of the Grass Instrument Company, whose equipment for EEG recording and electrophysiological analysis became standard in laboratories in neurology and neuroscience in the United States and throughout the world for many decades. The Grass camera was the main means for recording oscilloscope traces of electrophysiological responses until the arrival of digital recording, storage, and playback in the 1990s. (I had a series of these cameras in my own laboratory beginning in the 1960s. The worst disaster was after a great experiment to discover that someone had forgotten to remove the lens cap.)

Epilepsy played an important role not only in enabling investigation of cerebral mechanisms but also as a means for organizing neurologists. The International League Against Epilepsy was constituted in modern form in 1935 and the National Epilepsy League in 1939 (see Aird, 12), bringing neurologists and lay groups together to fight social discrimination against people suffering from epilepsy (this association between clinicians, research workers, and the public would later play a role in establishing the Neurology Institute at the National Institutes of Health [NIH]). Lennox was involved in both these organizations, as well as establishing the American Epilepsy Society and its journal, *Epilepsia*. The *Atlas of Electroencephalography* by Gibbs and Gibbs (1950) and *Epilepsy and Related Disorders* by Lennox (1960) contributed greatly to defining epilepsy as a multiple clinical entity as well as to the emerging clinical specialty of neurology.

Another step forward was the discovery of drugs that could reduce or control seizures without unduly depressing mental function. This work began with Tracy Putnam, who trained under Harvey Cushing in neurosurgery at the Peter Bent Brigham Hospital in Boston and then joined Cobb in the Neurological Unit. Cobb became increasingly interested in the psychiatric aspects of his patients and in 1935 moved to the Massachusetts General Hospital (MGH) to bring his neurological approach to the new unit for psychiatry there.

Putnam replaced Cobb as director of the unit at the Boston City Hospital. At that time it was known that barbiturates had an effect of suppressing seizures, but it was at too great a cost of depressing mental activity (we have already encountered that problem in the story of H. M., Chapter 12). Putnam together with a young collaborator, Houston Merritt, began to test different phenyl derivatives of barbiturates for their differential effects on different types of seizures. This led to the identification of diphenylhydantoin (phenytoin, Dilantin) as an effective agent in 1938 (see Merritt and Putnam, 1984). The importance of this discovery for medicine, in general, and neurology, in particular, is shown by the following comments:

Dilantin became the first drug to inhibit epileptic seizures effectively in man.

(Vilensky et al., 2004)

The immediate success of phenytoin initiated the modern era of anti-epileptic drug therapy in epilepsy.

(Aird, 1994, 14–15)

Merritt went on to become briefly head of the unit while a search was conducted, which led to the appointment of Derek Denny-Brown in England. He arrived in 1941, and Merritt then followed Putnam to Columbia. Merritt's *Textbook of Neurology* (first published in 1958) helped to define the new field based on the scientific principles he and others had introduced.

Derek Denny-Brown. Derek Denny-Brown had been educated in his native New Zealand, then trained in spinal cord physiology at Oxford with Sherrington in the 1920s. He was one of the outstanding cohorts of Creed, Liddell, and Eccles who, with Sherrington, produced the classic *Reflex Activity of the Spinal Cord* in 1932 (see Creed et al., 1932). Denny-Brown and Sherrington in 1930 noted the apparent recruitment of larger motor units with increasing levels of excitation of afferent fibers, which has been regarded as the first evidence for the "size principle" later studied in depth and characterized as a general principle by Elwood Henneman and coworkers (Henneman, 1967) (see Chapter 9). Denny-Brown went on in London to develop the electromyograph (EMG) to diagnose muscle disorders and introduced muscle biopsy as an adjunct for this purpose. He also produced classic articles on the neural mechanisms controlling micturition (urination) and defecation, critical knowledge for the care of spinal injury patients.

In 1936 Denny-Brown was a Rockefeller Foundation Fellow with Fulton at Yale, where he began studies of the effects of precentral cortical ablations on motor function in monkeys. This was to become a major theme in his research at the Neurological Unit in the 1940s to 1960s. As noted by Vilensky et al. (2004, 510),

The goal was to understand how various levels of the nervous system control primate motor behavior and thereby how to develop therapies to ameliorate abnormal postures and movements in his patients.

This work produced many articles, several books, and hundreds of films (totaling 222,000 feet) on these disorders. (The films were an integral part of Denny-Brown's teaching, as I remember from lectures in the late 1950s and a rotation on his service. The monkeys in the films were as pathetic in their loss of motor functions as patients with corresponding lesions, which was of course Denny-Brown's point, though it made for difficult viewing. It is possible that today's mores, dictated by student sensitivities and anti-animal research extremists, would not permit this use of animals; but it was done in the belief that there is no better way to reveal the underlying nature of human disease than to see and understand it in another animal. This was one of the foundations of the rise of scientific medicine [see Warner, 1997; Dagi, 1997a].)

Vilensky et al. (2004) note that "Denny-Brown's writing ability was not on a par with his analytical skills," a comment that also applied to the occasional opacity of his lectures on complex neurological disorders. During my rotation on the service, I once asked one of the house staff if he could explain in simple terms Denny-Brown's theory of the neural basis of aphasia. He replied, "We don't understand it either, so don't worry."

Denny-Brown's training program included an emphasis on neuro-pathology. This was based on a weekly brain-cutting conference, in which house staff would present the history, physical, and neurological workup; discuss the differential diagnosis; and predict the neuropathological findings. This was an application of the clinical pathological case method of medical training that was a long tradition at Harvard. Denny-Brown would then discuss his own views and prediction, after which the formalin-fixed brain would be produced and the neuropathologist would cut the brain and describe the findings. Such was his aura that the joke was that if his prediction was incorrect, it was the brain that was wrong! As Vilensky et al. (2004) note, this anecdote indicates the rather authoritarian manner Denny-Brown had in running the unit. When he was not amused, the temporal vessels would start pumping. This happened frequently when Jerry Lettvin, the brilliant young neurologist and neurophysiologist, was on his service in the late 1940s. A well-known story was that, as a prank, Jerry arranged that all the Babinskis would have upgoing toes on one side of the ward and downgoing on the other. When Denny-Brown realized what was going on, the temporal vessels started pumping.

Denny-Brown's scholarship and leadership dwarfed these minor concerns. The Neurological Unit was extremely successful. Vilensky et al. (2004) note that by the early 1960s the chairs of almost half of the 41 departments of neurology in the United States had received training under Denny-Brown. In addition were visits from distinguished neurologists from around the world. He trained over 300 neurologists, thus playing a central role in the rise of modern neurology.

Raymond Adams. Among the trainees was Raymond D. Adams, who joined Denny-Brown to head neuropathology in the Neurological Unit in 1941. His early work was on experimental concussion in the cat and motor paralysis in the rat, indicating the empirical approach to neurological disease based on animal research that was providing a new scientific basis for clinical neu-rology. In patients, he studied acute necrotizing hemorrhagic encephalopathy with Denny-Brown and Jan Cammermeyer (Adams et al., 1949). His studies with Denny-Brown led to the classic monograph *Diseases of the Muscle* (Adams et al., 1954). Among other subjects studied were EEG changes in hepatic coma with Joseph Foley (Foley et al., 1950), congenital hydrocephalus, and ade-nomas of the pituitary. It was an early indication of the tremendous depth and range of subjects for which Adams became renowned as a consummate neurologist and educator.

(Cammermeyer was a meticulous histologist, who went on to identify and characterize the "dark neuron" [Cammermeyer, 1962], cells that degenerate because of hasty removal of a perfused brain. I knew him at NIH during the 1960s and drew on his experience for my own histological study of the olfactory bulb. Foley became a much loved figure in neurology and medical education. I remember a rounds with him at the Neurological Unit during which he described a patient with a diagnosis of psychopathic [now termed "socio-pathic"] personality as a person with a "moral blind spot," the kind of insight that stays with one the rest of one's life.)

In 1951 Adams became chief of the neurological service at the MGH in Boston. Starting with a foundation in neuropathology, he extended the service to include laboratories of neurochemistry, immunology, and behavior (Aird, 1994, 238). Neural fine structure was added with the advent of the electron microscope in the middle 1950s (see Chapter 4). The service helped to define the multidisciplinary nature of modern neurology. Studies followed on a wide range of neurological disorders. This range was well reflected in his textbook of neurology. In addition, he became a master organizer of related neurological laboratories and departments in sister institutions. According to Aird (1994, 238–39),

> As a teacher, Ray Adams stood apart. His vast knowledge and in-depth discussion often bordered on the incredible. [As a pioneer of modern neurology] Adams especially well illustrates the combination of superb clinical teacher with neurological research . . .

C. Miller Fisher. One of Adams' colleagues at the MGH was C. Miller Fisher, who early became interested in cerebral circulation and cerebrovascular accidents (Fisher and Adams, 1951). This led to a lifelong interest in the vascular and neurological basis of *stroke*, the sudden attacks of loss of blood supply to the brain that are the cerebral counterpart of heart attacks. The early interest in this problem led to a series of conferences on "cerebral vascular disease," sponsored by the American Heart Association, of which the first was held in January 1954 at Princeton University (Appendix 13.1). Analysis of the events leading up to a stroke indicated that there were brief periods of "intermittent cerebral ischemia," which often appeared to precede the advent of a full stroke. These periods came to be called "transient ischemic attacks" (TIAs). Lectures by Fisher on TIAs were part of our medical undergraduate curriculum in neurology at the MGH in the late 1950s.

A controversy soon arose as to the duration of a TIA. At the second conference (Classication, 1958), Fisher characterized TIAs as episodes that "may last from a few seconds up to several hours, the most common duration being a few seconds up to 5 or 10 minutes" (reported in Mohr, 2004, online); anticoagulant therapy was also discussed at this early stage (see Fisher, 1958). Subsequently, the duration as a defining characteristic of a TIA was loosened, particularly in the United Kingdom, to be up to 24 hours (see Mohr, 2004). A rule of thumb emerged that Mohr (2004) describes as follows:

> Dr Fisher recalled some time ago that it was generally decided that, if roughly 24 hours passed and there was still evidence of neurologic injury, the event was probably a stroke. And that if, in a time period short of that the neurologic disturbance had cleared, no one could say for sure that it was a stroke. The emphasis that he put on it, which has remained with me ever since, was that this was a *negative* definition. Again, there was at the time no imaging available to help distinguish these events, and the 24-hour rule was established simply to ensure, as much as possible, that if there was a disturbance lasting at least 1 day everyone would agree that it was serious and represented some injury to the brain.

The realization, starting in the 1980s, that anticoagulant treatment can be effective in stroke if started within 2–3 hours gave a new urgency to the problem of discriminating TIAs without neurological sequelae from those that constitute small strokes or prestrokes. Since then there has been an evolution in the definition of transient ischemic attack, summarized in the New England Journal of Medicine as follows (Albers et al., 2002, adapted from 1715):

> Current time-based definition: A transient ischemic attack is a sudden focal neurologic deficit lasting for less than 24 hours, of presumed vascular origin, and confined to an area of the brain or eye perfused by a specific artery.
>   Proposed tissue-based definition: A transient ischemic attack is a brief episode of neurologic dysfunction caused by focal brain or retinal ischemia, with clinical symptoms typically lasting less than one hour, and without evidence of acute infarction.

The 1950s can thus be seen as containing the first steps in diagnosing and treating one of the most frequent and debilitating of nervous disorders. In this way, it played a critical role in defining the new specialty of neurology.

(Adams and Fisher were still active in the 1980s and 1990s, so our son Gordon had the privilege of undergraduate as well as house staff training by them on the MGH neurological service in the 1980s and 1990s. Adams was still awe-inspiring as a teacher, and Fisher was still the authority on TIAs.)

Montreal Neurological Institute

Another important contributor to the rise of neurology was the neurosurgeon Wilder Penfield, whom we have already met in Chapter 10 and elsewhere.

Penfield trained with Sherrington in Oxford, Gordon Holmes at Queen Square, Ramón y Cajal in Madrid, and Ottfried Foerster in Breslau, Germany— a very distinguished pedigree. In 1928, through his acquaintance with Alan

Greg at the Rockefeller Foundation, he was encouraged to found a new neurological institute. Through another acquaintance, Edward Archibald, he settled on McGill University in Montreal, Canada. Begun in 1934, the Montreal Neurological Institute rapidly established itself as a leading institution for neurological and neurosurgical research in the world.

Penfield himself focused his research on studying and relieving chronic epilepsy.

> This involved careful initial neurological, psychological, and EEG studies, followed by his cortical stimulatory studies on conscious patients. This resulted in several classical reports on brain localization and function (15–17). Electrocorticography and neuropathological studies aided in the understanding of the underlying neuropathophysiology of symptomatic forms of epilepsy. His recruitment of Herbert Jasper...led, not only to thorough EEG studies before, during, and after surgery, but also to basic neurophysiological studies in the different forms of epileptic seizures.... This comprehensive approach inevitably attracted a host of trainees in the clinical and preclinical specialties—many of whom went on to professorships in the United States, Canada, and other countries.
>
> (Aird, 1994, 18–19)

This reiterates that a careful workup of patients was a hallmark of the new neurology. The focus on epilepsy shows that the early advances by the neurologists also carried over into the rise of modern neurosurgery.

Penfield's contributions to neurology and neuroscience, apart from his work as a neurosurgeon, were many. During training with Ramon y Cajal in the 1920s he carried out studies characterizing different types of neuroglial cells. We have discussed his pioneering studies of the human cortex, with its elucidation of the homunculus in humans (Chapter 10). The training that Brenda Milner received there was to prove invaluable in laying the foundations of cognitive neuroscience through her study of H. M., as recounted in Chapter 12.

Penfield's admirable personal qualities showed that high standards could be attained by a person with a "normal" life and personality, in contrast to the all-consuming drive of Cushing and others.

Aird (1994, 19) comments that

> Penfield always struck me as somewhat of a saintly person; this went beyond his Bible reading on Sunday evenings. He was a thoughtful and kindly person in his relations with his patients and colleagues. At the same time, his critical mind demanded the best of himself and his staff in both his research and the operation of the institute.

There were others like Penfield. "God grant that the human race will produce more men like William Lennox: men of wisdom, patience, kindness, and dedication" (Aird, 1994, 13).

Cerebral Circulation: Historical Background

One of the most interesting developments in the 1950s, not widely recognized, is how brain circulation and metabolism were explored and how this laid the basis for the development of brain imaging. The story, as usual, has deep roots.

The idea that brain metabolism can be used to observe the brain in action arose from observations of changes in blood vessels in the brain during mental activity. As reported by William James in his *The Principles of Psychology* (1890, 98–99), the Italian neurologist Mosso made extensive observations in patients after head trauma of pulsations of the brain during mental activity. In his book Ueber den Kreislauf des Blutes im Menschenlichen Gehirn (*On the Circulation of the Blood in the Human Brain*) Mosso (1881) noted (translation by Christiane Nockels Fabbri, 121):

> The intra-cranial blood-pressure rose immediately whenever the subject was spoken to, or when he began to think actively, as in solving a problem in mental arithmetic.... We must suppose a very delicate adjustment whereby the circulation follows the needs of the cerebral activity. Blood very likely may rush to each region of the cortex according as it is most active.... the primary congestions which we have been considering follow the activity of the brain-cells by an adaptive reflex vaso-motor mechanism doubtless as elaborate as that which harmonizes blood-supply with cell-action in any muscle or gland.

These observations 130 years ago are as true now as they were then. Mosso was widely regarded in his time. He was one of the special invited guests, together with Ramón y Cajal, at the inauguration of Clark University in 1904 (see Haines, 2007).

Remarkably similar conclusions were drawn by Charles Sherrington, the English physiologist, in the same period. C. S. Roy and Sherrington carried out a study (1890) of the cerebral cortex of the monkey in which changes were observed in superficial cerebral vessels with electrical stimulation of local areas of the cortex. They postulated that the brain has

> ...intrinsic mechanisms by which its vascular supply can be varied locally in correspondence with local variations of functional activity... [we postulate that] chemical products of cerebral metabolism...cause variations of caliber of the cerebral vessels.

This study was forgotten, to be re-discovered in the early years of brain imaging. "[Their] work on cerebral circulation...is only today being acclaimed by experts armed with sophisticated techniques" (Eccles and Gibson, 1979, 5). It is recognized now for its pioneering insights (see Raichle, 2009).

Sherrington's student John Fulton, working with Harvey Cushing, reported on a patient in whom, during brain surgery, one could observe an increase in blood flow in the occipital lobe during visual stimulation (Fulton, 1928). This too was forgotten but now is also regarded as a seminal observation along the path to brain imaging.

(I recall the radiologist Merrill Sossman telling us at Harvard Medical School in the late 1950s that, during visual stimulation of a patient, head X-ray angiography showed dilatation of blood vessels along the visual projection from the lateral geniculate nucleus to the occipital lobe.)

From Cerebral Circulation to Brain Metabolism

The "sophisticated techniques" referred to began with the use of radioactive tracers to study cerebral blood flow by Seymour Kety and his colleagues (Kety and Schmidt, 1948). Louis Sokoloff, a student of Kety and a pioneer in the development of brain imaging methods, tells the story (see http://www.nap. edu/html/biomems/skety.html):

> In the U.S., casualties in World War II (1941–1945) brought a heightened interest in circulatory physiology and the mechanisms by which the body defended blood flow to the brain in response to trauma. Carl Schmidt at the University of Pennsylvania began developing methods to measure quantitatively cerebral blood flow in humans. He was joined by Seymour Kety, a young instructor, and together they invented a method for measuring arterio-venous differences in N_2O and applying them to oxygen, carbon dioxide, glucose and lactate.

Their experiments around 1950 and beyond with different tracers enabled them to distinguish between regional blood flow, glucose uptake, and oxygen consumption (Kety and Schmidt, 1948) (Fig. 13.1, Appendix 10.2). They were able to show that the three properties are closely coupled: When a local brain region is active, all three increase. As Mosso (1881) first observed, this is like the increased supply of blood that goes to an active muscle, except that muscle, like most other organs of the body, is not so dependent on oxygen for aerobic metabolism because it can also obtain its energy by anaerobic metabolism.

The impact of this work is described by Sokoloff:

> This ingenious conceptual approach resulted in the Kety-Schmidt method for the quantitative determination of cerebral blood flow and metabolism in unanesthetized man. The experimental work that led to its development was supported by a grant from the Scottish Rite and carried out on conscientious objectors who had volunteered to be used as subjects in medical research rather than to be inducted into the armed forces during the war. The N_2O method and five of its applications in various physiological and disease states were published in a single issue of the *Journal of Clinical Investigation* in 1948. Its impact was like a thunderclap that revolutionized research on the human brain.

Numerous applications in neurology, psychiatry, and medicine led to much of our knowledge of the normal physiology, pathophysiology, and pharmacology of the circulation and metabolism of the human brain in health and disease. Carl Schmidt, in whose department Seymour [Kety] developed the method, wrote,

Now, for the first time, the clinical physiologist is no longer at a disadvantage in studying the circulation in the human brain. As a matter of fact he is now able to learn more about this, and its relation to the metabolic functions of the organ supplied, than about any other organ of the body. The change is one of the small profits of the research activities of the war years and is one more example of the benefits to be expected from giving brilliant young men opportunities to develop and test out original ideas.

This work led in the 1970s to the development of the 2-deoxyglucose (2-DG) activity mapping method used to map patterns of brain activity in animals and positron emission tomography (PET) for the same purpose in humans. Kety was a leader in this effort. His personal low-key approach to doing science was an inspiration to his colleagues, as recalled by Sokoloff:

It was a fantastic experience. Seymour was an inspiring leader. Despite his towering intellect, he never allowed it to overwhelm us. He was always humble and unpretentious and listened to everything we had to say. Often he would raise questions and patiently consider our comments even though, as we would later learn, he already knew the answers. His attitude stimulated us to think critically and deeply. A frequent comment of his was, "Well, think about it." He valued conceptualization, originality, and uniqueness above all. In my very first project as a research fellow . . . we were scooped in the publication. . . . He consoled me with the comment, "Don't feel bad. It must not have been such a great idea. Someone else thought of it too"—a sentiment typical of his attitude.

The Clinical Center of NIH was under construction when he arrived, and Seymour, as scientific director, had what he considered almost unlimited resources in space, budget, and positions to organize the intramural research programs of the NIMH [National Institute of Mental Health] and NINDB [National Institute of Neurological Diseases and Blindness]. He approached this responsibility in characteristic Kety fashion: cautiously, deliberately, systematically, studiously, and with great humility. He had no preconceived notions about how best to study mental and neurological diseases but had faith that more basic, fundamental knowledge of the structure and functions of the nervous system would be needed. He therefore emphasized the basic sciences and relegated most of his resources to laboratories organized along more or less traditional disciplinary lines.

...Seymour collaborated with several biochemists in Europe and the United States (e.g., Heinrich Waelsch, Paul Mandel, Derek Richter, Henry McIlwain) in efforts to bring greater recognition and respect to and interest in the field of neurochemistry. Their efforts resulted in the initiation in 1954 of biennial neurochemical symposia, later transformed into the International Society for Neurochemistry, the founding of the *Journal of Neurochemistry* in 1956, and the establishment of the International Brain Research Organization (IBRO) in 1960.

Seymour allocated to his own Section on Cerebral Metabolism a modest amount of laboratory space in which to conduct his own research. Because his nitrous oxide method measured only average blood flow and metabolic rates in the brain as whole, it could not localize changes in these functions in discrete regions of the brain. He therefore undertook the development of a method to measure local cerebral blood flow based on his theory of inert gas exchange between blood and tissues that he had previously developed and published in 1951. With the help of several research fellows (i.e., William Landau, Walter Freygang, Lewis Rowland, and myself) he ingeniously translated his theories into an operational method for measuring local CBF. The method could be used with any chemically inert tracer that could diffuse freely across the blood–brain barrier, but they selected ^{131}I-labeled trifluoroiodomethane ($[^{131}I]CF3I$), a gas with the requisite properties. Localization within the brain was achieved by a unique quantitative autoradiographic technique that limited its use to animals. The method and its use to determine local CBF in individual structural and functional units of the brain in conscious and anesthetized cats was first reported in 1955. When used to examine the effects of visual stimulation, the autoradiograms clearly visualized the increases in CBF in the various structures of the visual pathways and led to the very first published demonstration of functional brain imaging, a field now enjoying enormous popularity.

A comprehensive account of the historical development of the modern array of methods for functional brain imaging is described by Raichle (2009).

Spreading Depression of Leão and Migraine

We cannot leave midcentury neurological research without including "spreading depression," always associated with the name of its discoverer, Aristides Leão.

Leão was born in 1914 in Rio de Janeiro, Brazil, of well-to-do parents. While a medical student, he contracted an illness which caused him to withdraw from school. After recovering, and being of independent means, he decided he would take some time out and in 1940 went on a study trip to the United States. While there, he was accepted into the degree program in physiology at Harvard Medical School under Hallowell Davis and Arturo Rosenblueth. It had been observed that electrical stimulation of the exposed cerebral cortical surface of an experimental animal can lead to a spread of activity through the surrounding cortex, a phenomenon called "cortical epilepsy." They suggested that Leão study its mechanism for his degree project.

Leão soon observed in his experiments that, rather than a spread of excitatory activity through the cortex, the most noteworthy feature of the cortical response to a local electric shock was a spread of depression of the surrounding ongoing electrical wave activity. His basic findings were published in an instantly classical paper in 1944 (Leão, 1944a; Appendix 13.3). As indicated in the introductory paragraph (359):

> This study originated in an attempt to secure more data for the understanding of the cortical electrogram which occurs in "experimental epilepsy," and of the conditions in which it is brought forth by electrical stimulation. Early in the development of the study an interesting response, elicited by electrical stimulation, was noticed in the cortex of rabbits. The distinctive feature of this response was a marked, enduring reduction of the "spontaneous" electrical activity of the cortex. We have endeavored to define experimentally some of the characteristics of this response.

His results were remarkable in their elegance and clarity. As shown in Figure 13.2, the response took the form of a suppression of the electrical activity, which spread at a steady rate of a millimeter or so per minute in an enlarging circle around the stimulation point. After the depression, there could ensue alternating "tonic–clonic" activity reminiscent of epileptic seizures. He noted that

> ...the depression and "tonic–clonic" activity of experimental cortical epilepsy seem to be closely related phenomena. The spread of tonic–clonic responses is probably mediated by the same cortical elements which are involved in the spread of depression. The two processes are mainly or exclusively cortical, i.e., they do not require a contribution from sub-cortical centers.

Vasodilation and increased blood flow in the pial blood vessels were shown to occur in association with the spreading depression (Leão, 1944b). According to a later observer, this was the first demonstration of increased cerebral blood flow that was not in response to an increase in cerebral neural activity (Somjen, 2005). In 1945, Leão and Morrison suggested that the slow rate of spread of the depression could be related to the slow drifting movement of the area of temporary blindness (scotoma) associated with migraine.

In 1944 Leão returned to Rio to set up his own laboratory and continue his experiments. Initially, there was some skepticism about his findings, particularly as they came from a young PhD student. It began with his original mentors: Davis is reported to have observed of the initial findings that "nothing resembles a new phenomenon as much as a good artifact" (quoted in Teive et al., 2005) (a healthy attitude, it may be noted, for any mentor and student). However, skepticism in the epilepsy research community gradually gave way to acceptance as an increasing number of investigators tested the finding not only in the cortex but in other tissues as well, finding it among others in the hippocampus, striatum, and cerebellum.

As a further comment on the question of language in international scientific communication, I met Leão at a meeting of the Swedish Physiological Society in the mid-1970s when we both happened to be in Stockholm and were guests of the then president, Carl Gustav Bernhard. Bernhard insisted that the meeting be given exclusively in English. During the banquet at the end of the meeting, as one speaker after another spoke in English, I looked around and realized that Leão and I were the only non-Swedes present for whom this effort was being made. Goran Liljestrand, then well into his eighties, was the only Swedish speaker who spoke in Swedish, explaining that he was of an earlier generation that learned German as its international scientific language.

The retina in many animals turned out to provide particularly dramatic demonstrations of spreading depression. I saw this myself on a visit to Rio a few years ago, when one of my hosts was Hiss Martins-Ferreira, a long time colleague of Leão and one of the great contributors to our understanding of spreading depression. "Come," he said, "I will show you that I can produce spreading depression at will." He and his assistant set up a preparation of the exposed retina of a frog. On a signal, the assistant lightly jabbed a sharp point into the middle of the retina and invited me to watch what happened under the microscope. Immediately, beginning at the site of the jab, I observed a tiny dark spot, which grew into a dark disk that enlarged relentlessly to engulf the entire retina. Its borders were incredibly sharp, like the opening aperture of a camera. I had to admit it was an amazing phenomenon.

The discovery of spreading depression illustrates several themes of our review of neurological research in the mid-twentieth century. There are always discoveries to be made by observant graduate students. Real phenomena have to be discriminated from artifacts. You don't have to be medically trained to make discoveries relevant to clinical disorders. Animal research gives valuable clues to mechanisms that underlie human function and neurological disorders.

The connection to migraine became accepted after Peter Milner in 1958 pointed out the correlation between spreading depression of Leão and the description by Karl Lashley in 1941 of the rate of movement of the scotomas he observed associated with his migraine headaches. Since the 1950s the correlation between spreading depression and the aura of migraine has become established. Spreading depression has also attracted attention for its possible relation to transient global amnesia and to cerebral vascular disorders. Recent studies have tracked spreading depression in human patients using diffusion-weighted functional magnetic resonance imaging and magnetoencephalography.

Those first observations of a graduate student continue to give insights into the complex physiology and pathology of cortical tissues.

The Eradication of Polio

No account of advances in neurology in the 1950s would be complete without including mention of the eradication of poliomyelitis. Although this arose as a problem in virology and required the development of a vaccine, it belongs in this account of neurology because "infantile paralysis" was one of the most feared of the neurological diseases.

Anyone from infancy to adulthood was at risk. We have noted that the neurophysiologist Birdsey Renshaw was a victim (Chapter 9). Perhaps the most famous of the patients who survived was the future president of the United States, Franklin D. Roosevelt, stricken at the age of 41. Anyone from the author's generation, born before around 1950, knew the anxiety in every family during the late summer and early fall, when a sniffle might lead to the dreaded diagnosis and life-changing or life-ending result. The annual number of cases in the United States ranged from 20,000 to 50,000 (see "polio" article on Wikipedia).

The cure for the disease depended on the development of tissue culture methods to grow the virus in monkey cells so that the virus could be identified and grown in quantities in test tubes, enabling a vaccine to be developed against it. The basic research was carried out in the late 1940s in the laboratory of John Enders at Harvard by Thomas Weller and Frederick Robbins with Enders. Their successful isolation of the virus led to its isolation from fecal samples, and the way was paved for the development of a vaccine.

(The last polio epidemic in the United States was in the fall of 1955; as a first-year medical student I volunteered for all-night duty at the MGH to assist with new patients on life support in the emergency ward. There was a delay in making the vaccine accessible around the globe. On an externship in the American Hospital in Beirut, Lebanon, in the summer of 1957, I helped with the care of a British woman who was brought in to the neurology service of Dr. Fuad Sabra (a Denny-Brown trainee) from an oil company in Iran in an iron lung. She had been to a square dance, come home, felt ill the next day, and suddenly become paralyzed, unable to breathe on her own. She was eventually transferred home to the United Kingdom. She was one of the last of the iron-lung survivors. This experience has made many of us feel that it is easy to defend the funding of biomedical research: Would you rather put your money in more sophisticated iron lungs or in the development of methods for tissue culture of viruses?)

The development of the vaccine proceeded in a rush in the early 1950s, with Jonas Salk producing an injected inactivated virus and Albert Sabin promoting an oral attenuated virus. Salk was widely celebrated for his achievement, though the Nobel fame went to the three who had isolated the virus. His name lives on through the establishment in the 1960s of the Salk Institute for Biological Studies, an elite research institute, with buildings designed by Louis Kahn, on a beautiful site in San Diego overlooking the Pacific Ocean.

Chapter 14

Neurosurgery: From Cushing to Penfield

The brain had from earliest times presented severe challenges to surgery. Neurosurgery did not begin to emerge as a specialty until around 1900. Harvey Cushing at Hopkins and Harvard led the way, based on meticulous surgical technique and combinations of technical approaches. Surgery for pituitary tumors was among his best-known advances, including the identifi- cation of "Cushing disease." Visualization of the brain was attempted by pneumoencephalography and cerebral angiography, the latter much improved in the 1950s by the introduction of femoral injections, which stimu- lated the rise of neuroradiology. Cerebral stereotaxy allowed the placement of deep electrodes according to precise coordinates, leading to the Talairach brain atlas, a foundation for current brain imaging atlases. The first deep- electrode procedures for relief of Parkinson disease were introduced. Wilder Penfield in Canada led the way in surgery for relief of epilepsy, now among the brain procedures with the highest success rates. Psychosurgery had a brief period of flourishing before being abandoned when the negative outcomes became apparent and drug therapies became available.

The history of neurosurgery can be considered to be either very long or very brief. It is very long if one's perspective includes the evidence for trepanning (opening) of the skull as part of ancient rituals going back to the Egyptians and before. It is very brief if the perspective is of the emergence of neurosurgery as a subdiscipline of surgery in the twentieth century. It is the latter which will be relevant to understanding the role of neurosurgery in the history of neuroscience and our modern understanding of the brain (Greenblatt, 1997a; Spencer, 1997).

For this purpose, the story begins with two discoveries that were essential to the establishment of surgery in general: the advent of general anesthesia in the 1840s and the introduction of aseptic and antiseptic techniques in the 1860s.

After that, the first great advance toward surgery of the brain was the discovery of cerebral localization of function. This came, on the one hand, from the identification from clinical cases by Paul Broca and Karl Wernicke of the cortical centers for speech in the 1860s and 1870s and, on the other hand, from evidence for cortical centers for motor control. This began in 1870 with the experiments of Gustav Fritsch and Eduard Hitzig in Berlin, using electrical stimulation of the cortical surface of the dog, an approach that was pursued energetically by David Ferrier in London in the 1870s and after in a variety of animal species. Thus was revealed the motor strip, the band of cortex in the precentral gyrus along which the movements of different muscles in the body were represented. Hughlings Jackson's concepts of cerebral foci for the motor convulsions accompanying epileptic seizures during this period contributed to this concept of the orderly representation of body muscles and movements in cortical motor control. Also in this period, forgotten until recently, was the work of Angelo Mosso on patients with skull trauma, which allowed observations of changes in cerebral blood flow under different behavioral conditions (see Chapter 13).

Despite these advances, few surgeons dared to undertake operations on the brain because of the still great ignorance about the localization of function in different brain regions, the lack of special instruments, and the high risks involved in operative and postoperative management of the patients. A few were emboldened. The first surgeon to use these advances to carry out operations for removal of brain tumors was William MacEwen in Glasgow, as he initially reported in 1879. More operations were reported by Bennett and Godlee in London in 1884. In 1886 Victor Horsley was appointed in Queen's Square, London, the great neurological hospital, as the surgeon for the paralyzed and epileptic. This is regarded as the beginnings of neurosurgery as a subspecialty of surgery (Greenblatt, 1997a, 1997b). Horsley's first series of patients was reported in 1890: 43 operations for removal of tumors of the brain, with 10 deaths.

This report and the renown of Queen's Square stimulated a number of surgeons around the world to follow in Horsley's footsteps. In 1903, a young surgeon, Antony Chibault, edited a three-volume handbook entitled *L'Etat Actuel de la Chirurgie Nerveuse*, containing articles by 50 surgeons around the world (Walker, 1997, xiii). However, the results were disappointing; the mortality was high, and improvements in the health of the patients were limited. Horsley, as well as most other surgeons, continued their general surgical practice, incorporating brain surgery on a case-by-case basis.

Harvey Cushing

The person who more than any other led the way forward was Harvey Cushing (Fig. 14.1). So central was he that a summary of his life is a summary of the establishment of neurosurgery as a clinical discipline.

Born in Cleveland, Ohio, in 1869, he was an undergraduate at Yale and trained in medicine at Harvard. There, he began to be interested in patients with brain injuries and began to consider surgery as a career. While interning at the Massachusetts General Hospital, he was drawn to the exciting clinical environment of Johns Hopkins Medical School and Hospital and entered there as a resident in 1896. He received his training in surgery under William Halsted, then renowned in the world for putting surgery on a new plane of rigor and sophistication.

> ...a spirit of thoughtful investigation pervaded the place. For surgery, this scientific attitude had two practical aspects. The more obvious part was Halsted's commitment to improving clinical surgery by advancing the science on which it is based, especially physiology and pathology. But the same investigational spirit was also applied to everything that surgeons did, including their manual techniques and perioperative care. If there was clear evidence for a better way to do something, nothing was sacred.
>
> (Greenblatt and Smith, 1997, 171)

Stimulated by this environment, Cushing's appetite for prodigious workloads was soon evident. Quickly becoming Halsted's chief resident, and with it an instructor in surgery, Cushing carried much of the surgical load at Hopkins for the remainder of his training, to 1900. During this time he began to take on neurological cases, with a particular interest in operations for relief of trigeminal neuralgia.

Among his many new colleagues and friends at Hopkins was the chief of Internal Medicine, William Osler. Osler was also a legend in his time, combining high clinical standards with a friendly personality and a broad interest in history and culture—a contrast with Cushing's monomaniacal focus on his work. However, opposites seemed to attract, and Osler took a special interest in the career of his younger colleague. His most important advice was that at the end of his training Cushing should take a year of travel in Europe to visit and become acquainted with the leading scientists, clinicians, and scientific institutions of Europe. This reflected the fact that the Hopkins system had been modeled on the new science and medicine, and ways of teaching them, in Europe.

It was thus that Cushing spent from July 1900 to August 1901 in Europe. In London he met Horsley but was disappointed in the lack of the standards of practice that he was used to from Hopkins. He worked with Kronecker in Berne, Switzerland, on brainstem control of blood pressure under conditions of increased cranial pressure, a critical problem with practical applications in identifying pathology affecting the brain. He visited Mosso in Turin, Italy, working on the same problem, taking advantage of Mosso's extensive observations of cerebral blood flow in trauma victims. Finally, he worked briefly with Sherrington in Liverpool on mapping motor areas of the cortex in anthropoid apes. The research endeavors and personal contacts greatly extended the experience and cultural appreciation of the committed clinician.

Returning to Hopkins, he was given a position as a surgeon under Halsted. In 1903 he was one of a small number of surgeons who founded the Society of Clinical Surgery. At the same time, Cushing pressed Halsted hard for an appointment as a neurosurgeon, despite the fact that there were practically no patients requiring brain surgery at that time. Halsted finally told him, "All right, the field is yours" (Greenblatt and Smith, 1997, 173). On the basis of a dozen cases of removal of intracranial tumors, he delivered an address at a medical meeting, to which he gave the title "The Special Field of Neurological Surgery," which was published in the *Bulletin of the Johns Hopkins Hospital* in early 1905. That might seem like an obscure journal, but in those days it was widely read—as it continued to be into the 1950s, when Vernon Mountcastle published his monumental four articles on cortical columns there (see Chapter 10).

In his article, Cushing lamented the fragmented state of surgery on the brain, with its lack of expertise and coordination during the operations. He proposed that specialization in brain surgery was necessary, built on a systematic training in clinical neurology, neuropathology, and experimental neurophysiology (Greenblatt and Smith, 1997, 175). This was his vision for the future, which constituted the clearest call for the creation of the subspecialty of neurosurgery. However, to be effective, such training required a sufficient body of knowledge in each of these areas. Cushing, and those who heard his call, knew they lacked that foundation and that they had their work cut out for them.

In 1912 Cushing moved to Harvard to head surgery at the Peter Bent Brigham Hospital, a commanding position in American medicine. When the Great War of 1914–18 broke out, Cushing immediately organized a surgical unit to support the war effort in France and was himself in the field in 1917–18 to lead this effort. His war experience of dealing with a range of kinds of trauma, including especially head trauma, convinced him that the time had come for the independent development of neurosurgery. In a meeting in 1919 he presented the results of a series of brain operations with a mortality of only 7.4% (at a time when mortality was running up to 50% in other centers). It is recorded that, after this presentation, another leading surgeon, William Mayo, rose in the audience and declared, "Gentlemen, we have this day witnessed the birth of a new specialty—neurological surgery." (Greenblatt and Smith, 1997, 187) Cushing was ready with a proposal for a society for the new specialty, and in 1920 the Society of Neurological Surgeons was founded, the first such society in the world.

As observed by Saris (1997, 249),

It is rare in the history of medicine for one individual to almost single-handedly develop and advance a specialty, but such can be said of Harvey Cushing in the years approximately from 1900 to 1930. During this three-decade interval, Cushing established that brain tumors could be resected [removed] with reasonable safety and helped to design and implement the equipment and techniques that made this possible. . . . In these three [decades], his success is reflected in the operative mortality rate for tumors such as meningiomas, which dropped from 25% to 12% to 4%.

At the end of his active career, in *Intracranial Tumours* (1932), Cushing identified the innovations which made this and related advances in the surgery of the brain possible:

(1) the generally accepted methods of decompression to relieve tension, (2) such irreproachable wound healing that secondary infections are practically unknown [this purely through aseptic and antiseptic techniques, before the advent of antibiotics in the 1940s], (3) the separate closure of the galea by buried, fine-black silk sutures which has made the once dreaded *fungus cerebri* nigh forgotten, (4) in place of ether inhalation, the introduction by [Thierry] de Martel of local anaesthesia ... [this allowed the patient to remain conscious during the operation, used to great effect by Penfield in his explorations of the human cortex in the 1940s and 1950s], (5) the more precise tumour localisation which in obscure cases Dandy's ventriculography permits us to make, (6) the use of a motor driven suction apparatus as an indispensable adjunct to every operation and (7) the successive improvements in methods of hemostasis which since 1927 have been most advantageously supplemented by the introduction of electrosurgical devices [here he refers to electrocautery, which through small pincers quickly coagulates small bleeding vessels].

These advances not only were to the benefit of human patients but carried over into the neurosurgical operations on nonhuman primates as well. When John Fulton, for example, came from Oxford to Harvard Medical School to be trained by Cushing in the late 1920s, he observed and learned these techniques at the side of the master. Together with his training with Sherrington in Oxford, they became the foundation for his research on nonhuman primates at Yale in the 1930s to 1960s. (In the mid-1950s I observed these surgical approaches by one of Fulton's students, Karl Pribram, at the Hartford Hospital.) In this way, human neurosurgery, with the standards of meticulous care established by Cushing for the experimental animal as well as the human patient, contributed to the rise of behavioral neuroscience.

In these early years the main areas in which surgical intervention could be effective were explored. Several areas related most closely to the emergence of neuroscience may be mentioned.

Pituitary Surgery

As we have seen in Chapter 11, until late in the nineteenth century little was known about the pituitary; for most practical purposes, it was regarded as a vestigial structure. The first operation for removal of a pituitary tumor was performed by Victor Horsley in 1886 (Landolt, 1997, 376). Despite the difficulties of the surgical approach to the pituitary at the base of the brain, a number of surgeons tried the approach by reflecting the temporal lobe. This early work in humans was supported by parallel laboratory experiments in dogs, though the results were often confounded by sepsis and trauma to the reflected brain tissue. An important innovation was by rhinological surgeons, one of whom, Oskar Hirsch in Vienna, introduced a direct approach through the nose to the pituitary, the transsphenoidal approach, in 1912. (Hirsch emigrated to the United States in 1938 and was active at the Massachusetts General Hospital in the 1950s. I was amazed to see him among the audience at one of our teaching sessions in surgery at the Massachusetts General Hospital in 1959.)

Neurosurgery on the human pituitary contributed to the work in the early twentieth century that lay on the path much later to revealing the functions of the pituitary body as a master control center for the endocrine system (Chapter 11). Cushing took a particular interest. In 1912, he operated on a female patient with obesity, hairiness, and overdeveloped secondary sexual characteristics. He collected a number of these cases, attributing them either to primary adrenal tumors or to adrenal hyperplasia secondary to stimulation by pituitary tumors, a condition that has come to be called "Cushing disease" (Landolt, 1997, 375). For his operations, Cushing initially adopted Hirsch's approach, then abandoned it for the transcranial approach, though it subsequently, in the 1950s and later, has become the favored technique.

Visualization of the Human Brain

The initial surgical approach to understanding brain physiology utilized electrodes to stimulate the surface of the cortex. In the hands of David Ferrier and other pioneers of the late nineteenth century, this provided a map of the areas that were involved in motor control, because of the ability to observe the elicited movements, but could provide no insight into sensory areas or the majority of the cortex devoted to association areas and higher mental functions, especially in the human. The other main method was that of *ablation* (resection)—removing an area and observing the effect on behavior. This led to the identification of areas involved in perception in vision, hearing, and touch. But what about the remaining vast areas of the cortex as well as the rest of the "subcortical" brain? By the early twentieth century the main brain regions and many of the main pathways between them had been identified by anatomical means, but the normal physiology was unknown. Above all, the surgeon wanted to avoid disrupting or ablating an area that would turn out to be essential for the normal mental and emotional function of the patient; we have seen the disastrous effects that could ensue in the case of H. M. (Chapter 12).

In exploring the brain of other animals and relating the results to humans, it was necessary to have maps with reproducible landmarks. This had to be based initially on the use of topographical landmarks, that is, easily observable and agreed-on landmarks for relating one map to another. Early attempts were guided by topographical landmarks on the cortical surface, mainly the presence of folds (gyri) and valleys (sulci). In the human, the central sulcus dividing the motor gyrus from the posterior brain was especially prominent, but this was so variable in different individuals as to provide no guide to the location of other brain structures.

A significant advance came with the ability of X-rays to visualize deeper structures through air or contrast encephalography. This procedure was introduced in 1918 by one of the pioneers in neurosurgery, Walter Dandy (1918). Although pneumoencephalography became an established procedure for localization of brain pathology, in humans it carried a high risk of up to 10% mortality.

Another approach was cerebral angiography, introduced by the Portuguese neurologist Antonio de Egas Moniz and his neurosurgical colleague Pedro Almeida Lima in 1927 (Moniz, 1931). In their original procedure a contrast agent was injected into the carotid artery for visualization by X-ray. This carried with it a significant risk of embolism into the brain.

In 1953 angiography was rendered much safer and more effective by injection of the agent into the femoral artery. This innovation was due to Sven Seldinger, who, at a critical moment in developing the method to decide on the sequence of injections, reported that "I had a sudden attack of common sense" (Gobo, 1997). Removal of the injection site away from the brain rendered cerebral angiography much safer, effective for bilateral visualization of the brain from a single injection, and repeatable from the indwelling catheter. As a consequence, "The aftermath of the Seldinger technique saw the advent of neuroradiology as a subspecialty" (Gobo, 1997, 231) (Fig. 14.2, Appendix 14.1)—another testimony to the importance of new methods in biology and medicine.

Both of these visualization methods, however, had serious drawbacks: For pneumoencephalography it was the high mortality, and for cerebral angiography it was the lack of effectiveness in identifying deep brain structures. These shortcomings would be overcome by brain imaging introduced in the 1970s.

Stereotaxy

In parallel with these methods, another approach for this purpose was cerebral stereotaxis (*stereo*, "solid, three dimensions"; *taxis*, "arrangement"; *tango, tangere*, "touch"). Among the technical approaches to standardizing surgery on the brain, stereotaxy (in practice, orienting the tip of a probe within three coordinates in the volume of the brain) was especially important.

> Because so many early neurosurgeon-scientists were trained in physiology, it was natural for them to try to apply techniques that proved less physiologically disruptive in the study of subcortical structures to other purposes. Thus, from the outset, stereotaxis in

humans was directed at the same goals that had stimulated its development for use in laboratory animals: access to deep structures without cortical disruption, recording from neural structures, and lesioning with precision.

The four clinical areas that initially attracted stereotactic interest were the treatment of psychiatric disease, the treatment of movement disorders, the treatment of pain syndromes, and the drainage of cysts and cystic tumors.

(Dagi, 1997b, 423)

Although early attempts were made, the first practical stereotaxic device was built and used by Horsley and his colleague Robert Clarke at Queen's Square in the early 1900s. The utility of the device was that it enabled deep probing of the brain of a research animal, a cat, without ablation of the overlying cortical areas. In addition, Clarke and Elizabeth Henderson published an atlas of the cat brain that was organized in relation to the coordinate grid of the stereotaxic device. Together, the instrument and the atlas were the first step toward quantitating the landscape of the brain.

Application to the human brain was slow in coming. Horsley considered it only a tool for animal research. Clarke developed a device for humans, followed by several others; but in the absence of deep landmarks and knowledge of the functions of most brain regions, the practice declined. In the 1930s, Stephen Ranson and Franc Ingraham at Northwestern University in Chicago built a copy of the Horsley-Clarke apparatus for use in neurophysiological experiments, which popularized its use for research in the United States for many decades to come.

Human cerebral stereotaxy was revived after World War II: "After 1948, activity in the field exploded" (Dagi, 1997b, 406). This built on increased knowledge of deep structures, improved angiography for localization and landmarks, and new methods for effecting changes in the deep structures against brain pathology and dysfunction. Dagi (1997b, 406) identifies 14 devices introduced between the late 1940s and 1960. Among these may be noted one of the first, the Spiegel-Wycis rectilinear device; the Leksell polarimetric device; and the Talairach device combined with angiography. Each of these was designed to implement a particular kind of therapy, such as introduction of radioactive material into a tumor or electrical cautery of a deep structure. The Leksell device used polar coordinates (in other words, orientation by a circular ring with the electrode aimed at the center of the circle) to produce lesions of affected brain regions. Leksell used this device to make precise lesions in the globus pallidus, a basal ganglia structure, an operation termed "pallidotomy" (*palli*, "pallidum"; *otomy*, "opening"). Through this work he is regarded as among the pioneers in the surgical treatment of Parkinson disease (see Wikipedia). We have already encountered him in his basic discovery of the gamma innervation of the muscle spindle (Chapter 7) and will note his development of radiosurgery (the gamma knife) later.

Along with the rise of stereotaxy was the preparation of brain atlases to provide the coordinates for electrode placement. Spiegel et al. (1952) was among the first of a series of atlases from a number of laboratories over the following decades. It was soon realized that, despite the quantitation of position within the coordinate system, variability was still significant, due to several factors: inherent variability of brain regions from individual to individual, interactions of tissue with probes, and shrinkage artifacts during histological preparation. Among the early atlases, the Talairach atlas (Talairach et al., 1952) (Fig. 14.3) from France has come down to modern times through its use as a reference basis for analysing brain imaging data by different laboratories.

As noted earlier, stereotaxy has been used for amelioration of several types of neurological disorders. A cryoprobe (a needle that can be cooled and warmed rapidly) was introduced in 1948 (Haas and Taylor) and used by Irving Cooper in New York in the 1950s and 1960s for creating deep lesions for the relief of movement disorders. This and other means for focal irreversible ablations showed some effectiveness. In Parkinson disease this approach has been combined with the use of L-dopa (see Chapter 12). In the relief of pain, psychiatric disorders, and treatment of tumors, stereotaxy was initially little better than open surgical approaches; However, with the revolution in brain imaging and the advent of molecular probes, the future looks brighter.

An important advance was the development in Stockholm of "radiosurgery" by Lars Leksell, whom we met as a young neurosurgeon revealing the motor system to the muscle spindles (Chapter 9). In 1951, Leksell and physicist Borje Larsson reported operations carried out at a site near a cyclotron, enabling them to focus proton beams on target areas in the brain—first in experiments on animals, followed by operations in human patients. This led later to the development of the gamma knife, using radioactive cobalt instead. This is used as an effective treatment for a number of specific conditions, including vascular abnormalities, benign tumors (mengiomas), acoustic neuromas, and trigeminal neuralgias.

Epilepsy

A field of significant progress was the surgical treatment of epilepsy. This began with one of Hughlings Jackson's patients, who as a child suffered a unilateral brain wound producing hemiplegia on the opposite side and "Jacksonian march" motor seizures involving successively the affected leg, upper arm, wrists, fingers, and face. Jackson predicted that the seizures were due to a focal lesion over the motor strip and in 1886 persuaded Horsley to open the skull to cure the epilepsy by removing the irritating focus. Horsley, though only a 29-year-old surgeon at the very start of his career, agreed; at operation he discovered a vascular scar in the motor area, which on removal cured the seizures. It was a spectacular opening of the field of brain surgery for relief of epilepsy (summarized in Feindel et al., 1997).

Unfortunately, few cases proved as simple, and further progress was slowed by the usual lack of precision in cortical localization, the frequent presence of complications, as well as inadequate operative and postoperative care. In a series of patients in the early twentieth century, Fedor Krause in Berlin carried out careful studies with electrical stimulation of the human cortex, providing the first evidence for the motor strip in humans and ameliorating epileptic seizures by removal of irritation due to tumors or other local pathology (Feindel et al., 1997). After the Great War of 1914–1918I, Ottfried Foerster of Breslau became one of the leaders in surgery of the brain, including relief of epilepsy. In 1935 he introduced *electrocorticography*, the electrical recording of local cortical potentials produced by stimulation of sensory inputs or mental activity, thereby complementing the identification of cortical motor areas by local electrical stimulation. As in the latter, electrocorticography in humans benefited by previous and concurrent experiments in laboratory animals.

In the late 1920s a young Wilder Penfield joined with Foerster in Germany to carry out an in-depth study of cerebral scars as a cause of posttraumatic focal epilepsy. This led to a deeper understanding of the local effects of a scar, including the concept of "cerebral vasospasm." Penfield drew on this training when he moved to Montreal and became head of the new Montreal Neurological Institute in 1934. He established himself as a leader in surgery for the relief of epilepsy, combining focal electrical stimulation with local anesthesia to be able to interrogate the patient on the mental effects of the stimulation (see Chapter 10). Localization of epileptic foci was greatly aided by the introduction of electroencephalography (EEG) in 1937. In Montreal this came under the direction of Herbert Jasper, who carried out parallel electrophysiological investigations in animals (Chapter 10).

With the institute as a center for leadership and training, epilepsy neurosurgery flourished in the 1950s. Penfield's own series of studies were well publicized, including his books, which brought his studies on the representation of movements in the cortical homunculus and the use of tiny shocks to elicit the reporting of memories by conscious patients to a wider audience. The memory studies were carried out in the temporal lobe, which attracted increasing interest as the site of origin of generalized seizures. A number of neurosurgeons took up this challenge, and resection of the temporal lobe for relief of epileptic seizures quickly became a widespread procedure in the 1950s. All of these were unilateral, until William Scoville, in 1953, carried out a bilateral temporal lobe resection in one patient for relief of debilitating epilepsy, producing a profound loss of recent memory. The story of the patient, H. M., and the founding of a new field, cognitive neuroscience, is told in Chapter 12.

In recent years, operations for relief of epilepsy have become one of the success stories of neurosurgery. Relief by modern methods now involves teams of investigators and achieves success rates of 80%–90%

Psychosurgery

As soon as surgery on the brain began with the earliest operations of Victor Horsley, the possibility of operations to relieve psychiatric disorders was raised.

Gottlieb Burkhardt in Switzerland developed the hypothesis that schizophrenic symptoms were due to excessive excitatory spread from sensory to motor cortical areas, which could be alleviated by an ablation between them. Beginning in 1888, he began a short series of operations on schizophrenic patients, removing small parts of the temporoparietal cortex. He reported that the patients were rendered calmer and no longer required isolation (Valenstein, 1997, 502).

Operations such as this continued sporadically over the next several decades but were generally considered too risky. In the mid-1930s insulin shock therapy was introduced, involving large doses of insulin, which sent the patient into convulsion and shock, as was electroconvulsive therapy, involving excessive electrical shocks delivered across the head, which sent the patient into convulsions and unconsciousness. These systemic disturbances were not well controlled but had some success; in fact, electroconvulsive therapy continues as an option for severe depression to this day.

Several neurosurgeons began to consider or carry out operations on the frontal lobe for relief of psychotic symptoms, on the rationale that this was the part of the brain most developed in humans and most associated with mental abilities. But, as mentioned in Chapter 10, the lore of the field traces its beginnings to a meeting in 1935 at which Carlyle Jacobsen, a student of John Fulton at Yale, presented the results of experiments in extirpating the frontal lobe of a chimpanzee, Lucy, changing her behavior from aggressive to docile. Antonio de Egas Moniz, a 61-year-old Portuguese neurologist, at the sight of the results, rose in the audience and exclaimed, "It's a patient." Returning to Lisbon, he engaged his neurosurgical colleague Pedro Almeida Lima, then 33, to carry out a series of operations on psychiatric patients (no permissions necessary!), which he called "prefrontal leucotomy," involving insertion of a wire loop (a "leucotome") into the prefrontal cortex to sever a core of tissue. The first series was reported within a year, in 1936. Although this haste aroused skepticism, de Egas Moniz's reputation as the neurologist who had introduced angiography into neurosurgery meant that the results were taken seriously.

de Egas Moniz coined the term "psychosurgery" for this procedure. He did not hold back on performing more operations and widely publicizing the approach. Others were soon on his heels, chief among them an American, Walter Freeman, and his neurosurgical colleague, James Watts. Within 3 months of reading de Egas Moniz's results, they were reporting the first of what became a rapidly increasing patient population; and the practice rapidly spread around the world. Between 1946 and 1956, some 60,000–80,000 psychosurgery operations were performed worldwide. This rapid spread can be largely ascribed to the almost complete absence of any other credible form of therapy for severe and debilitating mental disorders such as depression and bipolar disorder (then called "manic-depressive illness"). Moreover, the procedure was given a theoretical rationale, of correcting imbalances in thalamocortical relations, that seemed to give it scientific credence.

The operation that spread in this way could no longer be regarded as true surgery. Freeman streamlined the operation so that it became an outpatient procedure that could be performed by any medical or paramedical personnel who could insert an icepick through the upper orbit of the eye, give it a few twists, and send the patient home, at a rate of up to 20 patients in a morning (see Valenstein, 1997). Not only was there lack of follow-up on patient outcomes, but the ease of the procedure encouraged Freeman and others to apply it to patients, particularly young people, who were merely hyperactive or considered to have "behavioral difficulties." The dubious outcomes began to be of open concern; the director of the New York State Psychiatric Institute in 1949 told *Newsweek* (Valenstein, 1997, 510),

> It disturbs me to see the number of zombies that these operations turn out. I would guess that lobotomies going on all over the world have caused more mental invalids than they've cured....I think it should be stopped before we dement too large a section of the population.

It was, in other words, a procedure that was a rejection of all the meticulous care behind the Cushing standards that had been the foundation of neurosurgery.

Continued opposition within the profession itself would likely have had limited success but for the appearance of psychopharmacological drugs in the mid-1950s, which transformed the treatment of psychiatric disease, as discussed in Chapter 15. By the 1960s, psychosurgery was largely abandoned in favor of pharmaceutical treatments. However, more precise methods by neurosurgeons, involving careful placement of probes and local lesions, often under stereotaxic control, continued to be applied in specific cases. This has continued to the present as success rates are improving with modern methods. It is estimated that significant psychiatric improvement can be obtained in some two-thirds of patients. The uncontrolled excesses of the 1950s nonetheless provided valuable guidelines to lead the way toward more effective means for neurosurgeons, using the methods that Cushing introduced, to ameliorate the most challenging of human diseases, the disorders of the mind.

Summary

Most would agree that the era of modern neurosurgery began in the decade of the 1970s, with the introduction of noninvasive brain imaging and the use of the operating microscope. It is of interest to ask what occurred during the 40 years between the end of Harvey Cushing's career in the 1930s and the start of our current modern era.

Over these four decades, there were minor steps, but not quantum leaps, as neurosurgery advanced (Saris, 1997, 249). By 1950, the history and physical examination were highly sophisticated and still the mainstay of localization of cerebral pathology, whereas imaging, mainly by ventriculography and to some extent by angiography, was still relatively crude. In the next 20 years, angiography was used increasingly but was still invasive, risky, and imprecise by current standards.

> ... it was still the day when the neurosurgeons called the shots as to where the tumor was and where to cut. Now the radiologists seem to tell everybody what to do ...
>
> (Hugh Wisoff, quoted in Sari, 1997, 256)

After 1970, the advances were "spectacular" (Sari, 1997, 256). They included, first and foremost, the use of brain scans for localization of tumors and other brain pathology. The operating microscope has allowed fine control of local details in removing tumors. Angiography has become more sophisticated and less risky, as have anesthetic techniques. Ultrasonic instruments for tumor removal have supplemented electrocautery and suction apparatus. Power tools rapidly turn bone flaps. Residency programs provide training across all of these many methods and disciplines. And the applications of molecular methods for localizing and treating brain pathology are only beginning.

Why did not neurosurgery share more fully in the revolutions that affected so many of the fields of biology and neuroscience in the 1950s? From the perspective of the last century, one can say that surgery on the brain had its first revolution when Cushing laid its foundations early in the century. We have seen that essential to those foundations was simply meeting the highest standards of surgical practice in order to reduce mortality and enhance outcome with the methods at hand. As he observed, "there is no field of surgery in which fastidiousness is more essential to success" (Cushing, 1920, 611).

Fastidiousness ensures the standards of a field, but it does not make a revolution; that can only come about by new methods, often from outside the field. That is what brain imaging has done since the 1970s and what molecular tools are beginning to do and promise for the future—applied with the fastidiousness on which Cushing would have insisted.

Chapter 15

Neuropsychiatry: The Breakthrough in Psychopharmacology

Before 1950 the means to ameliorate psychiatric disorders were limited to psychoanalysis, on the one hand, and extreme treatments such as psychosurgery or electrical stimulation of the brain to produce convulsions, on the other. Mind was still conceived to be separate from body. This situation was radically changed by drug discoveries in the 1950s. The antischizophrenic drugs chlorpromazine, reserpine, and butyrophenones (haloperidol) caused dramatic quieting of schizophrenic patients, resulting in reduction or elimination of violent patients from hospital wards. Several classes of antidepression drugs (iproniazid, monoamine oxidase inhibitors, and tricyclics) were discovered, which gave the first relief from this debilitating mental and emotional disorder. The efficacy of lithium in the treatment of depression and bipolar disorder was also established. Drugs to treat neuroses, such as anxiety states, were also discovered, beginning with meprobamate and the benzodiazepines. These discoveries defined the three main classes of drugs for psychiatric use for the next half-century. Taken together, these discoveries made the 1950s revolutionary not only for psychiatry but also for all of humanity. A separate line of work characterized the nature of stress and identified the central role of the hypothalamic–pituitary axis.

We have already touched on advances in understanding the signaling molecules underlying normal brain function in earlier chapters (Chapters 4 and 9). We now consider the advances made in discovering molecules that could be used in treating mental disorders. Here again, the major breakthroughs occurred in the 1950s:

All prototypes of modern psychopharmaceuticals (lithium, chlorpromazine, meprobamate, imipramine and chlordiazepoxide) were discovered in a period of about 10 years [1948/49–58]. Neither before nor since has such a series of therapeutic advances been made in psychiatry.

(Spiegel, 45)

This work revolutionized the treatment of mental illness, as well as providing new insights into neurotransmitters and neurotransmitter systems. Through these and related discoveries, psychiatry—and humanity—may have benefited the most from the revolutions of those few short years in the 1950s.

Antipsychotic Drugs

The discovery of manufactured chemicals that can be useful in clinical medicine to bring order to disordered minds began, as so often happens, with drugs that had been developed by pharmaceutical companies for other purposes. In this case it was drugs for treating the effects of histamine. Among its actions, histamine is released in the body during hypersensitivity reactions, some serious, such as anaphylactic shock which affects the whole body, and some annoying, such as the allergic reactions that cause sneezing associated with the common cold. During the 1940s, pharmaceutical laboratories in the United States and France (working independently of each other because of the disruption of the Second World War) were interested in synthesizing antihistamine compounds for these purposes.

The possibility of drugs like these to treat the common cold created great demand by the public; it is from that time that still popular medications, such as diphenhydramine (Benadryl), originated. This led Paul Charpentier, a chemist with the Rhone-Poulenc pharmaceutical company in France, in 1950 to synthesize a number of compounds with antihistamine actions. One of these was promethazine (Phenergan), which had the apparently undesirable side effect of making patients sleepy (an action that is still present with many antihistamine drugs today).

Chlorpromazine (Largactil, Thorazine)

The discovery that was to start the revolution in psychiatry began with a French naval surgeon stationed in Malta.

Henri Laborit. Promethazine attracted the interest of Henri Laborit (Fig. 15.1A) for both its sedating actions, which he found useful in calming patients when preparing them for surgery, and its antihistamine actions, on the theory that histamine release might be responsible for surgical shock (a sudden loss of blood pressure while under general anesthesia). He called the sedating action "potentiated anesthesia" and "artificial hibernation." He asked the company for more compounds to test further. Among these, Charpentier had synthesized a compound, 4560RP (called "chlorpromazine"), which the company had put on the shelf because it had little potency as an antihistamine and was thought to be too powerful as a sedative. Laborit found that chlorpromazine induced a state of "quiétude béatifique" ("beautiful calm") in his patients. He therefore suggested to his colleagues in psychiatry that it might be useful in calming agitated patients. However, most found it to be ineffective.

Pierre Deniker and Jean Delay. The breakthrough came in 1951–52 when two psychiatrists in Paris, Pierre Deniker and Jean Delay (Fig. 15.1B, C), tried an approach in which they started with small doses and built up slowly to relatively large doses. Dramatically, the agitated patients became calm. Further testing showed that the drug worked to reduce anxiety and even to bring about improvement in paranoia and manic psychotic symptoms. The news spread rapidly, through a series of 11 publications, beginning with Laborit in February and continuing with Delay and Deniker and four other French groups, over a period of only 6 months in 1952 (Deniker, 1983).

As with every drug, there were side effects. The most serious was that higher doses induced a syndrome resembling Parkinson disease, including muscle rigidity, slowness of movement, and a resting tremor of the extremities. The treatment therefore had to titrate the parkinsonian effects against the calming effects. As we shall see, the parkinsonian effects in fact became one of the keys to understanding the mechanisms of the action of drugs on the brain.

The many actions of chlorpromazine prompted Rhone-Poulenc to market the drug under the name "Largactil" ("large actions"). A young Swiss, F. Labhardt, learned of the drug while doing postdoctoral training in Paris in 1951–52. Back in Basel, he and his colleagues carried out trials with the drug in early 1953, demonstrating its effectiveness in depression, addiction, withdrawal, and particularly schizophrenia. The First Largactil Symposium was held in Basel in November 1953, where the reports of the drug stimulated wide interest.

Chlorpromazine was first tested in North America in 1954, and by 1955 the drug had been adopted in the United States under the name "Thorazine." There, as in Europe, its effect on the practice of psychiatry was immediate and dramatic. Patients with severe mental illness that made them manic, threatening, violent, withdrawn, screaming, and generally unmanageable became quiet, cooperative, and able to begin to function normally. I saw these quiet and cooperative patients myself as a medical student on our rounds through the wards of psychiatric hospitals in the Boston area in 1956; we were told that a year before it would have been impossible to walk through the wards because of the physical danger from these same patients.

All of this occurred long before there was a field called neuroscience, but few advances since then can match the revolutionary and beneficial impact on mental health. "It was ... the first time that a single drug was active in the treatment of the major psychoses" (Deniker, 1983, 166).

Reserpine

The next drug discovered to affect the mind came from a plant called the snakeroot (*Rauwolfia serpentina*), known in India as a traditional folk remedy.

In the 1930s it was introduced clinically in India for reducing high blood pressure. The active principal, reserpine, was isolated by the Ciba Drug Company in 1950, and clinical trials began for treatment of hypertension. It was soon noted that, like chlorpromazine, reserpine had calming effects on the mental state and could bring relief to schizophrenic patients. As in the case of chlorpromazine 2 years earlier, a rapid series of reports in 1954, by Nathan Kline in the United States, Delay and Deniker in France, H. Steck in Switzerland, and others, established these effects.

Careful studies by Steck showed that high doses of reserpine caused parkinsonian motor symptoms like those of chlorpromazine (stiff and slow movements, tremor of the hands, etc.). In assessing these results, Delay and Deniker (1955) imagined that it was as if the brain had been seized and held by the drugs, and they introduced the term "neuroleptic" (*neuro*, "neuron"; *lepti*, "take hold of") to describe the effect. This term came to be applied to all drugs that "counteract marked inner unrest, psychomotor agitation and severe insomnia," symptoms that characterize schizophrenic psychoses, mania, paranoia, and depression (Spiegel, 1997, 3).

Reserpine was found to have a very slow action, and with higher doses the parkinsonian symptoms interfered with the antipsychotic actions. The drug fell into disuse in psychiatry, though it continued to be used as an antihypertensive agent. Its mechanism of action was to provide important clues in the further development of neuroleptic drugs.

Butyrophenones: Haloperidol

Another important class of neuroleptics produced during the 1950s was the butyrophenones. This work began in 1953 with research by P. A. J. Janssen and J. P. Tollenaere and their colleagues on compounds that might be even more effective than chlorpromazine and reserpine (recounted in Janssen and Tollenaere, 1983). They started with completely unrelated chemicals in the diphenylpropylamine series, with the objective of increasing the analgesic (pain-reducing) power of a member of the series called "pethidine." They persisted in their synthesizing efforts through a series of derivatives with decreasing morphinomimetic (pain-dulling, like the action of morphine) and increasing chlorpromazine-like (making animals calm) properties to compound R 1625 (R standing for "research," 1625 being the number of compounds synthesized in the study).

R 1625, named "Haloperidol," was synthesized in February 1958 and patented in April of that year. Its potency was several times greater than that of chlorpromazine, it was faster and longer-lasting, and it had fewer side effects. "Haloperidol was by far the most active neuroleptic known in 1958" (Janssen and Tollenaere, 1983, 189).

"Today one can only guess as to what guided us to pick up that particular combination of molecular fragments out of many thousands of possible combinations we could have synthesized. A certain insight in the structure-activity relationships, luck and serendipity were definitely important factors on our side." (Janssen and Tollenaere, 1983, 188)

Haloperidol was subsequently valuable as a research tool. With radioactive labeling, it was shown that of the two types of receptors for dopamine in the brain, D1 and D2, haloperidol binds to the D2 receptor. This was important evidence indicating the action of neuroleptics in general, that is, blocking the dopaminergic D2 receptors (summarized in Snyder, 1996).

Antidepression Drugs

During the first part of the twentieth century, a consensus emerged among psychiatrists on the two major types of severe mental disorders. On the one hand were the *psychoses,* often grouped under the term "schizophrenia," characterized by disturbances of thought so severe that a person is disconnected from reality (*schizo*, "divided"; *phrenia*, "mind"). As we have seen, these were the disturbances ameliorated by chlorpromazine. On the other hand was *depression,* characterized by feelings of sadness and hopelessness so painful and profound that a person can lose all desire to live. Paradoxically, depression often alternates with *mania*, the overexcited feeling that one can do anything and everything. In normal life everyone experiences periods of feeling depressed or elated, but the severe forms are incapacitating and when occurring in a pattern together are termed "manic-depressive disorder," or *bipolar disease.*

The most effective treatment for severe depression was electric shock therapy(EST), involving delivering repeated large voltages across the head. EST was a crude method that was and is little understood but continues to be used in severe cases, with often relatively good results. However, it was a situation that demanded an alternative in the form of drug therapy.

Psychiatrists at midcentury were on the lookout for antidepressant effects of drugs, but chlorpromazine was disappointing in this respect. Pharmaceutical companies produced many variations on the antihistamines but with little success.

The breakthrough came from several unexpected sources.

Iproniazid

One was tuberculosis, which at midcentury was still a big public health problem. Patients were treated with largely palliative measures at sanitariums around the United States and the world. Pharmaceutical companies actively tried to develop specific antitubercular drugs, and in 1952 Hoffman-LaRoche began marketing two such drugs, iproniazid (Marsalid) and isoniazid. As a treatment for tuberculosis iproniazid had mixed results, but clinicians noted that patients on the drug became cheerful, even euphoric, more so than one would expect from any improvement in their condition. Several groups had tested iproniazid on psychiatric patients, but no one had looked specifically at its possible use as an antidepressant.

During this time, Nathan Kline, the psychiatrist who had introduced reserpine in the United States for treatment of schizophrenia, was developing the idea that if reserpine could have a calming effect on agitated patients, there should be another drug that would have a stimulating effect. In 1956 he learned from Charles Scott and Max Chessin at Warner laboratories of their experiments showing that if animals were given iproniazid before reserpine, it converted the reserpine effect from hypoactivity to hyperactivity (Lehmann and Kline, 1983, 218). Similar results had been obtained independently by Bernard Brodie (Fig. 15.1D) and Parkhurst Shore at the National Institutes of Health.

There were few regulations of drug development at that time. Kline quickly got approval for the first clinical trial, which he launched, together with John Saunders and Harry Loomer, at Rockland Hospital, in November 1956. By February 1957 it seemed clear that iproniazid (as "Marsalid") had a specific action in relieving depression. This was reported at meetings in April and May (the first paper, by Loomer et al., appeared in 1957). Thus, from hypothesis to successful completion of the first clinical trial took exactly 1 year (Lehmann and Kline, 1983). For better or for worse, those were the days!

Monoamine Oxidase Inhibitors

Insight into the mechanisms of action of iproniazid came from another line of work with its own long history. In the 1930s an enzyme that degrades the amino acid tyramine (by removing the terminal hydroxyl group) in the liver of the rat was discovered. A large family of amine compounds was identified, and the enzyme that degraded them came to be called "monoamine oxidase" (MAO) (Zeller et al., 1939; Zeller, 1983, 224). Among the compounds tested for anti-MAO properties were the hydrazides, the class containing iproniazid and isoniazid.

The new availability of radioactively labeled ^{14}C amines enabled animal studies by Albert Zeller and colleagues at Northwestern University to be carried out on amine metabolism, which showed that degradation by MAO was involved. They further found that iproniazid was the most effective substance known in blocking monoamine turnover (Zeller, 1983, 227). The amines tested included norepinephrine, known to be a neurotransmitter in the autonomic nervous system, and serotonin. On the basis of these results, Zeller and his colleagues initiated their own clinical studies of iproniazid in the treatment of depression. The results were consistent with the more extensive and widely known results of Kline et al.

Their work on MAO suggested at first the hypothesis that, in analogy with the action of acetylcholinesterase in terminating the action of acetylcholine at cholinergic synapses (see Chapter 4), MAO might terminate the action of epinephrine and other monoamines at adrenergic synapses. Later studies showed that the actions of monoamines are in fact terminated mainly by a different mechanism, reuptake into the presynaptic terminal (Zeller, 1983, 224; Axelrod, 1965).

The metabolic pathway for synthesis of monoamines, from tyrosine hydro-xylase through dopamine and norepinephrine to epinephrine, had been iden-tified in the classical work of Hugh Blashko in 1939 (Chapter 4). Analysis of this pathway was made possible by two key steps: the advent of MAO inhibitors, which blocked the degradation of the monoamine under study, and reserpine, which depleted the monoamines. Aided by these two tools in the early 1950s, plus radioactive labeling of the compounds, the monoamines were launched as a major area of research in neurochemistry and psychiatry, which continues today.

Depletion of monoamines by reserpine was first reported by Bernard Brodie and Parkhurst Shore in 1957, who found that reserpine depleted the amount of serotonin that could be measured in the whole brain. A similar effect was then found on the neurotransmitter norepinephrine. In 1958 whole-brain assays showed the presence of the related amine dopamine, and it was soon demon-strated that it too was depleted by reserpine (Snyder, 1996). Thus, while reser-pine was ceasing to be useful clinically, it was having a second life as a valuable tool in animal research.

Much of this early research in the United States emanated from Brodie's Laboratory of Chemical Pharmacology at the NIH. Brodie was a larger-than-life character, whose research was driven by both methods and ideas; as observed by his long-time collaborator Julius Axelrod (Healy, 2001, 43):

"He was very imaginative. . . . in order to be a productive scientist you have to have lots of ideas which you can try out. . . . If you have no novel ideas, nothing happens – you can do incremental work – that's just improving on something already known. But to do something original you have to have really bold ideas which Brodie had and he was also convincing. He was very stimulating and you wanted to rush to the lab to try out his ideas."

Imipramine and Tricyclic Drugs

After the introduction of chlorpromazine as an antipsychotic drug, chemists set out to search for chemically related drugs that might have similar effects. Among them were the iminodibenzyl compounds, which like chlorpromazine consist of a core of three benzine rings in a row, with an amine group several carbons long attached to the middle ring. Most of these sat on the shelf, so to speak, waiting for clinicians to test them.

Among the early clinicians testing chlorpromazine was Roland Kuhn at a psychiatric clinic in Switzerland. Not able to afford the expense of using chlor-promazine on a large scale, he inquired of the chemists at Geigy Pharmaceuticals in 1954 if they could provide him with a less expensive com-pound similar in structure to chlorpromazine. Compound G 22355, also called "imipramine," was provided. Kuhn tested it on a range of psychiatric patients with disappointing results, but he persisted. In the spring of 1957 it took success in only three patients to convince him that imipramine had a specific antide-pressant effect. His first report was delivered in September 1957 to an audience of about a dozen at the Second International Congress of Psychiatry in Zurich (see Kuhn, 1958).

Word spread quickly, and imipramine quickly became established in the treatment of endogenous (spontaneous) depression. It also became the proto-type of the class of tricyclic drugs that became not only a staple in clinical practice but also a powerful tool in animal experiments on the brain mechan-isms underlying depression. In recent years the tricyclic drugs have been increasingly replaced by selective serotonin reuptake inhibitors.

Lithium

A completely separate line of work involved the use of lithium against manic-depressive states. There had been anecdotal observations but no systematic study until John Cade (Fig. 15.2A) in Australia hypothesized that manic states might produce an excess of some body product which would be excreted in raised amounts in the urine. While testing the toxic effects of human urine on guinea pigs, he was led to the use of a soluble form of uric acid bound to lithium and eventually found that the protection against the toxic effects of urea was due to the lithium. Injection of lithium carbonate into guinea pigs caused lethargy. In 1949 he reported that lithium carbonate induced a reduction in excitable states of psychotic patients. Few psychiatrists took notice.

In 1954 Mogens Schou (Fig. 15.2B) in Denmark carried out a systematic clinical study that established the efficacy of lithium in the treatment of states of mania (Schou et al., 1954). Although there was initial skepticism that a simple metallic ion could have this effect, subsequent studies over several decades by Schou and others have gradually led to acceptance of lithium as a component in therapy for bipolar disorder.

One deterrent to the use of lithium was the fact that, as a common salt, it was not patentable; therefore, no pharmaceutical company was interested in devel-oping it for therapeutic uses. Yet the importance of lithium therapy should not be underestimated: according to Richard Restak (1995, 66–67): "His [John Cade's] discovery of the antimanic effects of lithium inaugurated the modern science of psychopharmacology".

"Minor Tranquillizers"

Distinct from the severe types of mental illness characterized by schizophrenia and depression are states of tension, anxiety, agitation, insomnia, headaches, gastrointestinal disturbances, and the like (Spiegel, 17) produced by the multi-tude of stresses of everyday life. In contrast to the psychoses, these go under the name of **neuroses**. They may vary from the annoying to the incapacitating.

Traditionally, people have sought to relieve these stresses by various means (Spiegel, 20). Alcohol is one of the main staples; however, as is all too well known, alcohol has only a general and transient calming action and with chronic use becomes addictive and harmful. Tobacco is also calming but addictive, with its own harmful effects on the body. Opiates have their well-known addictive qualities, as do drugs such as the barbiturates.

Meprobamate (Miltown)

Spurred on by the success of chlorpromazine in ameliorating psychoses, pharmaceutical companies and clinicians attempted in the early 1950s to test drugs for specific effects as calming agents (also called "anxiolytics") for neuroses. The line that eventually proved successful actually started with a research program at an English pharmaceutical company in the 1940s to develop drugs effective against penicillin-resistant bacteria (Spiegel and Markstein, 1997, 43; Snyder, 157).

The program was under Frank Berger, a Czechoslovakian who had escaped to England during World War II. One of the compounds produced was mephenesin. A side effect of this drug was that animals injected with high doses became limp due to muscle relaxation and sedation, though they remained fully conscious (Snyder, 157). Berger described the effect on animals as "tranquillization." Human tests also showed that it was muscle-relaxing as well as anxiety-relieving, without clouding consciousness.

Mephenesin breaks down rapidly in the body, so the chemists tested related compounds that would be more slowly metabolized. This led in 1954 to meprobamate, which fulfilled the desired criteria of relieving anxiety with a long duration of action and minimal side effects. Meprobamate was tested clinically by Berger in 1955 (Spiegel and Markstein, 1997, 45) and, introduced onto the American market in the same year under the name "Miltown," became the first widely used anti-anxiety drug. In contrast to chlorpromazine's action against psychoses (qualifying it as a "major tranquillizer"), meprobamate was referred to as a "minor "tranquillizer" in acting against neuroses. The barbiturates in turn were relegated to being "sedatives". However, meprobamate's success did not last long. Patients did become drowsy. Worse, patients became tolerant to the drug, requiring larger and larger doses, leading to addiction.

Benzodiazepines (Librium, Valium)

The initial success of meprobamate stimulated drug companies to get into this new field by directing their chemists to search for other compounds with "psychosedative" qualities. Among them was Leo Sternbach (Fig. 15.3) at Roche Laboratories. Sternbach had trained in Poland; he was working in Switzerland when World War II broke out and soon made his way to the United States. Instead of the usual strategy for drug development of building from known compounds, Sternbach decided on the more risky approach of striking out with entirely new compounds (Haefely, 1983, 272). He recalled some chemicals he had worked on in Poland as potential dyestuffs, including 3,1-4-benzoxadiazepines. These have a basic side chain, which is active in many drugs with biological activity (Haefely, 1983, 274).

Sternbach synthesized some compounds derived from this structure and tested them but obtained no interesting results in tests on animals. The work was laid aside, and he was told by the company to move on to other projects. While cleaning out his laboratory one day he noticed a last compound left over from the study and submitted it, labeled Ro 5-0690, to Lowell Randall, head of the pharmacology unit, for evaluation for its pharmacological effects. Several days later Randall reported that the compound showed all the desirable qualities: "a potent muscle relaxant and sedative with no general anaesthetic properties and apparently devoid of autonomic effects, and all this with a very low toxicity" (Haefely, 1983, 275).

Sternbach resynthesized Ro 5-0690 in larger quantities for further development. He found that the compound had the chemical structure of a quinazoline 3-oxide and belonged to the benzodiazepine class (Haefely, 1983, 277). It was eventually given the generic name "chlordiazepoxide." The pharmacological properties were reported in 1959 and published the year after (Randall et al., 1960). Clinical trials began in 1958 with discouraging results. The subjects felt sleepy and dizzy and had slurred speech, and the trials were stopped. Then it was realized the dose was too high; at lower doses the desired effects were produced. Acceptance spread quickly, and in February 1960, after 2 years of clinical trials, chlorazepoxide was introduced as a new (minor) tranquillizer on the U.S. market with the name "Librium." Further chemical tinkering with the molecule was carried out to find a compound less bitter to the taste, which resulted in 1963 in diazepam (Valium). Several dozen variations have appeared since then.

During the development of the benzodiazepines, no insights were gained into the pharmacological mechanisms. In contrast to the development of the antidepressant drugs, which early investigations showed were involved with the monoamine neurotransmitters, tests on acetylcholine and monoamine systems showed only negligible effects. It was not until later in the 1960s that the relation of the benzodiazepines to inhibitory synapses using the neurotransmitter γ-aminobutyric acid (GABA) was realized. Also, the actions of the benzodiazepines as anticonvulsant agents in the control of epileptic seizures awaited the future.

Stress

Few terms from biomedical research have entered the public vocabulary as widely as "stress," another product of the 1950s, for which **Hans Selye** was the originator.

Selye was born of Hungarian descent in Vienna in 1907. After obtaining his medical degree in Prague in 1929, he came to the United States to study at Johns Hopkins, then went to Canada at McGill University. He began by investigating the growth of bones and calcium metabolism and then carried out a project of injecting organ extracts into animals and observing the effects on different body organs. His initial findings were reported in a brief note in *Nature* in 1936, entitled "A Syndrome Produced by Diverse Nocuous Agents," which began as follows (p 32):

> Experiments on rats show that if the organism is severely damaged by acute nonspecific nocuous agents such as exposure to cold, surgical injury, production of spinal shock (transcision of the cord), excessive muscular exercise, or intoxications with sublethal doses of diverse drugs (adrenaline, atropine, morphine, formaldehyde, etc.), a typical syndrome appears, the symptoms of which are independent of the nature of the damaging agent or the pharmacological type of the drug employed, and represent rather a response to damage as such.

He described this syndrome as developing in three stages. In the first 2 days various body organs are affected: the thymus gland shrinks, the stomach and duodenum develop ulcers; there is widespread edema formation, and other effects. This is followed by swelling of the adrenal cortex and what appears to be a shift by the anterior pituitary to increased production of thyrotropic and adrenotropic hormones to deal with the body emergency. If this response is successful, it is called the "resistance stage." If not, the animal proceeds to the third stage, of exhaustion.

> We consider the first stage to be the expression of a general alarm of the organism when suddenly confronted with a critical situation, and therefore term it the "general alarm reaction." Since the syndrome as a whole seems to represent a generalized effort of the organism to adapt itself to new conditions, it might be termed the "general adaptation syndrome." It might be compared to other general defense reactions such as inflammation or the formation of immune bodies. The symptoms of the alarm reaction are very similar to those of histamine toxicosis or of surgical or anaphylactic shock; it is therefore not unlikely that an essential part in the initiation of the syndrome is the liberation of large quantities of histamine or some similar substance, which may be released from the tissues either mechanically in surgical injury, or by other means in other cases. It seems to us that more or less pronounced forms of this three-stage reaction represent the usual response of the organism to stimuli such as temperature changes, drugs, muscular exercise, etc., to which habituation or inurement can occur (32).

This 1936 article has been called "a cornerstone of neuropsychiatry because it led to the study of the effects of stress and hormones, particularly corticosteroids, on brain function" (Neylan, 1998, 230). Selye developed his idea of the "general adaptation syndrome" through a series of experiments on the effects on different body organs. By 1950 he had identified interconnected hormonal pathways that appeared to be involved. In so doing he is credited with identifying the hypothalamic–pituitary axis (HPA) as the central pathway for hormonal control, the physiological correlate of the anatomical and vascular pathway from hypothalamus to anterior pituitary identified by Harris and colleagues (1955) during this time period (see Chapter 11).

In 1949 he began to replace "alarm reaction" with "stress" in characterizing the syndrome, in research articles (Fortier and Selye, 1949) and soon thereafter in a massive monograph (Selye, 1956). These immediately gave stress wide currency among the lay public. I well remember this time, when the idea of a link between brain and body – often in the new context of "psychosomatic medicine" - was increasingly discussed. The 300 years of separation by Descartes between the two was being breached. It was during this time that the psychoactive drugs were coming on the market, promising alleviation or cures for many of the ills—anxiety, neurosis, depression—linked directly or indirectly to stress.

Selye churned out large numbers of papers and books on the subject. He became a charismatic figure in promoting this new kind of science, uniting the worlds of brains, bodies, and hormones, and how they cope with the stresses of life. By the time he died in 1982 he had published 1700 papers and 40 books. He was often mentioned as deserving the highest recognition for his achievements. There are several reasons he fell short. There was, to begin with, a problem with the definition of "stress." In physics, a *stress* is the agent, whereas the response is the *strain*, just the opposite of Selye's use. He was quoted later as regretting this terminological inconsistency. The all-embracing scale of his conception left it open to criticism of inaccuracies in representing specific aspects of the "stress" system, such as that the stress response was always the same regardless of the nature of the "stressor." Corticosteroids were an important part of the stress response and had already been oversold as a panacea for many inflammatory responses; this also encouraged a healthy skepticism about claims for the importance of the stress response. "Stress" soon became a blanket term, losing thereby its scientific value. Despite being a "cornerstone" of neuropsychiatry, stress is barely mentioned in a recent history of psychiatry, and Selye is forgotten (Shorter, 1997).

Modern research on stress is carried out mainly at the level of specific systems, such as the HPA axis, limbic systems for emotion and anxiety, and the cardiovascular systems underlying hypertension. However, from a longer perspective, "stress" is a among the important contributions of the 1950s, both for its impact on medicine and the general public and for its incorporation into daily thought about the human condition.

Chapter 16

Theoretical Neuroscience: The Brain as a Computer and the Computer as a Brain

The mid-twentieth century marked the emergence of several new fields that laid the foundations for general theories of brain function. McCulloch and Pitts applied the symbolic logic metaphor to nerve cell circuits, postulating that specific interconnections could perform basic logic functions such as AND, OR, and AND–NOT gates. John von Neumann drew on this idea of the brain in formulating the classical architecture of the digital computer. A new field of game theory arose from the seminal work of von Neumann and Morgenstern. Shannon and Weaver established the new discipline of information theory, which became the framework for the computer age. Developments in control theory, neurology, and adaptive behavior came together in the new field of cybernetics. The McCulloch-Pitts oversimplified neurons contributed to the rise of artificial intelligence and neural nets. von Neumann eventually realized that the fundamental computational elements of the nervous system are not over-simplified neurons but individual synapses distributed on dendritic trees. This insight anticipated current work on developing more realistic large-scale neural networks, drawing on studies at all the levels of organization covered in this book, to simulate how the brain actually carries out its functions.

The creation of modern neuroscience was obviously driven by experimental advances. However, the observant reader will have noticed that theory has in fact played a critical role. Some of the main advances that involved specific types of mathematical and/or theoretical models are summarized in Table 16.1.

In addition to these advances at specific levels of functional organization, the ultimate challenge in neuroscience is to build a theory that applies to the

Table 16.1 Contributions of Theory to Specific Functions of Nerve Cells

---

Physical model of DNA by Watson and Crick (Chapter 2)
Constant field membrane theory of Goldman-Hodgkin-Huxley (Chapter 4)
Mathematical model of the nerve action potential by Hodgkin and Huxley (Chapter 4)
Poisson/binomial theory for synaptic vesicle release by del Castillo and Katz (Chapter 5)
Dendritic branching theory of Rall (Chapter 6)
Synaptic learning theory of Hebb (Chapter 10)
Energy metabolism of the brain (Chapter 14)

Table 16.2 Initial Steps Toward a Theory of Brain Function

Symbolic logic (Boole, 1854; Shannon, 1937; McCulloch and Pitts, 1943)
The brain as a computer (von Neumann, 1945, 1957)
Game theory (von Neumann and Morgenstern, 1944)
Information theory (Shannon and Weaver, 1948)
Cybernetics (Wiener, 1948)
The "cell assembly" (Hebb, 1949)
Artificial intelligence and neural nets (1950s)

---

whole brain. If the impulse and the synapse are universal elements of the nervous system, how can we construct an overall theory of how they operate in an integrated manner to constitute the neural basis of behavior and, in particular, of human thought and feeling? Many feel that this is the holy grail of brain science.

It wasn't until the mid-twentieth century that this goal could even be formulated in a realistic manner and attempts to reach it could begin. Here, we summarize several of the most important initiatives during this period (Table 16.2). As we shall see, "giants walked the earth," as did so many others that we have discussed in this period. In this endeavor, the computer, heralding the new age of information, and the brain were intertwined in a remarkable manner.

The Metaphor of Symbolic Logic

A theory requires rigorous rules. How can the variety of human thought generated by the brain be expressed in a simple fashion?

The idea that thought could be characterized by logical rules was developed by George Boole (1815–64), a professor of mathematics in Ireland. His major treatise, entitled "An Investigation of the Laws of Thought, on Which Are Founded the Mathematical Theories of Logic and Probabilities" in 1854, set out in detail the rules by which combinations of simple propositions, such as "this and this," "this or this," and "this and not this," can be formalized into rules of AND, OR, and AND–NOT for logical inference.

Boole's extensive studies became well known among scholars in logical theory but otherwise remained relatively unknown and seemingly without much practical application in the real world. However, he took on new meaning when rediscovered in the 1930s by Claude Shannon (1916–2001) when taking a class in philosophy while an undergraduate at the University of Michigan:

> Shannon recognised that Boole's work could form the basis of mechanisms and processes in the real world. . . . Shannon went on to write a master's thesis at the Massachusetts Institute of Technology, in which he showed how Boolean algebra could optimize the design of systems of electromechanical relays then used in telephone routing switches. He also proved that circuits with relays could solve Boolean algebra problems. Employing the properties of electrical switches to process logic is the basic concept that underlies all modern electronic digital computers. . . . Boolean algebra became the foundation of practical digital circuit design; and Boole, via Shannon and Shestakov [in the Soviet Union], provided the theoretical grounding for the Digital Age.
>
> (http://en.wikipedia.org/wiki/George_Boole)

That dissertation has since been hailed as one of the most significant master's theses of the twentieth century. To all intents and purposes, its use of binary code and Boolean algebra paved the way for the digital circuitry that is crucial to the operation of modern computers and telecommunications equipment (Emerson, 2001).

Boole had also suggested that his approach had implications for understanding the brain:

> . . . no general method for the solution of questions in the theory of probabilities can be established which does not explicitly recognise . . . those universal laws of thought which are the basis of all reasoning . . .
>
> (http://www.kerryr.net/pioneers/boole.htm)

How such "universal laws of thought" might be implemented in the brain was the object of a study published by Warren McCulloch (1898–1969) and Walter Pitts (1923–69) in 1943, which played a seminal role in both computer development and theoretical neuroscience. We have already met them as collaborators much later in the study of what the frog's eye tells the frog's brain (Chapter 10).

Warren McCulloch majored in philosophy and psychology at Yale University, where he was inspired by Descartes and Leibniz to think about the physical basis of the brain and the mind. After earning an MD in the 1920s,

> . . . in spite of the busy life of the intern, I was forever studying anything that might lead me to a theory of nervous function. My fellow intern . . . accused me of trying to write an equation for the working of the brain. I am still trying to!
>
> (Morena-Diaz and Morena-Diaz, 2007)

When the Great Depression hit in the early 1930s he spent time teaching college psychology and studying mathematics and physics. In 1934 he turned to research in neurophysiology with a leading figure, Dusser de Barenne, at Yale. For several years they studied connections in the cerebral cortex using artificial activation by local application of strychnine, which blocked inhibition to cause intense activation of distant targets.

Walter Pitts was a child prodigy who by the age of 12, in 1935, had learned logic, mathematics, Latin, and Greek, among other subjects. Part of the Pitts legend is that he corresponded with Bertrand Russell, criticizing several aspects of his magnum opus, *Principia Mathematica*, written with Alfred North Whitehead. Deciding to become a logician, at 15 he ran away and, though homeless, hung around at the University of Chicago, attending the lectures of Rudolf Carnap on logic and logical positivism and engaging the philosopher in detailed discussions about his work. During this time he was befriended and helped by Jerry Lettvin (Chapter 10).

McCulloch moved from Yale to Chicago in 1941 and shortly thereafter met Pitts and Lettvin and invited them to live with him. Their conversations ranged over all the philosophers and scientists they had studied through the years. Leibniz's ideas of symbolic thought, anticipating Boole, particularly stimulated them. Out of their conversations came the idea of a paper: "A Logical Calculus of the Ideas Immanent in Nervous Activity," published in 1943 in the *Bulletin of Mathematical Biophysics* (McCulloch and Pitts, 1943).

They noted that "because of the all-or-none character of nervous activity, neural events and the relations among them can be treated by means of propositional logic." In this view the all-or-none property of the action potential (i.e., impulse) in the nerve axons represents a logic gate that is either on or off and thereby gives a two-valued logic underlying all mental activity. They illustrated this idea with diagrams of neurons that are interconnected in specific ways to generate the basic logic functions of AND, OR, and AND–NOT (see Fig. 16.1) as well as other more elaborate logic functions.

This conceptual framework was resisted as being too simple by most neurophysiologists, as they began learning of graded potentials at the synaptic junctions between nerve cells. Also, the idea of reducing a nerve cell to only a single node, representing the cell body, ignored the elaborate dendritic trees of most neurons that had been shown so elegantly in the studies with the Golgi stain by Golgi, Ramón y Cajal, and the classical histologists (Chapter 8). The logical calculus of McCulloch and Pitts therefore played little role in the rise of experimental neuroscience at midcentury. The development of the digital computer was another matter.

The Computer and the Brain

Midcentury saw the invention and rise of the digital computer, which has come to be one of the defining devices of modern life. The metaphor seemed, and seems, obvious: The brain processes information, and so does a computer. Indeed, the rise of the computer and the rise of theoretical neuroscience are closely intertwined. How this happened is little remembered today but is one of the most absorbing chapters in the revolution of midcentury neuroscience.

There are several claimants to inventing the digital computer, the clearest being **John Atanasoff** (1903–95). He was a physics professor at Iowa State College in Ames, Iowa. I grew up a block from his home. Like many other physicists, Atanasoff used the Bush differential analyzer to solve large sets of simultaneous equations. In the 1930s he began to develop the notion of replacing it with a faster, purely digital device. Struggling with unformed ideas, he went on a legendary automobile drive "at a high rate of speed" (Atanasoff, 1984) across the state in the middle of the night in 1939 and hit upon the main ideas of the new device: It would use electricity and electronics, calculations would use base-2 (binary) numbers, calculations would be stored in memory, and computations would be "by direct logical action, not by enumeration." Over the next 2 years he built a prototype of this computer with a graduate student, Clifford Berry; they called it, appropriately, the "ABC."

The official computer histories note that during this time several others were working to the same purpose. Konrad Zuse in Germany was one; his machine also was electronic, divided into a calculating unit, memory unit, control unit, and input (the "program") and output units. However, when Germany went to war in 1939, his project was ignored. Meanwhile, in England, Alan Turing, a young mathematician, wrote an article in 1936 entitled "On Computable Numbers, with an Application to the Entscheidungsproblem [decision-making problem]." In it he conceived of a machine that could read an infinitely long tape in a digital logical manner and in principle could compute any number. Although a "Turing machine" was never built, it became the symbol (and still is) of a digital computer with unlimited computing power.

While building his prototype, Atanasoff went to a meeting and met **John Mauchly**, who was also doing large-scale calculations, related to climate. He was much interested to hear of Atanasoff's project and made a visit of several days in early 1941 to go over the machine and read a lengthy description of it that Atanasoff was preparing for submission for a patent. The onset of the war intervened, and the patent was never applied for; but Mauchly had seen the future. He returned to Philadelphia and took a course in advanced electronics at the Moore School of Engineering at the University of Pennsylvania. There, he met **J. Presper Eckert**, a brilliant young graduate student in electrical engineering who was helping to teach the course.

They hit it off and developed plans together to build a completely electronic computer, using vacuum tubes instead of condensers for the memory. Such a machine would be of use to the Army for calculating ballistic trajectories for aiming artillery. In August 1942 Mauchly submitted a proposal to the Ordnance Department of the Department of War, proposing "The use of high speed vacuum tube devices for calculating." The proposal was finally adopted and funded in June of 1943. The machine to be built was called the "ENIAC," for

"Electronic Numerical Integrator and Computer." (It was another example of funding of new technology by the armed services.)

The new innovations were that the ENIAC was large (20,000 vacuum tubes), very fast (200,000 pulses per second), programmable, and general-purpose. It was 8 feet high and 80 feet long, foreshadowing the era of room-sized mainframe computers. The project was not completed until late 1945, so ENIAC didn't in fact contribute to the war effort as hoped. However, it was immediately viewed as a tremendous success, launching the computer age.

John von Neumann. Essential to the computer is the program, which is where John von Neumann and the brain enter the picture.

He was born in Budapest, Hungary, in 1903. A prodigy, he graduated in mathematics in Budapest and chemical engineering at the Eidgenössische Technische Hochschule (Federal Institute of Technology) in Zurich in 1925. He taught and published prolifically for a few years. In 1930 he emigrated to the United States and in 1933 was named one of the first of the faculty of the Institute for Advanced Study at Princeton. During his time there he became a leader in many fields, including set theory, functional analysis, quantum mechanics, numerical analysis, and statistics. With the outbreak of World War II, he became a member of the Manhattan Project to build the atomic bomb.

It was while engaged in the Manhattan Project that he heard about the ENIAC. As the ENIAC was getting under way, Mauchly and Eckert were already conceiving of the next generation of computer, which would have a stored program to run the calculations through the central processor and a memory for both the data from the calculations and the programs that ran them. Based on their plans, the head of the Ballistics Research Laboratory, Herman Goldstine, applied for a grant, again from the Ordnance Department, in October of 1944 to build the EDVAC ("Electronic Discrete Variable Computer").

When von Neumann, by chance, heard about the ENIAC and EDVAC projects, he was immediately interested in a key aspect: What was their logical structure? He brought considerable intellectual respectability to the projects, which were being harshly criticized by Vannevar Bush and other leading physicists as too slow and a waste of money (Augarten, 1984). This is ironic because of Bush's key role as science advisor to the president and a sage architect of government funding of science after the war. To keep von Neumann from meddling in the projects, Bush had tried to block any knowledge of them reaching him. However, von Neumann was not to be denied.

von Neumann became a consultant to the project and in June 1945 wrote a 101-page manuscript entitled *First Draft of a Report on the EDVAC* on the plans for the EDVAC and, in particular, on the logical control design:

> In brief, von Neumann recommended the construction of a computer based on a central control unit that would orchestrate all operations; a central processor unit that would carry out all arithmetical and logical operations; and a random-access read/write memory (this is a

contemporary term) that would store programs and data in such a way that any piece of information could be entered or retrieved directly (rather than sequentially). He also recommended the use of binary words in series rather than in parallel. In other words, instead of operating on every bit in a word at the same time, as ENIAC did, EDVAC would process every bit one at a time. All things being equal, a parallel computer is faster than a serial one, but it is more difficult to build—thus the reason for von Neumann's suggestion.

(Augarten, 1984, 140)

This was the first description of the design of a general-purpose digital electronic computer. Coming from von Neumann, it instantly gave him recognition as a creator of the modern computer, which led to years of controversy over his role vis-à-vis Mauchly and Eckert, including the inevitable issue of patent rights.

What was the source of von Neumann's ideas? There were his talents as a mathematician, obviously. But there were two additional possible sources not heretofore emphasized. One was Atanasoff. In 1946 Atanasoff had been put in charge of a new program to build a computer at the Naval Ordnance Laboratory. But after several months, he was informed at a meeting that the computing project was canceled. Atanasoff later recalled that von Neumann was at this meeting and praised Atanasoff for his competence in computing. One is left to speculate that von Neumann might have joined with Mauchly to quench any competition from another ordnance laboratory—also, that von Neumann, in recommending the use of binary logic to build EDVAC, must have been aware that he was following Atanasoff, who had built his early machine specifically on this basis.

The other source was the brain. von Neumann met McCulloch at a series of conferences organized by the Macy Foundation to bring together investigators from different fields working in the area of information and control theory. According to McCulloch (in Moreno-Diaz and Moreno-Diaz, 2007, 186), "von Neumann used our article in teaching the general theory of digital computers..." Evidence for this critical role of the brain as the model for the computer is found at several places in his "First Draft" (see also Burks, 2003):

2.6 The specific parts [central arithmetic, central control, memory] correspond to the *associative* neurons in the human nervous system. It remains to discuss the equivalents of the *sensory* or *afferent* and the *motor* or *efferent* neurons. These are the input and output organs of the device.

4.2 It is worth mentioning, that the neurons of the higher animals are definitely elements [for computing] in the above sense. They have all-or-none character, that is two states: Quiescent and excited.... An excited neuron emits the standard stimulus along many lines (axons). Such a line can, however, be connected in two different ways to the next neuron: First: In an excitatory synapse, so that the stimulus causes the excitation of the neuron. Second: In an inhibitory synapse, so that the stimulus absolutely prevents the excitation of the neuron by any stimulus on any other (excitatory) synapse. The neuron also has a definite reaction time, between the reception of a stimulus and the emission of the stimuli caused by it, the synaptic delay. [This was a decade before the work of Eccles revealed these properties in central neurons—Chapter 7].

Following W. S. MacCulloch [*sic*] and W. Pitts... we ignore the more complicated aspects of neuron functioning: Thresholds, temporal summation, relative inhibition, changes of the threshold by after-effects of stimulation beyond the synaptic delay, etc. It is, however, convenient to consider occasionally neurons with fixed thresholds 2 and 3, that is, neurons which can be excited only by (simultaneous) stimuli on 2 or 3 excitatory synapses (and none on an inhibitory synapse)....

It is easily seen that these simplified neuron functions can be imitated by telegraphic relays or by vacuum tubes. Although the nervous system is presumably asynchronous (for the synaptic delays), precise synaptic delays can be obtained by using synchronous setups.

4.3 It is clear that a very high speed computing device should ideally have vacuum tube elements. Vacuum tube aggregates like counters and scalers have been used and found reliable at reaction times (synaptic delays) as short as a microsecond.... It is interesting to note that the synaptic time of a human neuron is of the order of a millisecond....

5.0 Principles governing the arithmetical operation

... The analogs of human neurons, discussed in 4.2–4.3 are equally all-or-none elements. It will appear that they are quite useful for all preliminary, orienting, considerations of vacuum tube systems.... It is therefore satisfactory that here too the natural arithmetical system to handle is the binary one [as in Atanasoff's original machine but not ENIAC].

These passages make clear an intriguing irony: It was the unrealistic reduction by McCulloch and Pitts of the neuron to a single summing node that enabled von Neumann to use the brain as a model for constructing the computer.

Currently, neuroscientists analyze the brain as a computer. In the beginning, the computer was built to resemble the brain. We will see that von Neumann returned to consider in much greater detail the brain as a computer at the end of his life in 1957.

Game Theory

As an example of the tremendous range of von Neumann's accomplishments, in 1944 he co-authored with **Oskar Morgenstern** a thick book, full of equations, entitled *Theory of Games and Economic Behavior*. The reviews at the time heralded the importance of this book. Copeland, in the *Bulletin of the American Mathematical Society*, wrote that "Posterity may regard this book as one of the major scientific achievements of the first half of the twentieth century" (Kuhn, 2004, viii). Hurwitz, in the *American Economic Review*, wrote that "the techniques . . . are of sufficient generality to be valid in political science, sociology, or even military strategy" (Kuhn, 2004, viii). The importance is furthered described by Harold Kuhn (2004, xii-xiii) in his introduction to the Sixtieth Anniversary Edition:

> The period of the late '40s and early 50s was a period of excitement in game theory. The discipline had broken out of its cocoon and was testing its wings. Giants walked the earth. At Princeton, John Nash laid the groundwork for the general non-cooperative theory and for cooperative bargaining theory. Lloyd Shapley defined a value for conditional games, initiated the theory of stochastic games, coinvented the core with D. B. Gillies, and together with John Milner developed the first game models with an infinite number of players. Harold Kuhn reformulated the extensive form and introduced the concepts of behavior strategies and perfect recall. A. W. Tucker invented the story of the Prisoner's Dilemma, which has entered popular culture as a crucial example of the interplay between competition and cooperation.

With the development in recent years of methods for carrying out game theory paradigms in awake, behaving primates, these principles are extending deeply into current studies in behavioral and cognitive neuroscience. They not only give insight into neural mechanisms but also are contributing to new spin-off fields such as neuroeconomics. My colleague Daeyol Lee, who uses game theory paradigms to study decision making in single neuron activity in the prefrontal cortex of monkeys, maintains that von Neumann and Morgenstern's book is the greatest book in science in the twentieth century. We have seen (Chapter 12) that a strong case has also been made for Hebb's *Organization of Behavior*.

Information Theory

Yet another new field was about to be invented. Shannon's thesis on Boolean principles brought him instant recognition, opening doors for further training under the most stimulating circumstances. This involved a PhD at MIT, a National Research Fellowship at the Institute for Advanced Study at Princeton, and Bell Labs, the premier industry research institute of that time, in 1942.

The work for which he was most widely known was the book *The Mathematical Theory of Communication*, which he authored in 1948 together with Warren Weaver; it is said that Shannon supplied the math, and Weaver helped make it understandable to the general reader. Information was described in binary terms, a key step toward the era of modern telecommunications. The theory defines communication between a transmitter and a receiver in rigorous terms, characterizing information entropy as a measure of the uncertainty in the message. The book is regarded as a founding document of information theory and the information age. We knew at the time we were entering this age. The idea that electronic communication could be characterized in rigorous terms was iconic. In this sense this book is also a worthy competitor to von Neumann and Morgenstern's.

> The impact of this work was immediate and far-reaching. Lauded as "The Magna Carta of the information age," disciplines as diverse as computer science, genetic engineering, and neuroanatomy used Shannon's discoveries to solve puzzles as different as computer error correction code problems and biological entropy.
>
> (http://www.kerryr.net/pioneers/shannon.htm)

Shannon returned to MIT in 1956, where he stayed until retiring in 1978. His prodigious achievements were instrumental in founding and enriching many fields of science.

Analysis of encoding of messages in spike discharges in neurons, using the principles of information theory, was taken up later in the 1960s and 1970s by Juan Segundo and colleagues.

Cybernetics

Another mathematical prodigy during this period (it was a great era for mathematicians and opera singers, in addition to neuroscientists) was **Norbert Wiener** (1894–1964). The son of a Harvard professor, he was mostly home-taught, graduating from high school at 11, from Tufts College at 14, and obtaining his PhD from Harvard at 18 in mathematical logic. Further study abroad before the World War I gave him contacts with Russell, Hilbert, and other leading mathematicians and philosophers. After the World War I, he was denied a professorship at Harvard, as were most Jews at the time, there and elsewhere, and joined the faculty at MIT, where he remained for his career. The 1920s and 1930s were given over to a variety of problems in mathematics.

During the Second World War he refrained from joining the Manhattan Project on ethical grounds, working instead on problems related to ballistics and communication theory. This led him to work on control theory, having generally to do with feedback loops to control the output of a system at some desired set point. This in turn led him to thinking about how these principles might apply to human behavior.

For this purpose he gathered many influences, including the logical calculus of McCulloch and Pitts, the autonomous robots of Grey Walter, and the then current knowledge of neurophysiology and neuroanatomy. When he came to the point of weaving these strands into a book, he needed a term and invented "cybernetics," from the Greek meaning "steersman." The book, entitled

Cybernetics, or Control and Communication in the Animal and Machine, was actually published in France and came out in 1948.

Cybernetics fell on fertile soil. The neurologist Denny-Brown (Chapter 13) once described for me the ferment at the time, with investigators from Harvard, MIT, and other institutions gathering frequently at evening seminars throughout the Boston area to exchange data and ideas on the new concept and how it related to neurology, computer design, neuroanatomy, neurophysiology, etc. Wiener himself was an enthusiastic participant in all of this. One story was that when Wiener learned of the electroencephalogram (EEG), he postulated that prominent alpha rhythm would be correlated with intelligence. Unfortunately, his own EEG recordings failed to confirm his theory.

This ferment was still tangible well into the 1950s, when I worked under Walter Rosenblith in Wiener's old laboratory at the Research Laboratories in Electronics (the old World War II barracks that survived for decades) at MIT. My job was to run one of the early analog computers to carry out auto- and cross-correlations of evoked cortical potentials and cardiac rhythms (Angelakos and Shepherd, 1957). J. C. R. Licklider, the future architect of ARPANET, was around, as well as Lettvin, McCulloch, and collaborators. Oliver Selfridge gave a seminar on parallel vs. serial computer architectures. I once went to see McCulloch for advice about becoming a neurophysiologist. He sat in his office gazing off into space for several minutes, then murmured "I'm struggling with a problem that Johnny left me." I later told this story to a colleague, Jack Cowan, who had been at MIT at the time, and he immediately said, "Oh, that's von Neumann's problem of how do you get reliable brains from unreliable neurons!"

The basic idea of cybernetics and control theory was that when a system senses an input and generates an output to reach a goal, it also senses the output to compare it with the goal and adjust its action, which generates new input. The features of error signal, self-organization, self-reproduction, and goal-directed behavior are therefore what cybernetics is about, giving it a lasting legacy of fundamental relevance to understanding the brain, as well as to virtually all dynamic systems.

Artificial Intelligence

The idea of machines that can act like humans began with the ancients, but it was, again, not until mid-twentieth century that real solutions became practical through a merging of many of the developments described in this chapter. This meant essentially that investigators from different fields could combine their expertise to understand in general terms how information is handled by humans and to design machines to simulate them.

This process may be said to have begun with the Macy Conferences in the early 1940s, entitled "Conferences on Circular, Causal and Feedback Mechanisms in Biological and Social Systems." Some of the subjects covered were (see Moreno-Díaz and Moreno-Díaz, 2007) goal-directed activity, signal communication, neural nets, closed cortical loops (of Lorente de No), economics, psychiatry, reverberating and content-addressable memory, and learning theory. Attendees included W. Ross Adey, Y. Bar-Hillel, Julian Bigelow, Jan Droogleever-Fortuyyn, W. Grey Walter, Rafael Lorente de No, Donald MacKay, Warren McCulloch, J. M. Nielsen, F. S. C. Northrop, Linus Pauling, Antoine Remond, Arturo Rosenblueth, Claude Shannon, Heinz Von Forester, John von Neumann, and Norbert Wiener (Morena-Diaz and Morena-Diaz, 2007).

We have already seen that these conferences fostered the interactions that stimulated von Neumann's use of McCulloch-Pitts neurons in formulating his concept of digital computer architecture, Shannon's development of information theory, and Wiener's cybernetics.

In 1947 Pitts and McCulloch published a second paper entitled "How We Know Universals: The Perception of Visual and Auditory Forms." This addressed the problem of how to produce invariant recognition of a pattern despite distortions. It contributed to the emerging field of pattern recognition.

In the 1950s several papers, stimulated by McCulloch and Pitts, compared artificial systems with neuronal systems (see Cowan and Sharp, 1988, for summary and references). In 1954 A. M. Uttley drew on the recent ideas of Hebb (Chapter 12) to propose that neural nets with activity-dependent modifiable synaptic connections could learn the simple task of recognizing binary stimulus patterns. In 1955 neuroanatomist B. G. Cragg and physicist H. N. V. Temperley published a paper on the properties of spinning atoms in a ferromagnetic substance (later called "spin glass"). The atoms could be oriented up or down, depending on all-to-all interactions with neighbors, in order to minimize the total energy of the system. This was likened to the neurons that could be on or off depending on the interactions with other neurons. They suggested that analogous neural patterns stimulated by a sensory input could be stable and therefore function as a kind of memory of the imposed stimulus. In 1956 R. L. Beurle carried this kind of analysis further in terms of randomly connected neurons.

The different strands of research beginning in the 1940s in the logical formulations of McCulloch and Pitts, in control theory and cybernetics, the formulation of information theory, and the development of the digital computer, came together in the 1950s in a new field called "artificial intelligence" (AI). According to lore, the igniting event was a conference at Dartmouth in the summer of 1956. The most prominent names were John McCarthy, Marvin Minsky, Allen Newell, and Herbert Simon.

The new discipline appeared immediately. From the start, AI was promoted with considerable hype, similar to the hype used in promoting NASA after Sputnik appeared in 1957. It was going to replace human brains with artificial brains and change society forever. My close friend and colleague Robert Brayton came as a graduate student to MIT in 1956, with an interest in the new field of computer science, and had a choice between electrical engineering and the new field of AI. He chose electrical engineering to launch a distinguished career in computer science.

Perhaps the best-known early initiative in AI and pattern recognition with possible relevance to the nervous system was the "perceptron" of Frank Rosenblatt in 1958. This was a type of McCulloch-Pitts net with modifiable connections that could be "trained," by repeated exposures, to "learn" to discriminate between different patterns. The network consisted of a single layer of nodes representing the neurons, with connections that are adjusted according to their appropriate activity in responding to the stimulus. A similar system was described in 1960 by Widrow and Hoff, called "Adaline" (*ada*ptive *li*near *ne*uron). While these systems stimulated great interest in the AI community at the time, they were ultimately proven inadequate by Minsky and Papert (1969).

Toward Networks of Realistic Neurons: von Neumann's Last Word

For all of those working on the nervous system, the fundamental problem through all of these developments was that the representations of the nervous system were highly unrealistic: the glorious branching patterns of the dendrites were butchered down to the single cell body, the synaptic inputs distributed at specific levels of the dendritic tree were perforce all focused on the cell body node, the axonal connections onto specific target cell bodies and dendrites were exploded into random all-to-all interactions, and the differentiation into excitatory and inhibitory one-way synapses were replaced by adjustable synaptic weights in both directions.

Renewed interest in neural nets blossomed in the 1980s with parallel distributed networks (McClelland and Rumelhart, 1987) and Hopfield (1984) networks. This has led to a vast field of neural network–based devices, with many applications. However, for simulating how the brain actually does what it does, the same problems still apply. How do we build real neurons into networks, to give the depth of computational capacity of the real nervous system?

By the 1980s enhanced computer power enabled one to simulate a dendritic tree with excitatory and inhibitory inputs to different levels. Building on an early suggestion by Rall (1970) and earlier work by Koch et al. (1983), Robert Brayton, then at the IBM Watson Research Center, and I showed in realistic simulations that dendritic spines with active properties could function as McCulloch-Pitts-like nodes, with their responses to synaptic inputs interacting within the dendritic tree to generate the basic logic gates of AND, NOT, and AND–NOT (Shepherd and Brayton, 1987). This suggested that the computational power of a neuron is greatly amplified by hundreds of dendritic spines acting as local input–output units, leading up to the final output from the cell body and axon. This idea is summarized in Figure 16.2.

Based on this result, I reviewed the literature on the new generation of neural networks, pointing out their unrealistic nature. These networks have simple nodes compared with the highly branched architecture of a real neuron, random interconnections of the nodes compared with the specific connections of most real axons, and simulated synapses converging on the nodes compared with the distributed synapses on the dendrites of most real neurons (Shepherd, 1990).

In the course of that review I was amazed and delighted to find that von Neumann had in fact anticipated many of these arguments. In the mid-1950s he was invited to deliver the Silliman Lectures at Yale and chose as his subject "The Brain and the Computer." Unfortunately, he contracted cancer. With only a short time to live, he was not able to deliver the lectures; but he did gather enough of his thoughts to publish a short book by that title, which came out after he died in 1957.

In comparing the brain and the computer, he returned to the theme of his 1945 paper on computational architecture and asked again, What is the fundamental element that carries out the basic logical operations of the brain, corresponding to the transistor in a computer? He first considered the McCulloch and Pitts view that this fundamental element is the neuron (which he had used in his 1945 article):

> "And" and "or" are the basic operations of logic. Together with "no" (the logical operation of negation) they are a complete set of basic logical operations—all other logical operations, no matter how complex, can be obtained by suitable combinations of these . . . the neurons appear, when thus viewed, as the basic logical organs. . . . (53)

von Neumann then considered the actual structure of neurons and the many synaptic units converging on the soma and dendrites (obviously reflecting his many interactions with neuroanatomists and neurophysiologists in the intervening years):

> One may have to face situations in which there are, say, hundreds of synapses on a single nerve cell, and the combinations of stimulations on these that are effective are characterized not only by their number but also by their coverage of certain special regions on that neuron (on its body or on its dendrite system) by the spatial relations of such regions to each other, and by even more complicated quantitative and geometrical relationships that might be relevant (54).

He concluded by observing the following:

> All complications of this type mean, in terms of the counting of basic active organs as we have practiced it so far, that a nerve cell is more than a single basic active organ, and that any significant effort at counting has to recognize this. If the nerve cell is activated by the stimulation of certain combinations of synapses on its body and not by others, then the significant count of basic active organs must presumably be a count of synapses rather than of nerve cells (59).

This conclusion, that the synapse is the basic computational unit of the nervous system, not the whole neuron, anticipated the modern view of distributed synaptic units over the dendritic tree, as summarized in Figure 16.2. It is the real basis of the "microstructure of cognition." On this fundamental element is built the increasing levels of functional organization of the brain, from patterns of synaptic nodes to whole neurons (as in Fig. 16.2) to microcircuits of interconnected neurons within a region and finally to the extensive pathways and systems which constitute the neural basis of behavior. An overall theory of how our brains work, combining all of the breakthroughs documented in this book, lies in this direction. One feels that von Neumann would be leading the way.

Chapter 17

Summing Up

Every year, decade, or era in the history of science and study of the nervous system has had its signal achievements, generating benefits for science and for mankind. In that respect, the mid-twentieth century played its part. However, our account makes the case for considering it as a period of unusual fecundity.

We have focused on the people, ideas and methods of this period. By framing the account in relation to the levels of organization of the nervous system at which the work was carried out, we have been able to understand the context for the advances, as well as provide the means for comparing advances across different levels. For example, the breakthrough in the high level role of the hippocampus in memory from the case of HM (Chapter 12) can be seen in parallel with the breakthroughs in membrane physiology (Chapters 6 and 7) and in the cellular mechanisms underlying learning and memory (Chapters 7 and 9). Many other correlations can be identified across the levels in the various chapters.

For those interested in creativity in science, a perennial question is at what age and stage of one's career do the greatest advances occur? According to conventional wisdom, mathematicians and physicists make their major contributions early in their careers, whereas for biologists it is supposed to come later – Darwin at 50 being a prime example. Our account indicates that there is no rule in modern biology and modern neuroscience. An amazing number of the fundamental advances chronicled here were made by younger investigators: undergraduates (local currents by Alan Hodgkin – Chapter 6; master's student (boolean algebra for circuit design by Claude Shannon – Chapter 16; graduate students (REM sleep by Eugene Aserinsky – Chapter 11; operant conditioning by

James Olds – Chapter 11; spreading depression by Aristides Leão – Chapter 13); postdoctoral fellows (DNA by James Watson – Chapter 2). In contrast of course are many well-trained scientists in mid and later careers; John Eccles is a prime example (Chapters 7–9). Anyone interested in examples of the creative process at these different career stages in science has a rich lode to explore among these pioneers of the mid-twentieth century.

Although the pioneers were mostly male, reflecting the historical gender wall extending all the way into this period, our account shows that many women were among them: Rosalind Franklin for DNA, and Barbara McClintock for translocating genes (Chapter 2) Rita Levi-Montalcini for NGF (Chapter 3); Betty Geren for myelin fine structure (Chapter 5); Angelique Arvanitaki-Chalazonitis for Aplysia (Chapter 7), Denise Albe-Fessard for central nervous system electrophysiology (Chapter 10); Berta Scharrer for neuroendocrinology (Chapter 11); and Brenda Milner for cognitive neuroscience (Chapter 12). They were not only pioneers of neuroscience but also pioneers beginning the process of making science accessible as a career to all young people regardless of gender and race, a process that, though increasingly successful, is still a work in progress.

In this account we also gain more clearly an international perspective on this field. One is able to see for the first time in a more systematic fashion how the origins of modern neuroscience are truly international, with contributions that go beyond the United States to include investigators from around the world. This is the more surprising because this period, from the 1940s through the 1950s, was during and in the aftermath of the Second World War, when much of the rest of the world lay literally in ruins. Only neutral Sweden and Switzerland among the European countries survived intact.

Nevertheless, the reader will appreciate that many European scientists persisted tenaciously in their craft during the war (see Rita Levi-Montalcini's experiments in the face of the fascists in Italy – Chapter 3), and rebuilt their careers, in the late 1940s and through the recovery in the 1950s, despite the paucity of resources. An attempt has been made to communicate, for young readers especially, the huge obstacles of those years. Despite them, the United Kingdom was at the heart of the golden years of 1951–1952, when Hodgkin, Huxley, and Katz (and Eccles from the Commonwealth) built the new cellular neuroscience (Chapters 5–7). On the continent, even more devastated by occupation and demoralization, investigators in France showed enormous determination, as evidenced by the contributions of Rene Couteaux to the neuromuscular junction (Chapter 5), Arvanitaki-Chalazonitis for Aplysia (Chapter 7), Alfred Fessard and Denise Albe-Fessard in neurophysiology (Chapter 10), Jacques Le Magnen in feeding behavior (Chapter 11), and Henri Laborit, Pierre Deniker and Jean Delay for starting the revolution in psychiatric drug treatments (Chapter 15). In addition, the French had to learn to communicate in a new "lingua franca"; Denise Albe-Fessard (Chapter 10) gives vivid testimony to this added burden.

Among the topics not adequately covered here is the institutions which fund the research. Mention has been made (see Chapter 2) of the new climate in the aftermath of the Second World War, which ended in 1945, when the example of the effectiveness of science in helping to win the war was turned on health to understand better normal body function and prevent and cure disease. There had been foundations before then that assumed these responsibilities, most notably the Rockefeller Foundation, whose benignant hand was behind the establishment of many research institutes around the world and many travelling fellowships in the early part of the century. But after the war, broad and systematic support of biomedical science became possible with the enlargement of the National Institutes of Health to include institutes devoted to neurological diseases, mental health, vision, and many other areas of biomedical research. These institutes provided not only direct research grants to individual investigators, but also training grants for bringing successive generations of graduate students and post-doctoral fellows into the field. Similar strategies began to be used in other countries as well. Many would view this new type of support system as one of the great innovations of the 1950s.

A systematic review of these institutions is beyond the scope of the present account, and will reward much future study. However, it may be noted that the relation between levels of funding and levels of creativity is not a linear one. Many of the great advances recorded here were achieved with simple experimental equipment and minimal funding – the string and beeswax era described by Hodgkin (Chapter 6), and the discovery of REM sleep (Chapter 11). And there is further testimony to a bygone era when new drugs could be tested virtually immediately, sometimes by the investigators themselves, with few scientific or government standards, as in the revolution in psychopharmacology (Chapter 15). However, our account shows clearly the areas where funding makes an essential difference, as in creating new kinds of equipment, positions for investigators, and travel to exchange ideas.

Perhaps in all of this, the most critical constant was the freedom of the investigator to pursue his or her own belief in what was the key to solving the next problem. The reward for this we see repeated over and over, whether it was the elation of observing one night under the electron microscope the first sight of a synapse (Chapter 5), finally teasing out the first burst of impulses of a brain cell to a small bar of light (Chapter 10), or stumbling on a drug that cured schizophrenic patients of their uncontrollable violence (Chapter 15). The revolution documented here is testimony to the freedom of inquiry that lies at the heart of the scientific enterprise. Was that freedom better supported then than it is now? Keeping that question always alive may be the most important lesson we can learn from that revolutionary period.

Appendix A
Resources

The main resources for this account focused on the 1950s come from the primary articles of that time, from memoirs and commentaries, and from having lived through those times as a student and known many of the participants then and in my subsequent career. The literature is gathered in the following Reference List. In most chapters the background includes the earlier 20th century, and in some cases the late 19th century. To aid the modern student in understanding this earlier material I have provided some references in secondary sources which give the context of that time. Some of this literature is included in the Reference List; for others the reader has been directed to secondary sources, including my earlier "Foundations of the Neuron Doctrine". I use some of these secondary sources in my teaching; they are particularly valuable in the case of primary sources that are not accessible to busy modern readers, and for their modern perspectives on the relevance of this background material to the context of my modern focus in this book.

As a working scientist I have had limits on the time for the writing, so I'm keenly aware of deficiencies in a thorough documentation of all the relevant literature. I apologize especially to pioneers not adequately recognized. A mea culpa is raised on two counts. First, I want to keep the focus on this unusual period in and around the 1950s. I focus on how extraordinary this decade was in its outburst of creative talent, methodology, institutional support, and other factors. Second, I hope the limited relevant literature will serve as a stimulus to interest professional historians of science in a deeper analysis of this period.

We neuroscientists are only beginning to provide overall assessments of the origins of our field. A comprehensive background source for the older literature is "Origins of Neuroscience. A History of Explorations into Brain Function" by Stanley Finger (New York: Oxford University Press, 1994). The excellent volume by Horace Magoun, assisted by Louise Marshall ("American Neuroscience in the Twentieth Century". New York: Swets and Zeitlinger, 2003), has a broader focus on neuroscience in the entire twentieth century but narrower focus on the U.S. Eric Kandel has provided a deep and balanced view of the history behind his pioneering research contributions, in his early monograph "Cellular Basis of Behavior. An Introduction to Behavioral Neurobiology", San Francisco: Freeman (1976), especially good on the early work in psychology, and his recent "In Search of Memory", New York: Norton (2006). The review of Max Cowan, Donald Harter and Kandel: "Emergence of modern neuroscience. Some implications for neurology and psychiatry", in Annual Reviews of Neuroscience 23: 343–391 (2000) touches on some of the key work in the 1950s before going on to developments later in the twentieth century.

Valuable and readable sources for insights into the people who made the discoveries are provided by autobiographical accounts. These began in an organized way under the aegis of Frank Schmitt in "The Neurosciences: Paths of Discovery", edited by Frederic Worden, Judith Swazey and George Adelman. Cambridge MA: The MIT Press (1975), followed by "The Neurosciences: Paths of Discovery II", edited by Fred Samson and George Adelman. Boston: Birkhauser (1992). This autobiographical approach was institutionalized in a series of volumes initiated and edited by Larry Squire, supported by the Committee on the History of Neuroscience, and published by the Society for Neuroscience, as "The History of Neuroscience in Autobiography", which has now passed through its fifth volume. Various chapters are quoted in the present account, and will repay visiting by the interested reader. In addition to these volumes is a series of video interviews with these and other leading senior neuroscientists, also published by the Society for Neuroscience; details may be found on the Society for Neuroscience website (http://www.sfn.org/). Another source of neuroscience history is the International Brain Research Organization (IBRO) (http://www.ibro). Many other sources are listed in the References. Individual memoirs and commentaries are increasingly available on the internet, which place these historical figures and events literally at the fingertips of the modern student. Other information, such as the later awarding of prizes to the pioneers of the 1950s, can be found online (see e.g. http://nobelprize.org/).

I have drawn on several previous accounts of my own in some of the sections; in addition to historical background (Chapters 4 and 8), these include the synapse (Chapter 5), the work of Eccles (Chapters 7–9), and the role of computation and theory (Chapter 16), as noted in those sections.

Personal notes by the present author are included in many chapters. I hope they do not intrude, but rather help to indicate the impact of the events of the 1950s on a student at the time. I have not gone to the extent of conducting formal interviews. However, I have benefited from much advice from colleagues regarding specific areas covered in the different chapters, as noted in the Preface.

Appendix B
Supporting Material Available on the Web

As indicated in the Preface, this book is based on a course given for graduate students and advanced undergraduates at Yale in recent years entitled "History of Modern Neuroscience". The classes have been taught from the web using scans of the classical papers and with other digital materials such as video clips. The urls for these materials are indicated below. The easy access of online materials is the most effective means for making the past a part of the present.

2.1   Watson and Crick article, April 25, 1953:
      http://www.ncbi.nlm.nih.gov/pubmed/13054692

2.2   *New York Times* article, June 13, 1953
      New York Times (1953) Clue to chemistry of heredity is found. June 13.

3.1   Harrison growth cone article, 1910 Harrison RG (1910) The outgrowth of the nerve fiber as a mode of protoplasmic movement. J Exp Zool 9:787–846.

3.2   Hamburger and Levi-Montalcini article, 1949
      http://www.ncbi.nlm.nih.gov/pubmed/18142378

3.3   Sperry article, 1963
      http://www.ncbi.nlm.nih.gov/pubmed/14077501

3.4   Weiss and Hiscoe article, 1948
      http://www.ncbi.nlm.nih.gov/pubmed/18915618

4.1   Carlsson et al. article, 1959
      http://www.ncbi.nlm.nih.gov/pubmed/13483658

4.2   Karlson and Luscher article on pheromones, 1959
      Karlson P, Luscher M (1959) "Pheromones": a new term for a class of biologically active substances. Nature 183:55–56.

5.1   Sherrington letter on the synapse
      Shepherd GM, Erulkar SD (1997) Centenary of the synapse: from Sherrington to the molecular biology of the synapse and beyond. Trends Neurosci 20(9):387.

5.2   Palade abstract 110, 1954
      Palade GE(1954) Electron microscope observations of interneuronal and neuromuscular synapses. Anat Rec 118:335–336.

5.3   Palay abstract 111, 1954
      Palay SL(1954) Electron microscope study of the cytoplasm of neurons. Anat Rec 118: 336.

5.4 de Robertis and Bennett abstract 116, 1954
de Robertis E, Bennett HS (1954) Submicroscopic vesicular component in the synapse. Fed. Proc. 13:35.

5.5 de Robertis abstract 166, 1954
de Robertis E (1954) Changes in the "synaptic vesicles" of the ventral acoustic ganglion after nerve section (An electron microscopic study). Anat Rec 118: 284–285.

5.6 de Robertis and Bennett article, 1955
http://www.ncbi.nlm.nih.gov/pubmed/ 14381427

5.7 Palay article, 1956
http://www.ncbi.nlm.nih.gov/pubmed/13357542

5.8 Gray article, 1959
http://www.ncbi.nlm.nih.gov/pubmed/13829103

5.9 Furshpan and Potter article, 1957
http://www.ncbi.nlm.nih.gov/pubmed/13464833

5.10 Geren article, 1954
http://www.ncbi.nlm.nih.gov/pubmed/16589348

6.1 Adrian and Zotterman article, 1926b
http://www.ncbi.nlm.nih.gov/pubmed/16993780

6.2 Movie clip of Young dissecting squid axon
From movie *The Squid and Its Giant Nerve Fiber*
http://www.science.smith.edu/departments/NeuroSci/courses/bio330/squid.html

6.3 Cole and Curtis article, 1939
http://www.pubmedcentral.nih.gov/articlerender.fcgi?artid=2142006

6.4 Hodgkin and Huxley squid movie clip
From movie *The Squid and Its Giant Nerve Fiber*
http://www.science.smith.edu/departments/NeuroSci/courses/bio330/squid.html

6.5 Hodgkin and Huxley article, 1952d
http://www.ncbi.nlm.nih.gov/pubmed/12991237
Skou article, 1957
http://www.ncbi.nlm.nih.gov/pubmed/13412736

7.1 Ling and Gerard article, 1947
http://www.ncbi.nlm.nih.gov/pubmed/15410483

7.2 Fatt and Katz article, 1951
http://www.ncbi.nlm.nih.gov/pubmed/14898516

7.3 Miniature EPPs, del Castillo and Katz article, 1954b
http://www.ncbi.nlm.nih.gov/pubmed/13175199

7.4 Brock et al. article, 1952
http://www.ncbi.nlm.nih.gov/pubmed/13003921

8.1 Impulse initiation, Fuortes et al. article, 1957
http://www.ncbi.nlm.nih.gov/pubmed/13428986

8.2 Crayfish, Eyzaguirre, and Kuffler article, 1955b
http://www.ncbi.nlm.nih.gov/pubmed/13252237

8.3 Pop spike, Andersen article, 1959
http://www.ncbi.nlm.nih.gov/pubmed/13793335

8.4   Rall review, 1964
      Theoretical significance of dendritic trees for neuronal input-output relations.
      In: Neural Theory and Modeling (Reiss RF, ed), pp 122–146. Palo Alto: Stanford
      University Press.

8.5   Spines, Chang article, 1952
      http://www.ncbi.nlm.nih.gov/pubmed/13049166

8.6   Neuron doctrine, Bullock article, 1959
      http://www.ncbi.nlm.nih.gov/pubmed/13646634

9.1   Renshaw inhibition, Eccles et al. article, 1954
      http://www.ncbi.nlm.nih.gov/pubmed/13222354

9.2   Hartline and Graham article, 1932
      Hartline HK, Graham CH (1932) Nerve impulses from single receptors in the
      eye. J Cell Comp Physiol 1:227–295.

9.3   Center surround, Kuffler article, 1953
      http://www.ncbi.nlm.nih.gov/pubmed/13035466

9.4   Command neuron, Wiersma article, 1938
      Wiersma CAG (1938) Function of the giant fibres of the central nervous system
      of the crayfish. Proc Soc Exp Biol Med 38:6617–662.

9.5   Central pattern generator, Wiersma article, 1962
      Wiersma CAG (1962) The organization of the arthropod nervous system. Am
      Zool 2:67–78.

9.6   Barlow article, 1953
      http://www.ncbi.nlm.nih.gov/pubmed/13035718

10.1 Lorente de No chapter in Fulton, 1938
      Lorente de No R (1938) Cerebral cortex: architecture, intracortical connec-
      tions, motor projections. In: Physiology of the Nervous System (Fulton J, ed),
      pp 291–339. New York: Oxford University Press.

10.2 Powell and Mountcastle article, 1959
      http://www.ncbi.nlm.nih.gov/pubmed/14434571

10.3 Hubel and Wiesel article, 1959
      http://www.ncbi.nlm.nih.gov/pubmed/14403679

10.4 Lettvin et al. article, 1959
      Lettvin, JY, Maturana HR, McCulloch WS and Pitts WH (1959) What the frog's
      eye tells the frog's brain. Proc Inst Radio Engrs NY 47:1940–1951.

10.5 Phillips article, 1959
      http://www.ncbi.nlm.nih.gov/pubmed/13624009

10.6 Extract from Penfield and Rasmussen, 1950
      Penfield W, Rasmussen T (1950) The Cerebral Cortex of Man: A Clinical Study
      of Localization of Function. New York: Macmillan.

10.7 Odor patterns, Adrian article, 1953
      http://www.ncbi.nlm.nih.gov/pubmed/13104158

11.1 Moruzzi and Magoun article, 1949
      http://www.ncbi.nlm.nih.gov/pubmed/18421835

11.2 Aserinsky and Kleitman article, 1953
      http://www.ncbi.nlm.nih.gov/pubmed/13089671

11.3 Aserinsky and Kleitman article, 1955
      http://www.ncbi.nlm.nih.gov/pubmed/13242483

11.4 Olds and Milner article, 1954
http://www.ncbi.nlm.nih.gov/pubmed/13233369

11.5 Stellar article, 1954
http://www.ncbi.nlm.nih.gov/pubmed/13134413

11.6 Scharrer review, 1987
http://www.ncbi.nlm.nih.gov/pubmed/3551757

11.7 Extract from Harris, 1955
Harris GW (1955) Neural Control of the Pituitary Gland. London: Edward Arnold.

12.1 Extract from Hebb, 1949
Hebb DO (1949) The Organization of Behavior: A Neuropsychological Theory. New York: John Wiley and Sons.

12.2 Papez article, 1995
http://www.ncbi.nlm.nih.gov/pubmed/7711480

12.3 Bucy and Kluver article, 1955
http://www.ncbi.nlm.nih.gov/pubmed/13271593

12.4 MacLean article, 1949
http://www.ncbi.nlm.nih.gov/pubmed/15410445

12.5 Scoville and Milner article, 1957
http://www.ncbi.nlm.nih.gov/pubmed/13406589

13.1 C. Miller Fisher lecture, 1958
Fisher CM (1958) Intermittent cerebral ischemia. In: Transactions of the Second Conference Held Under the Auspices of the American Heart Association (Wright IS, Millikan CH, eds), pp 81–97. New York: Grune & Stratton, 1958.

13.2 Kety and Schmidt article, 1948
http://www.ncbi.nlm.nih.gov/pubmed/16695568

13.3 Leão article, 1944a
Leão AAP (1944a) Spreading depression of activity in the cerebral cortex. J Neurophysiol 7:359–390.

15.1 Delay and Denicker article, 1955
http://www.ncbi.nlm.nih.gov/pubmed/14392209

16.1 McCulloch and Pitts article, 1943
http://www.springerlink.com/content/xw16676748262521/

References

Adams, P. (1998) Hebb and Darwin. *J. Theor. Biol.* **195**, 419–438.

Adams RD, Cammermeyer J, Denny-Brown D (1949) Acute necrotizing hemorrhagic encephalopathy. J Neuropathol Exp Neurol 8:1–29.

Adams RD, Denny-Brown D, Pearson CM (1954) Diseases of the Muscle. New York: Hoeber.

Adrian ED (1926a) The impulses produced by sensory nerve endings: part I. J Physiol 61:49–72.

Adrian ED (1926b) The impulses produced by sensory nerve-endings: part IV. Impulses from pain receptors. J Physiol 62:33–51.

Adrian ED (1928) The Basis of Sensation: The Action of the Sense Organs. London: Christophers.

Adrian ED (1953) Sensory messages and sensation: the response of the olfactory organ to different cells. Acta Physiol Scand 29:5–14.

Adrian ED (1966) Thomas Graham Brown, 1882–1965. In: Biographical Memoirs of Fellows of the Royal Society, pp 23–33. London: Royal Society.

Adrian ED, Bronk DW (1928) The discharge of impulses in motor nerve fibres: Part I. Impulses in single fibres of the phrenic nerve. J Physiol 66:81–101.

Adrian ED, Matthews R (1927a) The action of light on the eye: part I. The discharge of impulses in the optic nerve and its relation to the electric changes in the retina. J Physiol 63:378–414.

Adrian ED, Matthews R (1927b) The action of light on the eye: part II. The processes involved in retinal excitation. J Physiol 64:279–301.

Adrian ED, Matthews R (1928) The action of light on the eye: part III. The interaction of retinal neurones. J Physiol 65:273–298.

Adrian ED, Zotterman Y (1926a) The impulses produced by sensory nerve-endings: part II. The response of a single end-organ. J Physiol 61:151–171.

Adrian ED, Zotterman Y (1926b) The impulses produced by sensory nerve endings: part III. Impulses set up by touch and pressure. J Physiol 61:465–483.

Advisory Council for the National Institute of Neurological Disease and Blindness (1958) A classification and outline of cerebrovascular diseases: a report by an ad hoc committee established by the Advisory Council for the National Institute of Neurological Disease and Blindness Public Health Service. Neurology 8:395–434.

Aird RB (1994) Foundation of Modern Neurology: A Century of Progress. New York: Raven Press.

Albe-Fessard D, Buser P (1954) Microphysiological analysis of the reflex transmission from the electric organ of the numbfish *Torpedo marmorata* [in French]. J Physiol (Paris) 46:932–946.

Albe-Fessard D, Buser P (1955) Intracellular activities collected in the sigmoid cortex of the cat; participation of the pyramidal neurons in the somesthetic evoked potential [in French]. J Physiol (Paris) 47:67–69.

Albe-Fessard D, Massion J, Meulders M (1960) Responses observed in the median center of the thalamus in the awakening and unconfined cat, carrier of permanently fixed electrodes [in French]. C R Hebd Seances Acad Sci 250:2928–2930.

Albe-Fessard D (1996) Denise Albe-Fessard. In: The History of Neuroscience in Autobiography (Squire LR, ed), pp 6–52. Washington DC: Society for Neuroscience.

Albers GW, Caplan LR, Easton JD, Fayad PB, Mohr JP, Saver JL, Sherman DG (2002) Transient ischemic attack—proposal for a new definition. N Engl J Med 347:1713–1716.

Albers RW (ed) (1972) Basic Neurochemistry. Boston: Little, Brown.

Alberts B (1983) Molecular Biology of the Cell. New York: Garland.

Alexandrowicz JS (1953) Nervous organs in the pericardial cavity of the decapod Crustacea. J Mar Biol Assoc UK 31:563–580.

Alexandrowicz JS, Carlisle DB (1953) Some experiments on the function of the pericardial organs in Crustacea. J Mar Biol Assoc UK 32:175–192.

Anand BK, Brobeck JR (1951a) Hypothalamic control of food intake in rats and cats. Yale J Biol Med 24:123–140.

Anand BK, Brobeck JR (1951b) Localization of a "feeding center" in the hypothalamus of the rat. Proc Soc Exp Biol Med 77:323–324.

Andersen P (1959) Interhippocampal impulses. I. Origin, course and distribution in cat, rabbit and rat. Acta Physiol Scand 47:63–90.

Andersen P, Lundberg A (1997) John C. Eccles (1903–1997). Trends Neurosci 20:324–325.

Angelakos ET, Shepherd GM (1957) Autocorrelation of EKG during ventricular fibrillation. Circ Res 5:657–658.

Angeletti RH, Bradshaw RA (1971) Nerve growth factor from mouse submaxillary gland: amino acid sequence. Proc Natl Acad Sci USA 68:2417–2420.

Araki T, Otani T (1955) Response of single motoneurons to direct stimulation in toad's spinal cord. J Neurophysiol 18:472–485.

Araki T, Otani T, Furukawa T (1953) The electrical activities of single motoneurones in toad's spinal cord, recorded with intracellular electrodes. Jpn J Physiol 3:254–267.

Arvanitaki A (1941) Les caracteristiques de l'activite rythmique ganglionnaire "spontanee" chez l'Aplysie. C R Seances Soc Biol Fil 135: 1207–1211.

Aserinsky E (1996) The discovery of REM sleep. J Hist Neurosci 5:213–227.

Aserinsky E, Kleitman N (1953) Regularly occurring periods of eye motility, and concomitant phenomena, during sleep. Science 118:273–274.

Aserinsky E, Kleitman N (1955) Two types of ocular motility occurring in sleep. J Appl Physiol 8:1–10.

Astrachan L, Volkin E (1958) Properties of ribonucleic acid turnover in T2-infected *Escherichia coli*. Biochim Biophys Acta 29:536–544.

Atanasoff JV (1984) Advent of electronic digital computing. Ann Hist Comput 6:229–282.

Augarten S (1984) Bit by Bit: An Illustrated History of Computers. New York: Ticknor & Fields.

Avery OT, MacLeod CM, McCarty M (1944). Studies on the chemical nature of the substance inducing transformation of pneumococcal types: Induction of transformation by a desoxyribonucleic acid fraction isolated from Pneumococcus Type III. J Exper Med 79: 137–158.

Axelrod J (1958) Presence, formation, and metabolism of normetanephrine in the brain. Science 127:754–755.

Axelrod J (1965) The metabolism, storage, and release of catecholamines. Recent Prog Horm Res 21:597–622.

Axelrod J (1996) Julius Axelrod. In: The History of Neuroscience in Autobiography. Vol 1 (Squire LR, ed), pp 50–78. Washington DC: Society for Neuroscience.

Bacq, ZM (1975). Chemical Transmission of Nerve Impulses. A Historical Sketch. New York: Oxford University Press.

Bacq ZM (1983) Chemical transmission of nerve impulses. In: Discoveries in Pharmacology. Psycho- and Neuro-Pharmacology. Vol. 1. (Parnham MJ, Bruinvels J, eds). Amsterdam: Elsevier, pp 49–104.

Bargmann W (1951) The midbrain and neurohypophysis; a new concept of the functional significance of the posterior lobe. Med Monatsschr 5:466–470.

Barker D (1948) The innervation of the muscle-spindle. Q J Microsc Sci 89:143–186.

Barlow HB (1953) Summation and inhibition in the frog's retina. J Physiol 119:69–88.

Barsa JA, Kline NS (1955) Combined reserpine–chlorpromazine therapy in disturbed psychotics. Am J Psychiatry 111:780.

Bartlett J (1982) Bartlett's Familiar Quotations. Boston: Little-Brown.

Bazemore AW, Elliot KA, Florey E (1957) Isolation of factor I. J Neurochem 1:334–339.

Bateson W (1906) An address on mendelian heredity and its application to man. Brain 29:157–179.

Beale G (1993) The discovery of mustard gas mutagenesis by Auerbach and Robson in 1941. Genetics. 134:393–399.

Beaufay H, De Duve C, Novikoff AB (1956) Electron microscopy of lysosomerich fractions from rat liver. J Biophys Biochem Cytol 2:179–184.

Bellisle F, Laffort P, Köster E (2003) Jacques Le Magnen (1916–2002). Chem Senses 28:85–86.

Bennett MV, Aljure E, Nakajima Y, Pappas GD (1963) Electrotonic junctions between teleost spinal neurons: electrophysiology and ultrastructure. Science 141:262–264.

Bennett MR, Balcar VJ (1999) Forty years of amino acid transmission in the brain. Neurochem Internat 35: 269–280.

Benoit J, Tauc L, Assenmacher I (1954) New results of photoelectric measurement of penetration of visible luminescent radiations to the brain by the side of the summit of the head in white and colored ducks [in French]. C R Hebd Seances Acad Sci 239:508–510.

Bernstein J (1902) Untersuchungen zur Thermodynamik der bioelekrischen Strome. Erster Theil. Pflug Arch ges Physiol 92: 521–562.

Berthet J, Rall TW, Sutherland EW (1957) The relationship of epinephrine and glucagon to liver phosphorylase. IV. Effect of epinephrine and glucagon on the reactivation of phosphorylase in liver homogenates. J Biol Chem 224:463–475.

Beurle RL (1956) Properties of a mass of cells capable of regenerating pulses. Phil Trans Roy Soc Lond B 240: 55–94.

Bishop GH, Clare MH (1955) Facilitation and recruitment in dendrites. Electroencephalogr Clin Neurophysiol 7:486–489.

Blaschko H (1939) The specific action of L-dopa decarboxylase. J Physiol (Lond) 96:50P–51P.

Blaschko H (1957) Formation of catechol amines in the animal body. Br Med Bull 13:162–165.

Blinks LR (1930) The direct current resistance of *Nitella*. J Gen Physiol 13:495–508.

Bliss TV, Lomo T (1973) Long-lasting potentiation of synaptic transmission in the dentate area of the anaesthetized rabbit following stimulation of the perforant path. J Physiol 232:331–356.

Block SM (1992) Biophysical principles of sensory transduction. In: Sensory Transduction (Corey DP, Roper SD, eds), pp 1–17. New York: Rockefeller University Press.

Boole G (1848) The calculus of logic. Cambridge and Dublin Mathematical Journal Vol. III, pp. 183–198.

Boring E (1950) A History of Experimental Psychology. New York: Appleton-Century-Crofts.

Bowery NG, Smart TG (2006) GABA and glycine as neurotransmitters: a brief history. British J Pharmacol 147: S109–S119.

Bowery NG et al. (eds) (1990) GABA Receptors in Mammalian Function. New York: Wiley.

Bowman WC (1983) Peripherally acting muscle relaxants. In: Discoveries in Pharmacology (Parnham MJ, Bruinvels J, eds), pp 105–162. Amsterdam: Elsevier.

Boyd IA, Martin AR (1956a) The end-plate potential in mammalian muscle. J Physiol 132:74–91.

Boyd IA, Martin AR (1956b) Spontaneous subthreshold activity at mammalian neural muscular junctions. J Physiol 132:61–73.

Bremer F (1937) L'activité cerebrale au cours du sommeil et de la narcose. Contribution à l'etude du mécanisme du sommeil. Bull Acad Med Belg 4:68–86.

Brock LG, Coomgs JS, Eccles JC (1952) The nature of the monosynaptic excitatory and inhibitory processes in the spinal cord. Proc R Soc Lond B Biol Sci 140: 170–176.

Brodie BB, Shore PA (1957) A concept for a role of serotonin and norepinephrine as chemical mediators in the brain. Ann N Y Acad Sci 66:631–642.

Brown, C. (2003) The stubborn scientist who unraveled a mystery of the night. Smithsonian October 92–97.

Brown RE, Milner PM (2003) The legacy of Donald O. Hebb: more than the Hebb Synapse. Nature Revs Neurosci 4:1013–1019.

Brown H, Sanger F, Kitai R (1955) The structure of pig and sheep insulins. Biochem J 60:556–565.

Brown KT, Wiesel TN (1961) Localization of origins of electroretinogram components by intraretinal recording in the intact cat eye. J Physiol 158:257–80.

Bruce HM (1959) An exteroceptive block to pregnancy in the mouse. Nature 184: 105.

Broca P (1878) Sur la convolution limbique et la scissure limbique. Bulletins de la Societe d"Antrhopiologie 12:646–657.

Bucy PC, Kluver H (1955) An anatomical investigation of the temporal lobe in the monkey (*Macaca mulatta*). J Comp Neurol 103:151–251.

Bueker ED (1948) Implantation of tumors in the hind limb field of the embryonic chick and the developmental response of the lumbosacral nervous system. Anat Rec 102:369–389.

Bugnard L, Hill AV (1935) Electric excitation of the fin nerve of sepia. J Physiol 83:425–438.

Bullock TH (1948) Properties of a single synapse in the stellate ganglion of squid. J Neurophysiol 11:343–364.

Bullock TH (1959) Neuron doctrine and electrophysiology. Science 129:997–1002.

Bullock TH (1977) Introduction to Nervous Systems. San Francisco: W. H. Freeman.

Bullock TH, Bennett MV, Johnston D, Josephson R, Marder E, Fields RD (2005) Neuroscience. The neuron doctrine, redux. Science 310:791–793.

Bullock TH, Hagiwara S (1957) Intracellular recording from the giant synapse of the squid. J Gen Physiol 40:565–577.

Burgen ASV, Terroux KG (1952) On the negative inotropic effect in a cat's auricle. J Physiol 120:449.

Burke RE (2006) John Eccles' pioneering role in understanding central synaptic transmission. Prog Neurobiol 78:173–188.

Burks AR (2003) Who Invented the Computer? The Legal Battle that Changed Computing History. Amherst, NY: Prometheus.

Buser P, Albe-Fessard D (1955) Activités intracellulaires reçeuilles dans la cortex sigmoide du chat: participation des neurones pyramidaux au potentiel évoque somesthestique. J Physiol (Paris) 47:67–69.

Butenandt A, Groschel U, Karlson P, Zillig W (1959) N-Acetyl tyramine, its isolation from *Bombyx* cocoons and its chemical and biological properties [in German]. Arch Biochem Biophys 83:76–83.

Byrne JH, Shepherd GM (2008) Information processing in complex dendrites. In: From Molecules to Networks. An Introduction to Cellular and Molecular Neuroscience (Byrne JH, Roberts JL, eds). New York: Academic Press, pp 489–512.

Cade J (1949) Lithium salts in the treatment of psychotic excitement. Med J N Z 2:349–352.

Cammermeyer J (1962) I. An evaluation of the significance of the "dark" neuron. Ergeb Anat Entwicklungsgesch 36:1–61.

Cannon WB (1945) The Way of an Investigator. New York: WW Norton.

Carey B (2008) H. M., whose loss of memory made him unforgettable, dies. New York Times, December 4, 1, 36.

Carlsson A, Falck B, Hillarp NA (1962) Cellular localization of brain monoamines. Acta Physiol Scand. 56: Suppl 196: 1–26.

Carlsson A, Lindqvist M, Magnusson T, Waldeck B (1958) On the presence of 3-hydroxytyramine in brain. Science 127:471.

Carlsson A, Rasmussen EB, Krist Jansen P (1959) The urinary excretion of adrenaline and noradrenaline by schizophrenic patients during reserpine treatment. J Neurochem 4:318–320.

Chang HT (1952) Cortical neurons with particular reference to the apical dendrites. Cold Spring Harb Symp Quant Biol 17:189–202.

Chang HT (1984) Pilgrimage to Yale. The Physiologist 27: 390–392.

Charcot JM (1868) Lecons sur les Maladies des Vieillards et les Maladies Chroniques. Paris: A. Delahaye.

Chen WR, Midtgaard J, Shepherd GM (1997) Forward and backward propagation of dendritic impulses and their synaptic control in mitral cells. Science 278: 463–467.

Chessin M, Kramer ER, Scott CC (1957) Modifications of the pharmacology of reserpine and serotonin by iproniazid. J Pharmacol Exp Ther 119:453–460.

Clare MH, Bishop GH (1955a) Properties of dendrites; apical dendrites of the cat cortex. Electroencephalogr Clin Neurophysiol 7:85–98.

Clare MH, Bishop GH (1955b) Dendritic circuits: the properties of cortical paths involving dendrites. Am J Psychiatry 111:818–825.

Claude A (1943) The constitution of protoplasm. Science 97:451–456.

Claude A (1946) Fractionation of mammalian liver cells by differential centrifugation. J Exp Med 84:51.

Coghill GE (1930) The structural basis of the integration of behavior. Proc Natl Acad Sci USA 16:637–643.

Cohen S (1960) Purification of a nerve-growth promoting protein from the mouse salivary gland and its neuro-cytotoxic antiserum. Proc Natl Acad Sci USA 46:302–311.

Cohen S, Levi-Montalcini R, Hamburger V (1954) A nerve growth-stimulating factor isolated from sarcomas 37 and 180. Proc Natl Acad Sci 40: 1012–1018.

Cohen-Gadol AA, Ozduman K, Bronen RA, Kim JH, Spencer DD (2004) Long-term outcome after epilepsy surgery for focal cortical dysplasia. J Neurosurg 101:55–65.

Cole KS, Curtis HJ (1939) Electrical impedance of the squid giant axon during activity. J Gen Physiol 22:649–670.

Cole KS (1975) Neuromembranes: paths of ions. In: The Neurosciences: Paths of Discovery (Worden FG, Swazey JP, Adelman G, eds), pp 143–158. Cambridge, MA: MIT Press.

Corkin S (2002) What's new with the amnesic patient H. M.? Nat Rev Neurosci 3:153–160.

Couteaux R (1944) Nouvelles observations sur la structure de la plaque motrice et interprétation des rapports myo-neuraux. C R Soc Biol 138:976–979.

Couteaux R (1946) Sur les gouttières synaptiques du muscle strié. C R Soc Biol 140:270–273.

Couteaux R (1951) Observations on the current methods of histochemical determination of cholinesterase activities [in French]. Arch Int Physiol 59:526–537.

Couteaux R, Nachmansohn D (1940) Changes of cholinesterase at end-plates of voluntary muscles following section of sciatic nerve. Proc Soc Exp Biol 43:177–181.

Couteaux R, Taxi J (1952a) Distribution of the cholinesterase activity at the level of the myoneural synapse [in French]. C R Hebd Seances Acad Sci 235:434–436.

Couteaux R, Taxi J (1952b) Recherches histochimiques sur la distribution des activités cholinestérasiques au niveau de la synapse myoneurale. Arch Anat Microsc Morphol Exp 41:352–392.

Cowan WM, Harter DH, Kandel ER (2000) The emergence of modern neuroscience: some implications for neurology and psychiatry. Annu Rev Neurosci. 23:343–91.

Cowan JD, Sharp DH (1988) Neural nets. Q Rev Biophys 21:365–427.

Cragg BG, Temperley HNV (1955) Memory: the analogy with ferromagnetic hysteresis. Brain 78: 304–316.

Cranefield PF (1957) The organic physics of 1847 and the biophysics of today. J Hist Med Allied Sci 12:407–423.

Cranefield PF, Bell C, Magendie F (1974) The Way In and the Way Out: François Magendie, Charles Bell and the Roots of the Spinal Nerves, with a Facsim. of Charles Bell's Annotated Copy of His Idea of a New Anatomy of the Brain. Mount Kisco, NY: Futura.

Creed RS, Denny-Brown D, Eccles JC, Liddell EGT, Sherrington CS (1932) Reflex Activity in the Spinal Cord. New York: Clarendon Press.

Creese I, Burt DR, Snyder SH (1996) Dopamine receptor binding predicts clinical and pharmacological potencies of antischizophrenic drugs. J Neuropsychiatry Clin Neurosci 8:223–226.

Cremer M (1929) Erregungsgesetze des nerven. Handb Norm Pathol Physiol 9:244–248.

Creutzfeldt O (1986) Richard Jung, 1911–1986. Exp Brain Res 64:1–4.

Crick F (1988) What Mad Pursuit: A Personal View of Scientific Discovery. New York: Basic Books.

Crick FH, Barnett L, Brenner S, Watts-Tobin RJ. 1961. General nature of the genetic code for proteins. Nature. 192:1227–1232.

Curtis DR, Koizumi K (1961) Chemical transmitter substances in brain stem of cat. J Neurophysiol 24:80–90.

Curtis DR, Phillis JW, Watkins JC (1960) The chemical excitation of spinal neurones by certain acidic amino acids. J Physiol 150:656–682.

Curtis DR, Watkins JC (1961) Analogues of glutamic and gamma-amino-*n*-butyric acids having potent actions on mammalian neurones. Nature 191:1010–1011.

Cushing H (1905) The special field of neurological surgery. Bull Johns Hopkins Hosp 16:77–87.

Cushing H (1920) The special field of neurological surgery after another interval. Arch Neurol Psychiat 4: 603–637.

Cushing H (1932) Intracranial tumors. Notes Upon a Series of Two thousand Verified Cases with Surgical-Mortality Percentages Pertaining Thereto. Springfield IL: Charles C Thomas.

Cushing H (1932) Further concerning a parasympathetic center in the interbrain: VII. The effect of intraventricularly-injected histamine. Proc Natl Acad Sci USA 18:500–510.

Cushing H, Goodrich JT (2000) Reprint of "Concerning surgical intervention for the intracranial hemorrhages of the new-born" by Harvey Cushing, M.D. 1905. Childs Nerv Syst 16:484–492.

Dagi TF (1997a) Philosophical currents in the history of neurosurgery. In: A History of Neurosurgery in Its Scientific and Professional Contexts (Greenblatt SH, ed), pp 561–578. Park Ridge, IL: American Association of Neurological Surgeons.

Dagi TF (1997b) History of stereotactic surgery. In: A History of Neurosurgery in Its Scientific and Professional Contexts (Greenblatt SH, ed), pp 401–438. Park Ridge, IL: American Association of Neurological Surgeons.

Dale HH (1909) The action of extracts of the pituitary body. Biochem J 4:427–447.

Dale HH (1914a) The occurrence in ergot and action of acetyl-choline. J Physiol 48:3.

Dale HH (1914b) The action of certain esters and ethers of choline, and their relation to muscarine. J Pharmacol Exp Ther 6:147–190.

Dale HH (1934) Pharmacology and nerve endings. Proc R Soc Med 28:319–332.

Dale HH, Feldberg W (1934) The chemical transmission of secretory impulses to the sweat glands of the cat. J Physiol 82:121–128.

Dale HH, Feldberg W, Vogt M (1936) Release of acetylcholine at voluntary motor nerve endings. J Physiol 86:353–380.

Dalton AJ, Felix MD (1954) Cytologic and cytochemical characteristics of the Golgi substance of epithelial cells of the epididymis in situ, in homogenates and after isolation. Am J Anat 94:171–207.

Dandy WE (1918) Ventriculography following the injection of air into the cerebral ventricles. Ann Surg 68:5–11.

Darwin C (1859) On the Origin of Species by Means of Natural Selection, or Preservation of Favoured Races in the Struggle for Life. London: John Murray.

David R, Thiery G, Bonveallet M, Dell P (1952) Effets de la stimulation des bulbes olfactifs sur le cycle sexuel de la chatte. C R Soc Biol (Paris) 146: 670–672.

Dean RB, Curtis HJ, Cole KS (1940) Impedance of bimolecular films. Science 91:50–51.

de Egas Moniz A (1927) La radioartériographie cérébrale. Bull Acad Méd (Paris) 98: 40–45.

Delay J, Deniker P (1955) Neuroleptic effects of chlorpromazine in therapeutics of neuropsychiatry. J Clin Exp Psychopathol 16:104–112.

Delay J, Deniker P, Harl JM (1952) Therapeutic use in psychiatry of phenothiazine of central elective action (4560 RP) [in French]. Ann Med Psychol (Paris) 110:112–117.

Delay J, Deniker P, Tardieu Y, Lemperiere T. (1954) Premiers essais en therapeutique psychiatrique de la reserpine, alkaloide nouveau de la Rauwolfia serpentina. C R 52e Congres des alienists et neurol de Langue Fse, pp 836–841.

Delay J, Deniker P, Tardieu Y, Lemperiere T (1955) Neuroplegic medications and cures in psychiatry: preliminary trials with reserpine; comparison with the effects of chlorpromazine. Presse Med 63:663–665.

Delay J, Deniker P, Wiart C (1956) Additions to our experience with reserpine. Encephale 45:1042–1048.

Delbrück M (1972) Signal transducers: terra incognita of molecular biology. Angewandte Chem (Int Ed Engl) 11:1–6.

Del Castillo J, Katz B (1954a) Changes in end-plate activity produced by presynaptic polarization. J Physiol 124:586–604.

Del Castillo J, Katz B (1954b) Quantal components of the end-plate potential. J Physiol 124:560–573.

Del Castillo J, Katz B (1954c) Potential and resistance changes at the motor endplate. J Physiol 123:70P–71P.

Del Cerro M, Triarhou LC (2009) Eduardo De Robertis (1913–1988). J Neurol 256(1):147–8.

Dement W, Kleitman N (1957a) The relation of eye movements during sleep to dream activity: an objective method for the study of dreaming. J Exp Psychol 53:339–346.

Dement W, Kleitman N (1957b) Cyclic variations in EEG during sleep and their relation to eye movements, body motility, and dreaming. Electroencephalogr Clin Neurophysiol 9:673–690.

Deniker P (1983) Psychopharmacology and biologic psychiatry. Historical review. Soins Psychiatrie 37:5–6.

De Robertis E (1954) Changes in the "synaptic vesicles" of the ventral acoustic ganglion after nerve section (An electron microscopic study). Anat Rec 118: 284–285.

De Robertis E (1959) Submicroscopic morphology of the synapse. Int Rev Cytol 8:61–96.

De Robertis E, Bennett HS (1954) Submicroscopic vesicular component in the synapse. Fed. Proc. 13:35.

De Robertis ED, Bennett HS (1954) A submicroscopic vesicular component of Schwann cells and nerve satellite cells. Exp Cell Res 6:543–545.

De Robertis ED, Bennett HS (1955) Some features of the submicroscopic morphology of synapses in frog and earthworm. J Biophys Biochem Cytol 1:47–58.

Detwiler S (1920) On the hyperplasia of nerve centers resulting from excessive peripheral loading Proc Natl Acad Sci USA 6:96–101.

Dixon WE (1907) On the mode of action of drugs. Med Mag (Lond) 16:454–457.

Dowling JE, Werblin FS (1969) Organization of retina of the mudpuppy, *Necturus maculosus*. I. Synaptic structure. J Neurophysiol 32:315–338.

Drimmie AM (1957) Cross-infection in a children's ward; the pneumococcus as a tracer organism. Scott Med J 2:288–292.

du Bois-Reymond EH (1848) Untersuchungen über thierische elektricität. Berlin: G. Reimer.

du Bois-Reymond EH (1877) Gesammelte abhandlungen zur allgemeinen muskel- und nervenphysik. Leipzig: Veit.

Dudel J, Kuffler SW (1960) Excitation of the crayfish neuromuscular junction with decreased membrane conductance. Nature 187:246–247.

Eccles JC (1953) The Neurophysiological Basis of Mind: The Principles of Neurophysiology. Oxford: Clarendon Press.

Eccles JC (1957) The Physiology of Nerve Cells. Baltimore, MD: Johns Hopkins Press.

Eccles JC (1964) Physiology of Synapses. New York: Academic Press.

Eccles JC (1997) My scientific odyssey. Annu Rev Physiol 39:1–18.

Eccles JC, Fatt P, Koketsu K (1954) Cholinergic and inhibitory synapses in a pathway from motor-axon collaterals to motoneurones. J Physiol 126:524–562.

Eccles JC, Gibson WC (1979) Sherrington, His Life and Thought. New York: Springer International.

Eccles JC, Ito M, Szentágothai J (1967) The Cerebellum as a Neuronal Machine. New York: Springer-Verlag.

Eccles JC, Libet B, Young RR (1958) The behaviour of chromatolysed motoneurones studied by intracellular recording. J Physiol 143:11–40.

Eccles JC, O'Connor WJ (1939) Responses which nerve impulses evoke in mammalian striated muscles. J Physiol 97:44–102.

Eccles JC, Sherrington C (1930) Numbers and contraction-values of individual motor units examined in some muscles of the limb. Proc Roy Soc B. 106: 326–357.

Edwards C, Ottoson D (1958) The site of impulse initiation in a nerve cell of a crustacean stretch receptor. J Physiol 143:138–148.

Edwards DH, Heitler WJ, Krasne FB (1999) Fifty years of a command neuron: the neurobiology of escape behavior in the crayfish. Trends Neurosci 22:153–161.

Elliott TR (1904). On the action of adrenalin. J Physiol 31:20–21.

Elliott TR (1905) The action of adrenalin. J Physiol 32:401–467.

Ellis EL, Delbruck M (1939) The growth of bacteriophage. J Gen Physiol 22: 365–384.

Emerson A (2001) Claude Shannon. Obituaries. Guardian (U.K.), March 8, http://www.guardian.co.uk/science/2001/mar/08/obituaries.news.

Eränkö O (1956) Histochemical demonstration of noradrenaline in the adrenal medulla of the hamster. J Histochem Cytochem 4:11–13.

Estable C, Reissig M, De Robertis E (1954) Microscopic and submicroscopic structure of the synapsis in the ventral ganglion of the acoustic nerve. Exp Cell Res 6:255–262.

Eyzaguirre C, Kuffler SW (1955a) Processes of excitation in the dendrites and in the soma of single isolated sensory nerve cells of the lobster and crayfish. J Gen Physiol 39:87–119.

Eyzaguirre C, Kuffler SW (1955b) Further study of soma, dendrite, and axon excitation in single neurons. J Gen Physiol 39:121–153.

Fahrenbach WH (1985) Anatomical circuitry of lateral inhibition in the eye of the horseshoe crab, *Limulus polyphemus*. Proc R Soc Lond B Biol Sci 225:219–249.

Farquhar MG, Palade GE (1981) The Golgi apparatus (complex)—(1954–1981)—from artifact to center stage. J Cell Biol 91:77s–103s.

Fatt P (1957a) Electric potentials occurring around a neurone during its antidromic activation. J Neurophysiol 20:27–60.

Fatt P (1957b) Sequence of events in synaptic activation of a motoneurone. J Neurophysiol 20:61–80.

Fatt P, Katz B (1951) An analysis of the end-plate potential recorded with an intracellular electrode. J Physiol 115:320–370.

Fatt P, Katz B (1952) The action of inhibitory nerve impulses on the surface membrane of crustacean muscle fibres. J Physiol 118:47P–48P.

Fawcett DW (1954) The study of epithelial cilia and sperm flagella with the electron microscope. Laryngoscope 64:557–567.

Fawcett DW, Porter KR (1954) A study of the fine structure of ciliated epithelia. J Morphol 94: 221–281.

Fawcett DW (1981) The Cell. Second Edition. Philadelphia: W.B. Saunders.

Feindel W, Leblanc R, Villemure J-G (1997) History of the neurological treatment of epilepsy. In: A History of Neurosurgery in Its Scientific and Professional Contexts (Greenblatt SH, ed), pp 465–488. Park Ridge, IL: American Association of Neurological Surgeons.

Feng TP (1941) Neuromuscular junction. XXVI. Changes of end-plate potential during and after prolonged stimulation. Zhongguo Shenglixue Zazhi 16:341–372.

Fisher M, Adams RD (1951) Observations on brain embolism with special reference to the mechanism of hemorrhagic infarction. J Neuropathol Exp Neurol 10:92–94.

Fisher CM (1958) The use of anticoagulants in cerebral thrombosis. Neurology 8:311–332.

Fisher CM (1958) Intermittent cerebral ischemia. In: Cerebral vascular disease (Wright IS, Millikan CH, eds). New York: Grune & Stratton:81–97.

Flemming W (1878) Zur Kenntniss der Zelle und ihrer Theilungs-Erscheinungen. In: Schriften des Naturwissenschaftlichen Vereins für Schleswig-Holstein 3: 23–27.

Flexner A (1910) Medical Education in the United States and Canada. Bulletin 4. New York: Carnegie Foundation.

Florey E (1954) An inhibitory and an excitatory factor of mammalian central nervous system, and their action of a single sensory neuron. Arch Int Physiol 62:33–53.

Foley JM, Watson CW, Adams RD (1950) Significance of the electroencephalographic changes in hepatic coma. Trans Am Neurol Assoc 51:161–165.

Forbes A (1939) Problems of synaptic functions. J Neurophysiol 2:465–472.

Fortier C, Selye H (1949) Adrenocorticotrophic effect of stress after severance of the hypothalamo-hypophyseal pathways. Am J Physiol 159:433–439.

Foster M (1897) A Text-book of Physiology. Part III. 7th Edition. London: Macmillan.

Foster M, Shore LE (1897) Physiology for Beginners, new ed. New York: MacMillan.

Frahm J, Krueger G, Merboldt KD, Kleinschmidt A (1997) Dynamic NMR studies of perfusion and oxidative metabolism during focal brain activation. Adv Exp Med Biol 413:195–203.

Frank K, Fuortes MG (1955) Potentials recorded from the spinal cord with microelectrodes. J Physiol 130:625–654.

Frank K, Fuortes MG (1956) Unitary activity of spinal interneurones of cats. J Physiol 131:424–435.

Frankel G (1980) D.C. neurosurgeon pioneered "Operation Icepick" technique. Washington Post, A1–A2.

Fulton JF (1928) Observations upon the vascularity of the human occipital lobe during visual activity. Brain 51: 310–320.

Fulton JF (1938) The Physiology of the Nervous System. New York: Oxford University Press.

Fuortes MG, Frank K, Becker MC (1957) Steps in the production of motoneuron spikes. J Gen Physiol 40:735–752.

Furshpan EJ, Potter DD (1957) Mechanism of nerve-impulse transmission at a crayfish synapse. Nature 180:342–343.

Gaddum JH (1953) Antagonism between lysergic acid diethylamide and 5-hydroxytryptamine. J Physiol 121:15P.

Gage FH (1998) Stem cells of the central nervous system. Curr Opin Neurobiol 8:671–676.

Galindo A, Krnjevic K, Schwartz S (1967) Micro-iontophoretic studies on neurones in the cuneate nucleus. J Physiol 192:359–377.

Gall JG, Porter KR, Siekevitz P (1981) Discovery in cell biology. J Cell Biol 91:3–300.

Galvani L (1791) De viribus electricitatis in motu musculari: Commentarius. Commentarius De Bononiesi Scientarium et Ertium Instituto atque. Academia Commentarii 7:363–416.

Gasser HJ, Erlanger J (1922) A study of the action currents of nerve with the cathode ray oscillograph. Am J Physiol 62:496–524.

Geison GL (1987) Physiology in the American context, 1850–1940. Bethesda, MD: American Physiological Society.

Geren BB (1954) The formation from the Schwann cell surface of myelin in the peripheral nerves of chick embryos. Exp Cell Res 7:558–562.

Geren BB, Schmitt FO (1954) The structure of the Schwann cell and its relation to the axon in certain invertebrate nerve fibers. Proc Natl Acad Sci USA 40:863–870.

Gerschenfeld H, Tauc L (1961) Pharmacological specificities of neurones in an elementary central nervous system. Nature 189:924–925.

Gibbs FA, Gibbs EL (1950) Atlas of Electroencephalography. Cambridge, MA: Addison-Wesley.

Gilbert SF (1991) Developmental Biology. Sunderland, MA: Sinauer Associates.

Glees P, Griffith HB (1952) Bilateral destruction of the hippocampus (cornu ammonis) in a case of dementia. Monatsschr Psychiatr Neurol 123:193–204.

Goldman DE (1943) Potential impedance and rectification in membranes. J Gen Physiol 27:37–60.

Goldman-Rakic PS (1981) Development and plasticity of primate frontal association cortex. In: The Organization of the Cerebral Cortex (Schmitt FO, Worden FG, Adelman G, Dennis SG, eds). Cambridge, MA: MIT Press, pp 69–97.

Goodman LS, Gilman A (1955) The Pharmacological Basis of Therapeutics, 2nd ed. New York: Macmillan.

Gopfert H, Schaefer H (1938) Über den direkt und indirekt erregten Aktionsstrom und die Funktion der motorischen Endplatte. Pflügers Arch 239:597–619.

Grafstein B (1967) Transport of protein by goldfish optic nerve fibers. Science 157:196–198.

Grafstein B (1999) Intracellular traffic in nerve cells. Brain Res Bull 50:311.

Graham Brown T (1911) The intrinsic factors in the act of progression in the mammal. Proc R Soc Lond 84:308–319.

Graham Brown T (1913) The phenomenon of "narcosis progression" in mammals. Proc R Soc Lond 86:140–164.

Graham Brown T (1914) On the nature of the fundamental activity of the nervous centres, together with an analysis of the conditioning of rhythmic activity in progression, and a theory of evolution of function in the nervous system. J Physiol (Lond) 48:18–46.

Granit R (1947) Sensory Mechanisms of the Retina; with an Appendix on Electroretinography. London: Oxford University Press.

Granit R (1950) The organization of the vertebrate retinal elements. Monatsschr Kinderheilkunde 46:31–70.

Granit R (1967) The development of retinal neurophysiology. From Nobel Lectures, Physiology or Medicine 1963–1970, Elsevier Publishing Company, Amsterdam, 1972 http://nobelprize.org/nobel_prizes/medicine/laureates/1967/granit-lecture.html.

Granit R, Svaetichin G (1939) Principles and technique of the electrophysiological analysis of colour reception with the aid of microelectrodes. Ups Läkareförenings Förh 65:161–177.

Granit R, Therman PO (1935) Excitation and inhibition in the retina and in the optic nerve. J Physiol 83:359–381.

Grauer NA (2007) The brain voyager: catching up with the "Jacques Cousteau of the cortex." Hopkins Med Winter 2007 online. http://www.hopkinsmedicine.org/hmn/W07/classnotes.cfm.

Gray EG (1959) Axo-somatic and axo-dendritic synapses of the cerebral cortex: an electron microscope study. J Anat 93:420–433.

Green JD, Harris GW (1949) Observation of the hypophysio-portal vessels of the living rat. J Physiol 108:359–361.

Greenblatt SH (1997) The historiograph of neurosurgery: organizing themes and methodological issues. In: A History of Neurosurgery in Its Scientific and Professional Contexts (Greenblatt SH, ed), pp 3–10. Park Ridge, IL: American Association of Neurological Surgeons.

Greenblatt SH (1997b) Cerebral localization: from theory to practice. Paul Broca and Hughlings Jackson to David Ferrier and William Macewen. In: A History of Neurosurgery in Its Scientific and Professional Contexts (Greenblatt SH, ed), pp 137–152. Park Ridge, IL: American Association of Neurological Surgeons.

Greenblatt SH, Smith DC (1997) The emergence of Cushing's leadership: 1901–1920. In: A History of Neurosurgery in Its Scientific and Professional Contexts (Greenblatt SH, ed), pp 167–190. Park Ridge, IL: American Association of Neurological Surgeons.

Griffith F (1928) The significance of pneumococcal types. J Hygiene 27:141–144.

Grof, P (2006) Mogens Schou (1918–2005) Neuropsychopharmacology 31:891–892.

Grunberg-Manago M, Oritz PJ, Ochoa S (1955) Enzymatic synthesis of nucleic acidlike polynucleotides. Science. 122:907–910.

Gurin S, Delluva A (1947) The biological synthesis of radioactive adrenalin from phenylalanine. J Biol Chem 170: 545–550.

Haas GM, Taylor CB (1997) A quantitative hypothermal method for the production of local injury of tissue. Arch Pathol 45: 563–580.

Haefely W (1983) Alleviation of anxiety—the benzodiazepine saga. In: Psycho- and Neuro-Pharmacology (Parnham MJ, Bruinvels J, eds), pp 270–279. Amsterdam: Elsevier.

Haider B (2008) Contributions of Yale neuroscience to Donald O. Hebb's Organization of Behavior. Yale J Bio Med 81: 11–18.

Halberstam D (1993) The Fifties. New York: Villard Books.

Haines DE (2007) Santiago Ramon y Cajal at Clark University, 1899; his only visit to the United States. Brain Res Rev 55:463–480.

Haldane JBS (1947) What Is Life? New York: Boni and Gaer.

Hamburger V (1934) The effects of wing bud extirpation on the development of the central nervous system in chick embryos. J Exp Zool 68:449–494.

Hamburger V (1979) Roger Sperry. Neurosci Newslett 10:5–6.

Hamburger V (1989) The journey of a neuroembryologist. Annu Rev Neurosci 12:1–12.

Hamburger, V. (1996). Viktor Hamburger. In: The History of Neuroscience in Autobiography (Squire, LR, ed), Washington DC: Society for Neuroscience, pp 222–250.

Hamburger V, Levi-Montalcini R (1949) Proliferation, differentiation and degeneration in the spinal ganglia of the chick embryo under normal and experimental conditions. J Exp Zool 111:457–501.

Hamburger V, Hamilton H (1951) A series of normal stages in the development of the chick embryo. J Morphol 88:49–92.

Hammond WA (1871) A Treatise on the Diseases of the Nervous System. New York NY: D Appleton.

Harris GW (1955) Neural Control of the Pituitary Gland. London: Edward Arnold.

Harrison RG (1910) The outgrowth of the nerve fiber as a mode of protoplasmic movement. J Exp Zool 9:787–846.

Hartline HK (1940) The receptive fields of optic fibers. Am J Physiol 130:690–699.

Hartline HK (1949) Inhibition of activity of visual perceptors by illuminating nearby retinal areas in the *Limulus* eye. Federation Proc 8:69.

Hartline HK (1967) Visual Receptors and Retinal Interaction. From Nobel Lectures, Physiology or Medicine 1963–1970, Elsevier Publishing Company, Amsterdam, 1972 The Lecture in Text Format.

Hartline HK, Graham CH (1932) Nerve impulses from single receptors in the eye. J Cell Comp Physiol 1:227–295.

Hartline HK, Wagner HG, Macnichol EF Jr (1952) The peripheral origin of nervous activity in the visual system. Cold Spring Harb Symp Quant Biol 17:125–141.

Hayashi T (1954) Effects of sodium glutamate on the nervous system. Keio J Med 3:192–193.

Hayashi T (1956) Inhibition and excitation due to gamma-aminobutyric acid in the central nervous system. Nature 182:1076–1077.

Hayashi T (1959) The inhibitory action of beta-hydroxy-gamma-aminobutyric acid upon the seizure following stimulation of the motor cortex of the dog. J Physiol 145:570–578.

Healy D (2001) The Psychopharmacologists. London: Arnold.

Hebb DO (1949) The Organization of Behavior: A Neuropsychological Theory. New York: John Wiley and Sons.

Hecht S, Shlaer S, Pirenne MH (1941) Energy at the threshold of vision. Science 93:585–587.

Hershey AD, Chase M (1952) Independent functions of viral protein and nucleic acid in growth of bacteriophage. J Gen Physiol. 36:39–56.

Hetherington A, Ranson S (1940) Hypothalamic lesions and adiposity in the rat. Nutr Rev 78: In: Nutrition classics. Nutr Rev (1983) 41:124–127.

Heuser JE, Reese TS, Landis DM (1974) Functional changes in frog neuromuscular junctions studied with freeze-fracture. J Neurocytol 3:109–131.

Hilgard ER, Marquis DG (1940) Conditioning and Learning. New York: Appleton-Century.

Hill AV (1936) Excitation and accommodation in nerve. Proc R Soc 119:305–355.

Himwich HE (1951) Brain Metabolism and Cerebral Disorders. Baltimore, MD: Williams & Wilkins.

His W (1880–1885) Die entwickelung des menschlichen rautenhirns vom ende des ersten bis zum beginn des dritten monats. Leipzig: Vogel.

His W (1886) Zur geschichte des menschlichen ruückenmarkes und der nervenwurzeln. Leipzig: S. Hirzel.

Hobson JA, McCarley RW (1977) The brain as a dream state generator: an activation–synthesis hypothesis of the dream process. Am J Psychiatry 134:1335–1348.

Hodgkin AL (1937a) Evidence for electrical transmission in nerve: Part I. J Physiol 90:183–210.

Hodgkin AL (1937b) Evidence for electrical transmission in nerve: Part II. J Physiol 90:211–232.

Hodgkin AL (1992) Chance and Design: Reminiscences of Science in Peace and War. New York: Cambridge University Press.

Hodgkin AL, Huxley AF (1939). Action potentials recorded from inside a nerve fibre. Nature 144: 710–711.

Hodgkin AL, Huxley AF (1945) Resting and action potentials in single nerve fibres. J Physiol 104:176–195.

Hodgkin AL, Huxley AF (1947) Potassium leakage from an active nerve fibre. J Physiol 106:341–367.

Hodgkin AL, Huxley AF (1952a) Currents carried by sodium and potassium ions through the membrane of the giant axon of *Loligo*. J Physiol 116:449–472.

Hodgkin AL, Huxley AF (1952b) The components of membrane conductance in the giant axon of *Loligo*. J Physiol 116:473–496.

Hodgkin AL, Huxley AF (1952c) The dual effect of membrane potential on sodium conductance in the giant axon of *Loligo*. J Physiol 116:497–506.

Hodgkin AL, Huxley AF (1952d) A quantitative description of membrane current and its application to conduction and excitation in nerve. J Physiol 117: 500–544.

Hodgkin AL, Huxley AF, Katz B (1952) Measurement of current–voltage relations in the membrane of the giant axon of *Loligo*. J Physiol 116:424–448.

Hodgkin AL, Katz B (1949a) The effect of sodium ions on the electrical activity of the giant axon of the squid. J Physiol 108:37–77.

Hodgkin AL, Katz B (1949b) The effect of calcium on the axoplasm of giant nerve fibers. J Exp Biol 26:292–294.

Hodgkin AL, Nastuk WL (1950) The electrical activity of single muscle fibers. J Cell Comp Physiol 35:39–73.

Hopfield JJ (1984) Neurons with graded response have collective computational properties like those of two-state neurons. Proc Natl Acad Sci USA 81:3088–3092.

Horsley V, Schafer EA (1886) Experiments on the character of the muscular contractions which are evoked by excitation of the various parts of the motor tract. J Physiol 7:96–110.

Horton JC, Adams DL (2005) The cortical column: a structure without a function. Philos Trans R Soc Lond B Biol Sci 360:837–862.

Houk J, Henneman E (1967a) Responses of Golgi tendon organs to active contractions of the soleus muscle of the cat. J Neurophysiol 30:466–481.

Houk J, Henneman E (1967b) Feedback control of skeletal muscles. Brain Res 5:433–451.

Hubel DH, Wiesel TN (1959) Receptive fields of single neurones in the cat's striate cortex. J Physiol 148:574–591.

Hubel DH, Wiesel TN (1962) Receptive fields, binocular interaction and functional architecture in the cat's visual cortex. J Physiol 160:106–154.

Hubel DH, Wiesel TN (2005) Brain and Visual Perception: The Story of a 25-Year Collaboration. New York: Oxford University Press.

Hunt CC, Kuffler SW (1951) Further study of efferent small-nerve fibers to mammalian muscle spindles; multiple spindle innervation and activity during contraction. J Physiol 113:283–297.

Huxley A (1980) Reflections on Muscle. Princeton, NJ: Princeton University Press.

Huxley AF (1999) Overton on the indispensability of sodium ions. Brain Res Bull 50: 307–308.

Huxley AF (2004) Andrew F Huxley. In: The History of Neuroscience in Autobiography. Vol 4 (Squire LR, ed), pp 282–318. Washington DC: Society for Neuroscience.

Huxley AF, Niedergerke R (1954a) Structural changes in muscle during contraction; interference microscopy of living muscle fibres. Nature 173:971–973.

Huxley AF, Niedergerke R (1954b) Measurement of muscle striations in stretch and contraction. J Physiol 124:46–47.

Huxley H, Hanson J (1954) Changes in the cross-striations of muscle during contraction and stretch and their structural interpretation. Nature 173:973–976.

Israel M (2000) Ladislav Tauc (1926–1999). Trends Neurosci 23:47.

Iversen LL, Glowinski J, Axelrod J (1965) The uptake and storage of H3-norepinephrine in the reserpine-pretreated rat heart. J Pharmacol Exp Ther 150:173–183.

Jacobsen CF (1934) Influence of motor and premotor area lesions upon the retention of acquired skilled movements in monkeys and chimpanzees. Res Publ Assoc Res Nerv Ment Dis 13:225–247.

Jacyna LS (1997) The neurosciences: 1800–1875. In: A History of Neurosurgery in Its Scientific and Professional Contexts (Greenblatt SH, ed), pp 131–136. Park Ridge, IL: American Association of Neurological Surgeons.

James W (1890) The Principles of Psychology. New York: H. Holt and Company.

Janssen PA, Tollenaere JP (1983) The discovery of the butyrophenone-type neuroleptics. In: Discoveries in Pharmacology, Vol. 1: Psycho- and Neuro-pharmacology (Parnham MJ, Bruinvels J, eds) pp 181–196. Amsterdam: Elsevier.

Jones EG (2006). Walle J. H. Nauta: June 8, 1916-March 24, 1994. Biogr Mem Natl Acad Sci. 88:284–302.

Jones EG, Burton H, Porter R (1975) Commissural and cortico-cortical "columns" in the somatic sensory cortex of primates. Science 190:572–574.

Jordan LM, Liu J, Hedlund PB, Akay T, Pearson KG (2008) Descending command systems for the initiation of locomotion in mammals. Brain Res Rev 57:183–191.

Judson HF (1996) The Eighth Day of Creation: Makers of the Revolution in Biology, exp ed. Plainview, NY: CSHL Press.

Jung, R; Kornmüller AE (1938). "Eine Methodik der ableitung lokalisierter Potentialschwankungen aus subcorticalen Hirngebieten". Arch Psychiat Nervenkr 109: 1–30.

Jung R, Baumgarten RV, Baumgartner G (1952) Microleads of single nerve cells in visual cortex of cat: photo-activated neurons [in German]. Arch Psychiatr Nervenkr Z Gesamte Neurol Psychiatr 189:521–539.

Junquera R (1992) Ramon y Cajal. In Facsimile Edition of the Textura del Systema Nerviosa del Hombre y de los Vertebros, by Santiago Ramon y Cajal, Madrid: Imprenta y Libreria de Nicolas Moya, 1904; Alicante: Graficas Vidal Leuka S.L., p. viii.

Kamm O (1928) The dialysis of pituitary extracts. Science 67:199–200.

Kandel ER (1964) Electrical properties of hypothalamic neuroendocrine cells. J Gen Physiol 47:691–717.

Kandel ER (2006) In Search of Memory: The Emergence of a New Science of Mind. New York: W. W. Norton.

Kandel ER, Spencer WA (1961a) Electrophysiology of hippocampal neurons. II. After-potentials and repetitive firing. J Neurophysiol 24:243–259.

Kandel ER, Spencer WA (1961b) Excitation and inhibition of single pyramidal cells during hippocampal seizure. Exp Neurol 4:162–179.

Kandel ER, Spencer WA (1961c) The pyramidal cell during hippocampal seizure. Epilepsia 2:63–69.

Kandel ER, Spencer WA, Brinley FJ Jr (1961) Electrophysiology of hippocampal neurons. I. Sequential invasion and synaptic organization. J Neurophysiol 24:225–242.

Kandel ER, Tauc L (1964) Mechanism of prolonged heterosynaptic facilitation. Nature 202:145–147.

Karlson P, Luscher M (1959) "Pheromones": a new term for a class of biologically active substances. Nature 183:55–56.

Katz B (1939) Electrical Excitation of Nerve: A Review. London: Oxford University Press.

Katz B (1950) Depolarization of sensory terminals and the initiation of impulses in the muscle spindle. J Physiol 111:261–282.

Katz B (1996) Sir Bernard Katz. In: The History of Neuroscience in Autobiography (Squire LR, ed). Washington DC: Society for Neuroscience, pp 346–381.

Katz B (1996) Neural transmitter release: from quantal secretion to exocytosis and beyond. The Fenn Lecture. J Neurocytol 25:677–686.

Katz B, Miledi R (1963) A study of spontaneous miniature potentials in spinal motoneurones. J Physiol 168:389–422.

Kebabian JW, Greengard P. (1972) Dopamine-sensitive adenyl cyclase: possible role in synaptic transmission. Science. 174:1346–1349.

Kety SS, Schmidt CF (1948) The nitrous oxide method for the quantitative determination of cerebral blood flow in man: theory, procedure and normal values. J Clin Invest 27:476–483.

Keynes RD (1951) The ionic movements during nervous activity. J Physiol 114:119–150.

Klein R (1999) The Hebb legacy. Canadian J Exptl Psychol online http://www.cpa.ca/cpasite/userfiles/documents/publications/cjep/special_eng.html. Adapted from Klein R (1999) Donald O Hebb. In: MIT Encyclopedia of the Cognitive Sciences (Wilson RA, Keil FC, eds). Cambridge MA: The MIT Press, pp 366–367.

Kline NS (1954) Use of *Rauwolfia serpentina* Benth. in neuropsychiatric conditions. Ann N Y Acad Sci 59:107–132.

Koch C, Poggio T, Torre V (1983) Nonlinear interactions in a dendritic tree: Localization, timing, and role of information processing. Proc Natl Acad Sci USA 80: 2799–280.

Koelle GB (1955) Neurohumoral transmission and the autonomic nervous system. In: The Pharmacological Basis of Therapeutics (Goodman LS, Gilman A, eds), pp 404–444. New York: MacMillan.

Koelle GB, Friedenwald JA (1949) A histochemical method for localizing cholinesterase activity. Proc Soc Exp Biol Med 70:617–622.

Kölliker A (1852) Handbuch der gewebelehre des menschen, für aerzte und studirende. Leipzig: W. Engelmann.

Korn H, Faber DS (2005) The Mauthner cell half a century later: a neurobiological model for decision-making? Neuron 47:13–28.

Krnjevic K, Schwartz S (1967) The action of gamma-aminobutyric acid on cortical neurones. Exp Brain Res 3:320–336.

Kuffler SW (1952) Neurons in the retina; organization, inhibition and excitation problems. Cold Spring Harb Symp Quant Biol 17:281–292.

Kuffler SW (1953) Discharge patterns and functional organization of mammalian retina. J Neurophysiol 16:37–68.

Kuffler SW, Hunt CC (1949) Small-nerve fibers in mammalian ventral roots. Proc Soc Exp Biol Med 71:256.

Kuffler SW, Hunt CC, Quilliam JP (1951) Function of medullated small-nerve fibers in mammalian ventral roots; efferent muscle spindle innervation. J Neurophysiol 14:29–54.

Kuhn HW (2004) Introduction. In: von Neumann J, Morgenstern O. Theory of Games and Economic Behavior. Sixtieth Anniversary Edition. Princeton NJ: Princeton University Press, pp vii-xiv.

Kuhn R (1958) The treatment of depressive states with G 22355 (imipramine hydrochloride). Am J Psychiatry 115:459–464.

Kuhne W (1869) On the origin and the causation of vital movement. Proc R Soc Lond Series B 44:427–447.

Kupfermann I, Weiss KR (1978) The command neuron concept. Behav Brain Sci 1:3–39.

Labhardt F (1954) Largactil therapy in schizophrenia and other psychotic conditions. Schweiz Arch Neurol Psychiatr 73:309–338.

Laborit H (1954) Some precautions in neuroplegic therapy with chlorpromazine (R.P. 4560 or largactil). Therapie 9:302–311.

Laborit H, Huguenard P (1952) Present technique of artificial hibernation [in French]. Presse Med 60:1455–1456.

Lambert KG (2003) The life and career of Paul MacLean: A journey toward biological and social harmony. Physiol Behavior 79: 343–349.

Land, LJ, Eager RP, Shepherd GM (l970). Olfactory nerve projections to the olfactory bulb in rabbit: demonstration by means of a simplified ammoniacal silver degenerative method. Brain Res. 23: 250–254.

Landolt AM (1997) History of pituitary surgery. In: A History of Neurosurgery in Its Scientific and Professional Contexts (Greenblatt SH, ed), pp 373–400. Park Ridge, IL: American Association of Neurological Surgeons.

Langley JN (1895) Note on regeneration of pre-ganglionic fibres of the sympathetic. J Physiol 18:280–284.

Lashley K (1950) In search of the engram. Symp Soc Exp Biol 4:454–482.

Lawler HC, Du Vigneaud V (1953) Enzymatic evidence for intrinsic oxytocic activity of the pressor-antidiuretic hormone. Proc Soc Exp Biol Med 84:114–116.

Leão AAP (1944a) Spreading depression of activity in the cerebral cortex. J Neurophysiol 7:359–390.

Leão AAP (1944b) Pial circulation and spreading depression of activity in the cerebral cortex. J Neurophysiol 7:391–396.

Leão AAP, Morison RS (1945) Propagation of spreading cortical depression. J Neurophysiol 8:33–46.

le Gros Clark, WE (1957) Inquiries into the anatomical basis of olfactory discrimination. Proc Roy Soc B 146: 299–318.

Lehmann HE, Kline NS (1983) Clinical discoveries with antidepressant drugs. In: Discoveries in Pharmacology (Parnham MJ, Bruinvels J, eds), pp 209–221. New York: Elsevier.

Lejeune J, Turpin R, Gautier M (1959) Mongolism; a chromosomal disease (trisomy) [in French]. Bull Acad Natl Med 143:256–265.

Leksell L (1945) The action potential and excitatory effects of the small ventral root fibres to skeletal muscle. Acta Physiol Scand 10(Suppl 31):1–84.

Le Magnen J (1999) Rôle de l'odeur ajoutée au régime dans la regulation quantitative à court terme de la prise alimentaire chez le rat blanc. C R Seances Soc Biol 150:136–139.

Le Magnen J (2001) My scientific life: 40 years at the College de France. Neurosci Biobehav Rev 25:375–394.

Lennox WG (1960) Epilepsy and Related Disorders. Boston: Little, Brown.

Lettvin, JY, Maturana HR, McCulloch WS and Pitts WH (1959) What the frog's eye tells the frog's brain. Proc Inst Radio Engrs NY 47: 1940–1951.

Levi-Montalcini R, Cohen S (1956) In vitro and in vivo effects of a nerve growth-stimulating agent isolated from snake venom. Proc Natl Acad Sci USA 42:695–699.

Levi-Montalcini R, Hamburger V (1951) Selective growth stimulating effects of mouse sarcoma on the sensory and sympathetic nervous system of the chick embryo. J Exp Zool 116:321–361.

Levi-Montalcini R, Hamburger V, Meyer H (1953) In vitro experiments on the effects of mouse sarcomas 180 and 37 on the spinal and sympathetic ganglia of the chick embryo. Cancer Res 14:49–57.

Levin EY, Levenberg B, Kaufman S (1960) The enzymatic conversion of 3,4-dihydroxyphenylethylamine to norepinephrine. J Biol Chem 235:2080–2086.

Li CL, Cullen C, Jasper HH (1956) Laminar microelectrode analysis of cortical unspecific recruiting responses and spontaneous rhythms. J Neurophysiol 19:131–143.

Lichtman JW, Sanes JR (2008) Ome sweet ome: what can the genome tell us about the connectome? Curr Opin Neurobiol. 18:346–353.

Liley AW (1956a) The effects of presynaptic polarization on the spontaneous activity at the mammalian neuromuscular junction. J Physiol 134:427–443.

Lillie RS (1935) The passive iron model of proto-plasmic and nervous transmission and its physiological analogues. Biol Rev 11:181–209.

Lillie FR (1952) The Development of the Chick: An Introduction to Embryology, 3rd ed. New York: Holt.

Ling G, Gerard RW (1947) The normal membrane potential of frog sartorius fibers. J Cell Physiol 34:383–396.

Loewi O (1921). Uber humorale Ubertragbarkeit der Herznervenwirkung. Pflugers Arch. 189: 239–242.

Loewenstein WR (1970) Input and output ends of transduction in Pacinian corpuscles. Neurosci Res Prog Bull 8:490–492.

Loewenstein WR, Rathkamp R (1958) Localization of generator structures of electric activity in a Pacinian corpuscle. Science 127:341.

Loomer HP, Saunders JC, Kline KS (1957) A clinical and pharmacodynamic evaluation of iproniazid as a psychic energizer. Psychiatr Res Rep Am Psychiatr Assoc 8:129–141.

Lorente de No R (1922) La corteza cerebral del raton. Trabajos del Laboratorio de Investigaciones Biológicas de la Universidad de Madrid 20:41–78.

Lorente de No R (1934) Studies on the structure of cerebral cortex: II Continuation of the study of the ammonic system. J Psychol Physiol 46:113–117.

Lorente de No R (1938) Cerebral cortex: architecture, intracortical connections, motor projections. In: Physiology of the Nervous System (Fulton J, ed), pp 291–339. New York: Oxford University Press.

Lorenz K (1952) King Solomon's Ring. London: Thomas J. Crewell.

Lyons AE (1997) The crucible years 1880–1900: Macewen to Cushing. In: A History of Neurosurgery in Its Scientific and Professional Contexts (Greenblatt SH, ed), pp 153–166. Park Ridge, IL: American Association of Neurological Surgeons.

Mach E (1897) Contributions to the analysis of sensations. Chicago: Open Court Publishing.

MacLean PD (1949) Psychosomatic disease and the visceral brain; recent developments bearing on the Papez theory of emotion. Psychosom Med 11:338–353.

MacLean PD (1952) Some psychiatric implications of physiological studies on frontotemporal portion of limbic system (visceral brain). Electroencephalogr Clin Neurophysiol 4:407–418.

MacLean PD (1990) The triune brain in evolution: role in paleocerebral functions. New York: Plenum.

MacLean PD, Delgado JM (1953) Electrical and chemical stimulation of frontotemporal portion of limbic system in the waking animal. Electroencephalogr Clin Neurophysiol 5:91–100.

Maddox B (2002) Rosalind Franklin: The Dark Lady of DNA. New York: HarperCollins.

Maranhao-Filho P, Vincent M (2009) Professor Aristides Leao. Much more than spreading depression. Headache 49:110–116.

Maynard DM (1955) Direct inhibition in the lobster cardiac ganglion. PhD Dissertation. University of California, Los Angeles.

Maynard LS, Cotzias GC (1955) The partition of manganese among organs and intracellular organelles of the rat. J Biol Chem 214:489–495.

Mazia D, Dan K (1952) The isolation and biochemical characterization of the mitotic apparatus of dividing cells. Proc Natl Acad Sci USA 38:826–838.

McClelland JL, Rumelhart DE (1987) Explorations in the Microstructure of Cognition. Parallel Distributed Processing, vol 2: Psychological and Biological Models. Cambridge MA: The MIT Press.

McClintock MK (1971) Menstrual synchrony and suppression. Nature 229:244–245.

McCulloch WS, Pitts WS (1943) A logical calculus of the ideas immanent in nervous activity. Bull Math Biophys 5:115–133.

McIlwain H (1955) Biochemistry and the Central Nervous System. London: J. A. Churchill.

McLennan H (1963) Synaptic Transmission. Philadelphia: Saunders.

Merritt HH. (1958) Textbook of Neurology. Philadelphia: Lea and Febiger.

Merritt HH, Putnam TJ (1984) Landmark article Sept 17, 1938: Sodium diphenyl hydantoinate in the treatment of convulsive disorders. JAMA 251:1062–1067.

Meyer nee Bjerrum K (1932) Hans Christian Oersted (1777–1815). In: Prominent Danish Scientists (Meisen V, ed), pp 89–93. Copenhagen: Munksgaard.

Milner PM (1999) Cell Assemblies: Whose Idea? Psycoloquy: 10(053) lashley hebb (4) http://www.cogsci.ecs.soton.ac.uk/cgi/psyc/newpsy?10.053.

Milner B, Penfield W (1955) The effect of hippocampal lesions on recent memory. Trans Am Neurol Assoc 80:42–48.

Milner PM (1958) Note on a possible correspondence between the scotomas of migraine and spreading depression of Leao. Electroencephalogr Clin Neurophysiol 10:705.

Minsky M, Papert S (1969) Perceptrons: An Introduction to Computational Geometry. Cambridge MA: The MIT Press.

Mitchell W (1864) Gunshot Wounds and Other Injuries of Nerves. Philadelphia PA: JB Lippincott.

Mohr JP (2004) Historical perspective. Neurology 62: 83–86. http://www.neurology.org/cgi/content/full/62/8_suppl_6/S3?cookietest=yes.

Mombaerts P, Wang F, Dulac C, Chao SK, Nemes A, Mendelsohn M, Edmondson J, Axel R (1996) Visualizing an olfactory sensory map. Cell 87:675–686.

Moniz, E (1931) Diagnostic Des Tumeurs Cerebrals Et Epreuve De L' encephalographie Arterielle. Paris: Masson.

Monnier AM, Lapicque L (1934) L'Excitation Electrique des Tissus: Essai d'Interpretation Physique. Paris: Hermann.

Moreno-Díaz R, Moreno-Díaz A (2007) On the legacy of W. S. McCulloch. Biosystems 88:185–190.

Morgan TH, Sturtevant AH, Muller HJ, Bridges CJ. (1915) The Mechanism of Mendelian Heredity. New York: Henry Holt. http://books.google.com/ books?id=GZEEAAAAYAAJ&d q=mechanism+of+mendelian+heredity+morgan.

Moruzzi G, Magoun HW (1949) Brain stem reticular formation and activation of the EEG. Electroencephalogr Clin Neurophysiol 1:455–473.

Mosso A (1881) Ueber den Kreislauf des Blutes im Menschenlichen Gehirn. Verlag von Veit:Leipzig. Translated from the original: Mosso A (1880) Sulla Circolazione del Sangue nel Cervello dell'Uomo; Ricerche Sfigmografiche. Rome: Salviucci.

Mountcastle VB (1957) Modality and topographic properties of single neurons of cat's somatic sensory cortex. J Neurophysiol 20:408–434.

Mountcastle VB, Davies PW, Berman AL (1957) Response properties of neurons of cat's somatic sensory cortex to peripheral stimuli. J Neurophysiol 20:374–407.

Mozell MM (1958) Electrophysiology of olfactory bulb. J Neurophysiol 21:183–196.

Muller HJ (1927) Artificial transmutation of the gene. Science. 66:84–87.

Nauta WJH (1993) Some early travails of tracing axonal pathways in the brain. J Neurosci 13: 1337–1345.

Nauta WJH (1994) MIT Tech Talk. 38:27.

Nauta WJH, Gvgax PA (1951) Silver impregnation of degenerating axon terminals in the central nervous system: (l) technic, (2) chemical notes. Stain Technol 26:5–l 1.

Nauta WJH, Gygax PA (1954) Silver impregnation of degenerating axons in the central nervous system: a modified technique. Stain Technol 29:91–93.

Nauta WJH, Ryan LF (1952) Selective silver impregnation of degenerating axons in the central nervous system. Stain Technol 27: 175–179.

Nernst W (1888) Zur kinetik der losung befindlichen korper: theorie der diffusion. Z Phys Chem 3:613–637.

New York Times (1953) Clue to chemistry of heredity is found. June 13, p. 18.

Neylan TC (1998) Hans Selye and the field of stress research J Neuropsych 10: 230–231.

Nicholls JG (1998) Stephen W. Kuffler: August 24, 1913–October 11, 1980. Biogr Mem Natl Acad Sci 74:193–208.

Nicholls JG, Quilliam JP (1956) The mechanism of action of paraldehyde and methylpentynol on neuromuscular transmission in the frog. Brit J Pharmacol Chemother 11: 151–155.

Nirenberg MW, Matthaei JH (1961) The dependence of cell-free protein synthesis in *E. coli* upon naturally occurring or synthetic polyribonucleotides. Proc Natl Acad Sci USA 47:1588–1602.

Novikoff AB, Beaufay H, DeDuve C (1956) Electron microscopy of lysosome-rich fractions from rat liver. J Biophys Biochem Cytol 2:Suppl 179–184.

Ochs S, Kachmann R, Demyer WE (1960) Axoplasmic flow rates during nerve regeneration. Exp Neurol 2:627–637.

O'Connor WJ (1991) British Physiologists 1885–1914. A Biographical Dictionary. New York: Manchester University Press.

Olds J, Milner P (1954) Positive reinforcement produced by electrical stimulation of septal area and other regions of rat brain. J Comp Physiol Psychol 47:419–427.

Oliver G, Schafer EA (1895) On the physiological action of extracts of pituitary body and certain other glandular organs: preliminary communication. J Physiol 18:277–279.

Orbach, J. (1999) Precis of: The Neuropsychological Theories of Lashley and Hebb. Psycoloquy 10(23). ftp://ftp.princeton.edu/pub/harnad/Psycoloquy/ 1999.volume.10/ psyc.99.10.029.lashleyhebb.1.orbach http://www.cogsci. soton.ac.uk/cgi/psyc/newpsy?10.029.

Osterhout WJ, Hill SE (1938) Reversal of the potassium effect in *Nitella*. Proc Natl Acad Sci USA 24:427–431.

Otsuka M, Iversen LL, Hall ZW, Kravitz EA (1966) Release of gamma-aminobutyric acid from inhibitory nerves of lobster. Proc Natl Acad Sci USA 56:1110–1115.

Ott I, Scott JC (1910) The galactagogue action of the thymus and corpus luteum. Proc Soc Exp Biol 8:49.

Ottoson D (1955) Analysis of the electrical activity of the olfactory epithelium. Acta Physiol Scand Suppl 35:1–83.

Ottoson D, Shepherd GM (1967) Experiments and concepts in olfactory physiology. In: Progress in Brain Research, vol. 23. Sensory Mechanisms (Zotterman Y, ed), pp 83–138. New York: Elsevier.

Ottoson D, Shepherd GM (1971) Transducer characteristics of the muscle spindle as revealed by its receptor potential. Acta Physiol Scand 82:545–554.

Overton E (1902) Beitrage zur allgemeinen Muskel- und Nervenphysiologie. 1 Mittheilung. Ueber die Unentbehhrlichkeit von Natrium (odor Lithium) Ionen fur den Contractionsact des Muskels. Pflugers Arch Gesamte Physiol 92: 346–386.

Palade GE (1953) An electron microscope study of mitochondrial structure. J Histochem Cytochem 1: 188–211.

Palade GE (1955b) A small particulate component of the cytoplasm. J Biophys Biochem Cytol 1:59–68.

Palade GE, Claude A (1949) The nature of the Golgi apparatus; parallelism between intercellular myelin figures and Golgi apparatus in somatic cells. J Morphol 85:35–69.

Palade GE (1954) Electron microscope observations of interneuronal and neuromuscular synapses. Anat Rec 118:335–336.

Palade GE, Porter KR (1954) Studies on the endoplasmic reticulum. 1. Its identification in cells in situ. J Exp Med 100: 641–656.

Palay SL (1954) Electron microscope study of the cytoplasm of neurons. Anat Rec 118: 336.

Palay SL, Palade GE (1954) The fine structure of neurons. J Biophys Biochem Cytol 1: 69–88.

Palay SL (1956) Synapses in the central nervous system. J Biophys Biochem Cytol 2 (Suppl): 193–202.

Palay SL (1958) The morphology of synapses in the central nervous system. Exp Cell Res 14:275–293.

Palay SL (1992) A concatenation of accidents. In: The Neurosciences: Paths of Discovery (Samson F, Adelman G, eds), pp 191–214. Boston: Birkhauser.

Palay SL, Palade GE (1955) The fine structure of neurons. J Biophys Biochem Cytol 1:69–88.

Papez JW (1995) A proposed mechanism of emotion. 1937. J Neuropsychiatry Clin Neurosci 7:103–112.

Passarge E (1995) Color Atlas of Genetics. Stuttgart: G. Thieme Verlag.

Paton WD (1958) Central and synaptic transmission in the nervous system; pharmacological aspects. Annu Rev Physiol 20:431–470.

Paul JR (1971) A History of Poliomyelitis. New Haven, CT: Yale University Press.

Pauling L, Delbrück M (1940) The nature of the intermolecular forces operative in biological processes. Science 92:77–79.

Pauling L, Itano HA, Singer SJ, Wells IC. 1949 Sickle cell anemia, a molecular disease. Science 110: 543–548.

Penfield W (1951) Epileptic Seizure Patterns: A Study in the Localizing Value of Initial Phenomena in Focal Cortical Seizures. Springfield, IL: Charles C. Thomas.

Penfield W (1959) The interpretive cortex; the stream of consciousness in the human brain can be electrically reactivated. Science 129:1719–1725.

Penfield W, Jasper H (1954) Epilepsy and the Functional Anatomy of the Human Brain. Boston, MA: Little, Brown.

Penfield W, Rasmussen T (1950) The Cerebral Cortex of Man: A Clinical Study of Localization of Function. New York: Macmillan.

Penfield W, Roberts L (1959) Speech and Brain Mechanisms. Princeton, NJ: Princeton University Press.

Peters A, Palay SL, Webster HD (1973) The Fine Structure of the Nervous System. The Cells and their Processes. New York: Oxford University Press.

Petty, GW, Duffy, J, Huston, J (1996) Cerebral ischemia in patients with hepatitis C virus infection and mixed cryoglobulinemia. Mayo Clin Proc 71:671–678.

Phillips CG (1955) The dimensions of a cortical motor point. J Physiol 129:20P–21P.

Phillips CG (1956a) Cortical motor threshold and the thresholds and distribution of excited Betz cells in the cat. Q J Exp Physiol Cogn Med Sci 41:70–84.

Phillips CG (1956b) Intracellular records from Betz cells in the cat. Q J Exp Physiol Cogn Med Sci 41:58–69.

Phillips CG (1959) Actions of antidromic pyramidal volleys on single Betz cells in the cat. Q J Exp Physiol Cogn Med Sci 44:1–25.

Pitts WS, McCulloch WS (1947) How we know universals: the perception of visual and auditory forms. Bull Math Biophys 9:127–147.

Pletscher A, Shore PA, Brodie BB (1955) Serotonin release as a possible mechanism of reserpine action. Science 122:374–375.

Ploog DW (2003) The place of the Triune Brain in psychiatry. Physiol Behav 79:487–93.

Popa G (1930) A portal circulation from the pituitary to the hypothalamic region. J Anat 65:88–91.

Popenoe EA, Du Vigneaud V (1953) Degradative studies on vasopressin and performic acid-oxidized vasopressin. J Biol Chem 205:133–143.

Popper K, Eccles JC (1977) The Self and Its Brain: An Argument for Interactionism. New York: Springer International.

Porter KR (1953) Observations on a submicroscopic basophilic component of cytoplasm. J Exp Med 97:727–750.

Porter KR (1955) The submicroscopic morphology of protoplasm. Harvey Lect. 51:175–228.

Porter KR, Bennett HS (1981) Introduction: recollections on the beginnings of the Journal of Cell Biology. J Cell Biol 91:IX–XI.

Powell TP, Mountcastle VB (1959) Some aspects of the functional organization of the cortex of the postcentral gyrus of the monkey: a correlation of findings obtained in a single unit analysis with cytoarchitecture. Bull Johns Hopkins Hosp 105:133–162.

Pribram KH, Kruger L (1954) Functions of the "olfactory brain". Ann N Y Acad Sci. 58:109–38.

Purves D, Lichtman JW (1985) Principles of Neural Development. Sunderland, MA: Sinauer Associates.

Raichle M (2009) A brief history of human brain mapping. Trends Neurosci. 2009 32:118–26.

Rall W (1957) Membrane time constant of motoneurons. Science 126:454.

Rall W (1959) Branching dendritic trees and motoneuron membrane resistivity. Exp Neurol 1:491–527.

Rall W (1960) Membrane potential transients and membrane time constant of motoneurons. Exp Neurol 2: 503–532.

Rall W (1964) Theoretical significance of dendritic trees for neuronal input-output relations. In: Neural Theory and Modeling (Reiss RF, ed), pp 122–146. Palo Alto: Stanford University Press.

Rall W (1970) Cable properties of dendrites and effects of synaptic location. In: Excitatory Synaptic Mechanisms (Andersen P, Jansen JKS, eds). Oslo: Universitetsforlag, pp 175–187.

Rall W (2006). Wilfrid Rall. In: The History of Neuroscience in Autobiography. Vol 5 (Squire LR, ed), pp 551–612. Washington DC: Society for Neuroscience.

Rall W, Shepherd GM, Reese TS, Brightman MW (1966) Dendrodendritic synaptic pathway for inhibition in the olfactory bulb. Exp Neurol 14:44–56.

Ramón y Cajal S (1891) Sur la structure de l'écorce cérébrale de quelques mammifères. Cellule 7:3–54.

Ramón y Cajal S (1892) El nuevo concepto de la histologia de los centros nerviosos. Rev Ciencias Med 18:457–476.

Ramón y Cajal S (1894) Les Nouvelles Idées sur la Structure du Système Nerveux chez l'Homme et chez les Vertébrés. Paris: C. Reinwald.

Ramón y Cajal S (1911) Histologie du Système Nerveux de l'Homme et des Vertébrés. Paris: Maloine.

Ramón y Cajal S (1928) Degeneration and Regeneration of the Nervous System. London: Oxford University Press.

Ramón y Cajal S (1933) Neuronismo o Reticularismo? Las Pruebas Objetivas de la Unidad Anatomica de las Celulas Nerviosas. Madrid: Consejo Superior de Investigaciones Cientificas, Instituto Ramón y Cajal.

Ramón y Cajal S (1937) Recollections of My Life. Philadelphia: American Philosophical Society.

Ramón y Cajal S (1954) Neuron Theory or Reticular Theory? Objective Evidence of the Anatomical Unity of Nerve Cells, Engl. Ed. Madrid: Consejo Superior de Investigaciones Cientificas.

Randall LO, Atkinson N, Iliev V (1960) The effect of psychostimulants and psychodepressants on DPN synthesis in the liver. Arch Int Pharmacodyn Ther 129:434–437.

Rapport MM, Green AA, Page IH (1948) Serum vasoconstrictor, serotonin; isolation and characterization. J Biol Chem 176:1243–1251.

Rashevsky N (1933) Outline of a physico-mathematical theory of excitation and inhibition. Protoplasma 20:42.

Ratliff F, Knight BW, Toyoda J, Hartline HK (1967) Enhancement of flicker by lateral inhibition. Science 158:392–393.

Reich P, Henneman E, Karnovsky ML (1967) Oxidative metabolism of glucose in resting and active sciatic nerve. J Neurochem 14:447–456.

Renshaw B (1941) Influence of discharge of motoneurons upon excitation of neighboring motoneurons. J Neurophysiol 4:167–183.

Renshaw B (1946) Observations of interactions of nerve impulses in the gray matter and on the nature of central inhibition. Am J Physiol 146:443–448.

Ressler KJ, Sullivan SL, Buck LB (1993) A zonal organization of odorant receptor gene expression in the olfactory epithelium. Cell 73:597–609.

Restak RM (1995) Receptors. New York: Bantam Books.

Revel JP, Karnovsky MJ (1967) Hexagonal array of subunits in intercellular junctions of the mouse heart and liver. J Cell Biol 33:C7–C12.

Ridley M (2006) Francis Crick: Discoverer of the Genetic Code New York: Atlas Books.

Rioch DM, Wislocki GB, O'Leary JL (1940) A précis of preoptic, hypothalamic and hypophysial terminology with atlas. Res Publ Ass nerv ment Dis xx: 3–30.

Roberts E (1998) Eugene Roberts. In: The History of Neuroscience in Autobiography (Squire, LR, ed), San Diego: Academic Press, pp 350–395.

Roberts RB (ed) (1958) Microsomal Particles and Protein Synthesis. New York: Pergamon.

Robertson JD (1955) The ultrastructure of adult vertebrate peripheral myelinated nerve fibers in relation to myelinogenesis. J Biophys Biochem Cytol 1:271–278.

Robertson JD (1956) Some features of the ultrastructure of reptilian skeletal muscle. J Biophys Biochem Cytol 2:369–380.

Robertson JD (1957a) New observations on the ultrastructure of the membranes of frog peripheral nerve fibers. J Biophys Biochem Cytol 3:1043–1048.

Robertson JD (1957b) Some aspects of the ultrastructure of double membranes. Prog Neurobiol 2:1–22, discussion 22–30.

Rosenblatt F (1958) The Perceptron, a probabilistic model for information storage and organization in the brain. Psych Rev 62: 386–408.

Rosenzweig MR, Leiman AL, Breedlove SM (1996) Biological Psychology. Sunderland, MA: Sinauer Associates.

Roy CS, Sherrington CS (1890) On the regulation of the blood-supply of the brain. J Physiol 11:85–158.

Rushton WAH (1937) Initiation of the propagated disturbance. Proc R Soc B 124:210–243.

Ryan J, Newman A, Jacobs M (eds) (2000) The Pharmacological Century. Ten Decades of Drug Discovery. Washington DC: American Chemical Society, Supplement to ACS Publications.

Ryle AP, Sanger F, Smith LF, Kitai R (1955) The disulphide bonds of insulin. Biochem J 60:541–556.

Sanger, F. and Tuppy, H. 1951 The amino-acid sequence in the phenylalanyl chain of insulin. 1. The identification of lower peptides from partial hydrolysates. Biochem. J. 49:463–481.

Saris S (1997) Intracranial tumors: the evolution of treatment. In: A History of Neurosurgery in Its Scientific and Professional Contexts (Greenblatt SH, ed), pp 247–258. Park Ridge, IL: American Association of Neurological Surgeons.

Sawyer CH. 1975. First Geoffrey Harris Memorial Lecture. Some recent developments in brain-pituitary-ovarian physiology. Neuroendocrinology 17:97–124.

Schaefer H (1936) Uber die mathematischen grundlagen einer spannungstheorie der elektrischen nervenreizung. Pflügers Arch 237:484–492.

Schafer EA (1928) Die lichtempfindlichkeit blinder elritzen (untersuchungen uber das Zwischenhirn der Fische). Z Vergl Physiol 7:1–38.

Scharrer B (1952) Neuroendocrine physiology of insects. Pflügers Arch 255:154–163.

Scharrer B (1987) Neurosecretion: beginnings and new directions in neuropeptide research. Annu Rev Neurosci 10:1–17.

Scharrer B, Scharrer E (1944) Neurosecretion, VI. A comparison between the intercerebralis–cardiacum–allatum system of the insects and the hypothalamo–hypophyseal system of the vertebrates. Biol Bull 87:242–251.

Scharrer E (1952a) Pituitary–diencephalic system of *Scyllium stellare*. Z Zellforsch Mikrosk Anat 37:196–204.

Scharrer E (1952b) The general significance of the neurosecretory cell. Scientia 46:177–183.

Scharrer E, Brown S (1961) Neurosecretion. XII. The formation of neurosecretory granules in the earthworm, *Lumbricus terrestris* L. Z Zellforsch Mikrosk Anat 54:530–540.

Scharrer E, Scharrer B (1963) Neuroendocrinology. New York: Columbia University Press.

Schmitt OH (1937) An electrical theory of nerve impulse propagation. Am J Physiol 119:399.

Schnapp BJ, Vale RD, Sheetz MP, Reese TS (1985) Single microtubules from squid axoplasm support bidirectional movement of organelles. Cell 40:455–462.

Schneider D (1957) Electrophysiolgical investigation on the antennal receptors of the silk moth during chemical stimulation. Experientia (Basel) 13: 89–91.

Schou M, Juel-Nielsen N, Stromgren E, Voldby H (1954) The treatment of manic psychoses by the administration of lithium salts. J Neurol Neurosurg Psychiatry 17:250–260.

Schrödinger E (1945) What Is Life? The Physical Aspect of the Living Cell. Cambridge: Cambridge University Press.

Scott GE, Toole JF (1998) 1860 – Neurology was there. Arch Neurol 12: 1584–1585.

Scoville WB, Dunsmore RH, Liberson WT, Henry CE, Pepe A (1953) Observations on medial temporal lobotomy and uncotomy in the treatment of psychotic states; preliminary review of 19 operative cases compared with 60 frontal lobotomy and undercutting cases. Res Publ Assoc Res Nerv Ment Dis 31:347–373.

Scoville WB, Milner B (1957) Loss of recent memory after bilateral hippocampal lesions. J Neurol Neurosurg Psychiatry 20:11–21.

Segev I, Rinzel J, Shepherd GM (1995) The theoretical foundations of dendritic function: the collected papers of Wilfrid Rall with commentaries. Cambridge, MA: MIT Press.

Seldinger SI (1953) Catheter replacement of the needle in percutaneous arteriography; a new technique. Acta Radiol 39:368–376.

Selverston AI (1985) Model Neural Networks and Behavior. New York: Plenum Press.

Selye H (1936) A syndrome produced by diverse nocuous agents. Nature 138: 32. Reproduced in: Neuropsychiatry Classics. J Neuropsych 10: 230–231.

Selye H (1950) The physiology and pathology of exposure to stress. Montreal: Acta Inc.

Selye H (1956) The Stress of Life. New York: McGraw-Hill.

Shannon CE (1937) Master's thesis. In: Shannon CE (1993) Collected Papers (Sloane NJA, Wyner AD, eds) IEEE press, ISBN 0-7803-0434-9.

Shannon CE, Weaver W (1948) The Mathematical Theory of Communication. Urbana: University of Illinois Press.

Sharp FR, Kauer JS, Shepherd GM (1975) Local sites of activity-related glucose metabolism in rat olfactory bulb during olfactory stimulation. Brain Res 98:596–600.

Shaw E, Woolley DW (1954) Pharmacological properties of some antimetabolites of serotonin having unusually high activity on isolated tissues. J Pharmacol Exp Ther 111:43–53.

Shepherd GM (1972) The neuron doctrine: a revision of functional concepts. Yale J Biol Med 45:584–599.

Shepherd GM (1990) The significance of real neuron architectures for neural network simulations. In: Computational Neuroscience (Schwartz E, ed), pp 82–96. Cambridge, MA: MIT Press.

Shepherd GM (1991) Foundations of the Neuron Doctrine. New York: Oxford University Press.

Shepherd GM (1994) Neurobiology. New York: Oxford University Press.

Shepherd GM (1994) Dedication of the first issue to Wilfrid Rall. Journal of Computational Neuroscience, Springer Netherlands 1:7–8.

Shepherd GM (2000) Complementarity beyond physics (1928–1962). Niels Bohr collected works. Endeavour 24:180–181.

Shepherd GM (2008) John Carew Eccles. In New Dictionary of Scientific Biography, pp 329–333. New York: Scribner's (Gale Cengage Learning).

Shepherd GM, Braun J (1989) The peak of electromechanical experimentation in physiology: a unique view through Walter Miles' "Report of a Visit to Foreign Laboratories" in 1920. Caduceus 5:1–84.

Shepherd GM, Brayton RK (1987) Logic operations are properties of computer-simulated interactions between excitable dendritic spines. Neuroscience 21:151–166.

Shepherd GM, Erulkar SD (1997) Centenary of the synapse: from Sherrington to the molecular biology of the synapse and beyond. Trends Neurosci 20:385–392.

Sherringon CS (1897) Spinal cord. In: A Text-Book of Physiology, 7th Edition (Foster M, ed), London and New York, NY: Macmillan, p 60.

Sherrington CS (1906) The Integrative Action of the Nervous System. New Haven, CT: Yale University Press.

Sherrington CS (1940). Personal letter to JF Fulton, in the Yale Medical Historical Library; reproduced in Shepherd and Erulkar (1997).

Sholl DA (1956) The Organization of the Cerebral Cortex. New York: Wiley.

Shore PA, Brodie BB (1957) LSD-like effects elicited by reserpine in rabbits pretreated with iproniazid. Proc Soc Exp Biol Med 94:433–435.

Shorey ML (1909) The effect of the destruction of peripheral areas on the differentiation of the neuroblasts. J Exp Zool 7:25–63.

Shorter E (1997) A History of Psychiatry. From the Era of the Asylum to the Age of Prozac. New York: John Wiley & Sons.

Siegel GJ, Agranoff BW, Albers RW, Fisher SK, Uhler MD (eds) (1999) Basic Neurochemistry. New York: Lippincott-Raven.

Siekevitz P, Zamecnik PC (1981) Ribosomes and protein synthesis. J Cell Biol 91:53s–65s.

Sjöstrand FS (1953) Electron microscopy of mitochondria and cytoplasmic double membranes. Nature 171:30–32.

Skou JC (1957) The influence of some cations on an adenosine triphosphatase from peripheral nerves. Biochim Biophys Acta 23(2):394–401.

Skrede KK, Westgaard RH (1971) The transverse hippocampal slice: a well-defined cortical structure maintained in vitro. Brain Res 35:589–593.

Smith DC (1997) The evolution of modern neurosurgery. In: A History of Neurosurgery in Its Scientific and Professional Contexts (Greenblatt SH, ed), pp 11–26. Park Ridge, IL: American Association of Neurological Surgeons.

Snyder SH (1996) Drugs and the Brain. New York: WH Freeman.

Snyder SH, Kandel ER, Nestler EJ, Nemeroff CB, Aghajanian G (2008) Science and Psychiatry: Groundbreaking Discoveries in Molecular Neuroscience. Arlington, VA: American Psychiatric Publishing.

Sokoloff L (2000) Seymour Kety. Biog Mem Natl Acads http://www.nap.edu/readingroom.php?book=biomems&page=skety.html.

Somjen GG (2005) Aristides Leão's discovery of cortical spreading depression. J Neurophysiol 94:2–4.

Spemann H, Mangold H (1924) Über induktion von embryonalanlagen durch implantation artfremder organisatoren. Arch Mikrosk Anat Entwicklungsmech 100:599–638.

Spencer DD (1997) Neurological surgery and biological science. In: Philosophy of Neurological Surgery (Awad IA, ed), pp 105–115. Park Ridge, IL: American Association of Neurological Surgeons.

Spencer WA, Kandel ER (1961) Electrophysiology of hippocampal neurons. IV. Fast prepotentials. J Neurophysiol 24:272–285.

Sperry RW (1943) Visuomotor coordination in the newt (*Triturus viridescens*) after regeneration of the optic nerve. J Comp Neurol 79:33–55.

Sperry RW (1948) Restoration of vision after crossing of optic nerves and after contralateral transplantation of eye. J Neurophysiol 8:17–28.

Sperry RW (1959) The growth of nerve circuits. Sci Am. 201:68–75.

Sperry RW (1963) Chemoaffinity in the orderly growth of nerve fiber patterns and connections. Proc Natl Acad Sci USA 50:703–710.

Spiegel EA, Wycis HT, Baird HW (1952) Studies in stereoencephalotomy. I. Topical relationships of subcortical structures to the posterior commissure. Confin Neurol 12:121–133.

Spiegel EA, Wycis HT (1952) Stereoencephalotomy. Part 1. (Thalamotomy and Related Procedures). New York: Grune & Stratton.

Spiegel R, (1996) Psychopharmacology. An Introduction. Third Edition. New York: John Wiley & Sons.

Starzl TE, Taylor CW, Magoun H (1951) Collateral afferent excitation of the reticular formation of the brain stem. J Neurophysiol 14:479–496.

Steck H (1954) Extrapyramidal and diencephalic syndrome in the course of largactil and serpasil treatments. Ann Med Psychol (Paris) 112(2):737–744.

Stellar E (1957) Physiological psychology. Annu Rev Psychol 8:415–436.

Stewart WB, Kauer JS, Shepherd GM (1979) Functional organization of rat olfactory bulb analysed by the 2-deoxyglucose method. J Comp Neurol 185:715–734.

Strasburger EA, Jost L, Schenck H, Karsten G (1894) Lehrbuch der Botanik für Hochschulen. English translation: A Text-Book of Botany. 1912 London: MacMillan and Co.

Stryer L (1988) Biochemistry, 3rd ed. New York: W. H. Freeman.

Stuart GJ, Sakmann B (1994) Active propagation of somatic action potentials into neocortical pyramidal cell dendrites. Nature 367:69–72.

Stuart DG, Pierce PA (2006) The contributions of John Carew Eccles to contemporary neuroscience. Prog Neurobiol 78:136–326.

Stuiver M (1960) An olfactometer with a wide range of possibilities. Acta Otolaryngol 51:135–142.

Summers WC (1999) Felix d'Herelle and the Origins of Molecular Biology, New Haven: Yale University Press.

Svaetichin G (1954) The cone action potential. Acta Physiol Scand 29:565–600.

Takeuchi A, Takeuchi N (1963) Glutamate-induced depolarization in crustacean muscle. Nature 198:490–491.

Talairach J, De Aljuriaguerra J, David M (1952) A stereotaxic study of the deep encephalic structures in man; technic, physiopathologic and therapeutic significance. Presse Med 60:605–609.

Talairach J, David M, Tournoux P (1957) Atlas d-Anatomic Stereotaxique. Paris: Masson et Cte.

Talbot SA, Kuffler SW (1952) A multibeam ophthalmoscope for the study of retinal physiology. J Opt Soc Am 42:931–936.

Talley CL (2005) The emergence of multiple sclerosis, 1870–1950: a puzzle of historical epidemiology. Perspect Biol Med 48:383–395.

Tatum EL, Lederberg J (1947) Gene recombination in the bacterium Escherichia coli. J Bacteriol. 53:673–684.

Teive HAG, Kowacs PA, Maranhão P, Filho E, Piovesan J, Werneck LC (2005) Leão's cortical spreading depression: from experimental "artifact" to physiological principle. Neurology 65:1455–1459.

Thudichum JLW (1884) Treatise on the Chemical Constitution of the Brain. London: Baillière, Tindall, and Cox.

Tinbergen N (1951) The Study of Instinct. Oxford: Clarendon Press.

Todman D (2008) History of neuroscience: Roger Sperry (1913–1994). In online: http://www.ibro.info/Pub/Pub_Main_Display.asp?LC_Docs_ID=3473.

Tsuji S (2006) René Couteaux (1909–1999) and the morphological identification of synapses. Biol Cell 98:503–509.

Tunturi AR (1952) A difference in the representation of auditory signals for the left and right ears in the iso-frequency contours of the right middle ectosylvian auditory cortex of the dog. Am J Physiol 168:712–727.

Turing A (1936) On computable numbers, with an application to the entscheidungsproblem. Proc Lond Math Soc 42: 230–265.

Uttley AM (1954) The classification of signals in the nervous system. EEG Clin Neurophysiol 6: 479–494.

Valenstein ES (1997) History of psychosurgery. In: A History of Neurosurgery in Its Scientific and Professional Contexts (Greenblatt SH, ed), pp 499–516. Park Ridge, IL: American Association of Neurological Surgeons.

Valléry-Radot P (ed) (1922–1939) Oeuvres de Pasteur. Paris: Masson.

Van der Lee S, Boot LM (1956) Spontaneous pseudopregnancy in mice. II. Acta physiol pharmacol neerl 5: 213–215.

Van der Loos H, Woolsey TA (1973) Somatosensory cortex: structural alterations following early injury to sense organs. Science 179:395–398.

Van Harreveld A, Mendelson M (1959) Glutamate-induced contractions in crustacean muscle. J Cell Comp Physiol 54:85–94.

Vassar R, Ngai J, Axel R (1993) Spatial segregation of odorant receptor expression in the mammalian olfactory epithelium. Cell 74:309–318.

Vilensky JA, Gilman S, Sinish PR (2004) Denny-Brown, Boston City Hospital, and the history of American neurology. Perspect Biol Med 47:505–518.

von Békésy G (1960) Experiments in Hearing. New York: McGraw-Hill.

von Frisch K (1967) The Dance Language and Orientation of Bees. Cambridge, MA: Harvard University Press.

von Helmholtz HLF (1850) On the rate of transmission of the nerve impulse. In: Preussische akademie der Wissenschaften, pp 14–15. Berlin: Berichtn. König.

von Neumann J (1945) First Draft of a Report on the EDVAC. http://en.wikipedia. org/wiki/First_Draft_of_a_Report_on_the_EDVAC.

von Neumann J (1957) The Brain and the Computer. New Haven: Yale University Press.

von Neumann J, Morgenstern O (1944) Theory of Games and Economic Behavior. Princeton NJ: Princeton University Press.

Von Waldeyer, W (1888) Über Karyokinese und ihre Beziehungen zu den Befruchtungsvorgängen. Archiv für mikroskopische Anatomie und Entwicklungsmechanik, 32: 1–122.

Waelsch H (ed) (1955) Biochemistry of the Developing Nervous System. International Neurochemical Symposium. New York: Academic Press.

Waldeyer HWG (1891) Uber einige neuere forschungen im gebiete der anatomie des zentralnervensystems. Dtsche Med Wochenschr 17:1213–1218.

Walker AE (1997) Preface. In: A History of Neurosurgery in Its Scientific and Professional Contexts (Greenblatt SH, ed), pp xiii–xiv. Park Ridge, IL: American Association of Neurological Surgeons.

Warner J (1997) The Therapeutic Perspective. Medical Practice, Knowledge, and Identity in America, 1820–1885. Princeton, NJ: Princeton University Press.

Watson JD, Crick FH (1953) Molecular structure of nucleic acids; a structure for deoxyribose nucleic acid. Nature 171:737–738.

Watson JD (1968) The Double Helix; A Personal Account of the Discovery of the Structure of DNA, 1st ed. New York: Atheneum.

Watts JW, Fulton JF (1935) The effect of lesions of the hypothalamus upon the gastro-intestinal tract and heart in monkeys. Ann Surg 101:363–372.

Weiner N (1948) Cybernetics: Or the Control and Communication in the Animal and the Machine. Paris, France: Librairie Hermann & Cie, and Cambridge, MA: MIT Press.

Weiss PA (1924) Die funktion transplantierter amphibienextremitaten. Aufstellung einer resonanztheorie der motorisschen nerventatigkeit auf grund abgestimmter endorgane. Arch Mikrosk Anat Entwicklungsmech 102:635–672.

Weiss PA (1934) In vitro experiments on the factors determining the course of the outgrowing nerve fiber. J Exp Zool 68:395–448.

Weiss PA (1939) Principles of Development. New York: H. Holt & Co.

Weiss P, Hiscoe HB (1948) Experiments on the mechanism of nerve growth. J Exp Zool 107:315–395.

Werblin FS, Dowling JE (1969) Organization of the retina of the mudpuppy, *Necturus maculosus*. II. Intracellular recording. J Neurophysiol 32:339–355.

Whitcomb BB (1979) William Beecher Scoville. Surg Neurol 12:109–110.

Whitten WK (1957) Effect of exteroceptive factors on the oestrus cycle of mice. Nature 186: 1436.

Whitten WK (1958) Modification of the oestrus cycle of the mouse by external stimuli associated with the male. Changes in the oestrus cycle determined by vaginal smears. J Endocrinol 17: 307–313.

Widrow B, Hoff Me (1960) Adaptive switching circuits. WESCON convention record IV: 96–104.

Wiener N (1948) Cybernetics, or Control and Communication in the Animal and Machine.

Wiersma CAG (1931) An experiment on the "resonance theory" of muscular activity. Arch Neerl Physiol 16:337–345.

Wiersma CAG (1938) Function of the giant fibres of the central nervous system of the crayfish. Proc Soc Exp Biol Med 38:661–662.

Wiersma CAG (1947) Giant nerve fibre system of the crayfish. A contribution to comparative physiology of synapse. J Neurophysiol 10:23–28.

Wiersma CA (1952) Neurons of arthropods. Cold Spring Harb Symp Quant Biol 17:155–163.

Wiersma CAG (1962) The organization of the arthropod nervous system. Am Zool 2:67–78.

Wiersma CA, Ikeda K (1964) Interneurons commanding swimmeret movements in the crayfish, *Procambarus clarki* (Girard). Comp Biochem Physiol 12:509–525.

Wilson E (1975) Sociobiology. Cambridge, MA: Harvard University Press.

Wilson CJ, Chang HT, Kitai ST (1990) Firing patterns and synaptic potentials of identified giant aspiny interneurons in the rat neostriatum. J Neurosci 10:508–519.

Wislocki GB, King LS (1936) The permeability of the hypophysis and hypothalamus to vital dyes, with a study of the hypophyseal vascular supply. Am J Anat 58:421–472.

Woodbury JW, Patton HD (1952) Electrical activity of single spinal cord elements. Cold Spring Harb Symp Quant Biol 17:185–188.

Woolley DW, Shaw E (1954) Some neurophysiological aspects of serotonin. Br Med J 2:122–126.

Woolsey TA, Van der Loos H (1970) The structural organization of layer IV in the somatosensory region (SI) of mouse cerebral cortex. The description of a cortical field composed of discrete cytoarchitectonic units. Brain Res 17:205–242.

Xu F, Greer CA, Shepherd GM (2000) Odor maps in the olfactory bulb. J Comp Neurol 422:489–495.

Yokota T, Reeves AG, MacLean PD (1970) Differential effects of septal and olfactory volleys on intracellular responses of hippocampal neurons in awake, sitting monkeys. J Neurophysiol 33:96–107.

Young JZ (1936) The giant nerve fibres and epistellar body of cephalopods Q J Micro Sci 78: 367–368.

Zeller EA (1983) Monoamine oxidase and its inhibitors in relation to antidepressive activity. In: Discoveries in Pharmacology (Parnham MJ, Bruinvels J, eds), pp 223–232. New York: Elsevier.

Zeller EA, Birkhuaser H, Mislin H, Wenk M (1939) Über das vorkommen der diamin-oxydase bei mensch, säugetier and vogel. Mit einem anhang über das vorkommen der cholinesterase beim vogel. Helv Chim Acta 22:1381–1395.

Zervas NT (1984) Neurosurgery at the Massachusetts General Hospital, 1909–1983. Boston: Massachusetts General Hospital.

ONLINE REFERENCES
http://en.wikipedia.org/wiki/Artificial_intelligence.
http://en.wikipedia.org/wiki/Cybernetics.
http://en.wikipedia.org/wiki/Norbert_Wiener.
http://en.wikipedia.org/wiki/Claude_Shannon.
http://en.wikipedia.org/wiki/George_Boole.
http://en.wikipedia.org/wiki/ENIAC.
http://www.kerryr.net/pioneers/boole.htm.
http://www.kerryr.net/pioneers/shannon.htm.
Biology 91:3–300J Exp Med 97:727–750.

Index

Note: Page numbers followed by *t* denote tables; *Fig* denotes illustrations in the insert.

Neuroleptics, 209. *See also* Neuropsychiatry
Neurological disorders, synaptic pathology and, 56. *See also names of specific disorders*
Neurology, clinical. *See* Clinical neurology
Neuromuscular junction (NMJ), 59–61, 66, 84, 85–86
Neuronal connections
  simplified, in logic operations, 221, *Fig 16.1*
  specificity of, theories on, 34–37
Neuron doctrine, 59, 60–61, 100–103, 112–113
Neurons
  complexity-within-unity concept, 112
  dynamic polarization of, 102–103, *Fig 8.1*
  excitability of, 69. *See also* Action potentials
  functional organization of. *See* Functional organization of neurons
  Golgi staining of, 100–101, 109, *Fig 8.1*
  integrative organization for action potential initiation, 105
  simplified, in logic operations, 221, *Fig 16.1*
  synaptic interactions of, 84
  theoretical contributions on function of, 218, 219t
Neuronism vs. reticularism, 59–61, 68
The Neurophysiological Basis of Mind: The Principles of Neurophysiology (Eccles), 94, 116
Neuropsychiatry, 206–217
  antidepressants, 206, 210–213
  antipsychotic drugs, 207
  benzodiazepines, 214–215
  chlorpromazine, 207–208
  emergence of, 177–178
  haloperidol, 209–210
  imipramine and tricyclic drugs, 212–213
  iproniazid, 210–211
  lithium, 213
  meprobamate, 214
  minor tranquilizers, 213–214
  monoamine oxidase inhibitors, 211–212
  reserpine, 208–209, 212

Neuroscience
  disciplines of, 4–5, 5t
  ethical issues and, 10–11, 10t
  factors producing discoveries in, 8–10, 8t
  hierarchical levels of organization, 7–8, 8t
  species investigated, 5–6, 6t
  systematic divisions of, 6–7, 7t
  as term, 4
  timetable of discoveries in the 1950s, 12t
Neurosecretory cells, discovery of, 152
Neuroses, treatment of, 213–215
Neurospora, 18
Neurosurgery, 193–205
  Cushing and, 194–197
  for epilepsy, 142, 193, 201–202
  history of, 193–194
  imaging developments and, 204–205
  on limbic lobe, 171–174, *Fig 12.6*
  on pituitary, 183, 197–198
  psychosurgery, 169, 193, 202–203
  stereotaxy, 115, 193, 199–201
  visualization of human brain during, 198–199
Neurotransmitters, 39–55
  acetylcholine, 42, 47
  in brain, 44–45
  catecholamine, 50–52
  "chemical mediators" and "receptive substances", 41
  criteria for identification of, 46
  Dale's law and, 46–47
  early experiments, 40
  GABA, 48–49
  Gerschenfeld–Tauc collaboration on, 96–97
  glutamate, 47–48
  hormones, 39, 53–54
  lock-and-key concept, 41–42
  monoamine histofluorescence, 52–53
  neuropeptides, 39, 54
  organ pharmacology, 42–43
  pheromones, 39, 54–55
  second messengers, 39, 53
  serotonin, 49–50, 52
  "soup vs. sparks" debate, 43–44
Newell, Allen, 229
NGF. *See* Nerve growth factor (NGF)
Nicholls, John G., 123
NIH (National Institutes of Health), 19